CW01376114

N. Hâncu · Cardiovascular Risk in Type 2 Diabetes Mellitus

Springer
*Berlin
Heidelberg
New York
Hong Kong
London
Milan
Paris
Tokyo*

Nicolae Hâncu (Ed.)

Cardiovascular Risk in Type 2 Diabetes Mellitus

Assessment and Control

With 55 Figures and 38 Tables

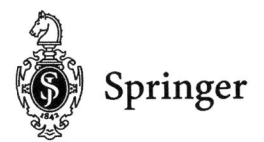

Springer

Prof. Dr. Nicolae Hâncu
Iuliu Hatieganu University of Medicine and Pharmacy
Diabetes Center and Clinic
2 - 4 Clinicilor St.
3400 Cluj Napoca / Romania

ISBN-13:978-3-642-63946-3 Springer-Verlag Berlin Heidelberg New York
Library of Congress Cataloging-in-Publication Data
Cardiovascular risk in type 2 diabetes mellitus : assessment and control / Nicolae Hâncu (ed.)
p. ; cm.
Includes biographical references and index.
ISBN-13:978-3-642-63946-3   e-ISBN-13:978-3-642-59352-9
DOI: 10.1007/978-3-642-59352-9

1. Diabetic angiopathies. 2. Cardiovascular system--Diseases. 3. Non-insulin-dependent diabetes--Complications. I. Title: Cardiovascular risk in type two diabetes mellitus. II. Hâncu, N.
[DNLM: 1. Cardiovascular Diseases--complications. 2. Cardiovascular Diseases--prevention & control. 3. Diabetes Mellitus, Non-Insulin-Dependent--complications. 4. Risk Factors. WG 120 C26777 2003]
RC700.D5 C375 2003
616.1'3--dc21   2002075765

This work is subject to copyright. All rights are reserved, whether the whole or part of the material is concerned, specifically the rights of translation, reprinting, reuse of illustrations, recitation, broadcasting, reproduction on microfilm or in any other way, and storage in data banks. Duplication of this publication or parts thereof is permitted only under the provisions of the German Copyright Law of September 9, 1965, in its current version, and permission for use must always be obtained from Springer-Verlag. Violations are liable for prosecution under the German Copyright Law.

Springer-Verlag Berlin Heidelberg New York
a member of BertelsmannSpringer Science+Business Media GmbH

http://www.springer.de/medizin

© Springer-Verlag Berlin Heidelberg 2003
Softcover reprint of the hardcover 1st edition 2003

The use of general descriptive names, registered names, trademarks, etc. in this publication does not imply, even in the absence of a specific statement, that such names are exempt from the relevant protective laws and regulations and therefore free for general use.
Product liability: The publishers cannot guarantee the accuracy of any information about the application of operative techniques and medications contained in this book. In every individual case the user must check such information by consulting the relevant literature.

Cover Design: design & production GmbH, 69121 Heidelberg
Typesetting: FotoSatz Pfeifer GmbH, D-82166 Gräfelfing
SPIN: 10755615   21/3130 - 5 4 3 2 1 0

Preface

A lot of time has been spent trying to convince health care providers and policy makers of the enormous importance of macrovascular disease in persons with type 2 diabetes. In this volume, we present facts that demonstrate how important it is to recognize macrovascular disease in these patients in daily practice.

This volume has been compiled to help those already involved in diabetes care, to be more involved in cardiovascular risk control, a task that is not easily achieved.

The area of cardiovascular risk in type 2 diabetes is heterogeneous. Trying to characterize it, we can only say: certainly we know more than we do, but for sure we do less than we could. Our challenge is to change this.

Nicolae Hâncu

Professor N. Hâncu was born in Romania in 1940. He studied medicine at the Iuliu Hatieganu University of Medicine and Pharmacy, Cluj-Napoca, and obtained his speciality in internal medicine in 1970, and in diabetes, nutrition and metabolic disease in 1986. He was appointed Professor and Head of the Department of Diabetes, Nutrition and Metabolic Diseases of the same university in 1993. He has been a full member of the Romanian Academy of Medical Sciences since 1995.

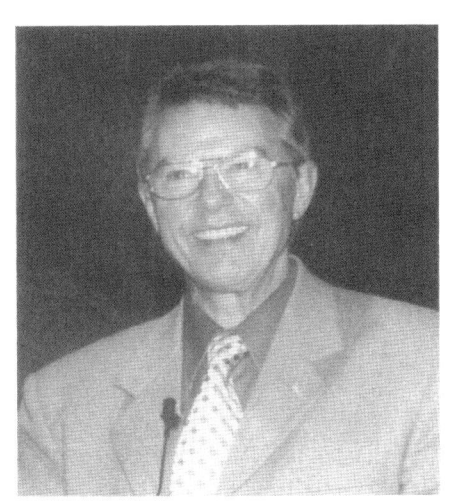

Professor Hâncu's major interest is related to clinical lipidology, visceral obesity, and cardiovascular risk in type 2 diabetes. He has published over 200 papers and 14 books in this area. He has been invited as Visiting Professor at many universities in Madrid, Valladolid, Barcelona, and Los Angeles.

Professor Hâncu is President of The Romanian Federation of Diabetes, Nutrition and Metabolic Disease and The Romanian Association for the Study of

Obesity, and is also a member of several international scientific societies in the field of diabetes, obesity and atherosclerosis. He coordinated the development of the "Romanian Recommendations for Prevention, Diagnosis and Treatment of Type 2 Diabetes and Obesity". He is involved in the European Task Force for the development of practical "Recommendations for Prevention, Diagnosis and Treatment of Obesity".

Professor Hâncu has received the Romanian Academy Award (1978), the Spanish Diabetes Society Award (1990), the "Iuliu Hatieganu Prize" of the Iuliu Hatieganu University of Medicine and Pharmacy, Cluj-Napoca (2001), and the "I. Pavel Prize" of the Romanian Academy of Medical Sciences (2002).

Since 1997, Prof. Hâncu has been President of the Ministerial Committee of Diabetes in Romania. In September 2001, he became Secretary of the Postgraduate Subcommittee of the European Association for the Study of Diabetes (EASD). He has given many lectures at the postgraduate courses organized by the EASD in Europe.

Contents

1. The Heavy Burden of Cardiovascular Disease in Type 2 Diabetes
   M. Laakso 1

2. Atherogenesis in Diabetes
   D. Dabelea 11

3. Hyperglycaemia as Cardiovascular Risk in Type 2 Diabetes
   P. Brunetti, G. Perriello 22

4. Gliclazide and Diabetic Angiopathy
   A.J. Weekes 28

5. Clinical Experience with Repaglinide, the First Prandial Glucose Regulator in Type 2 Diabetes
   K. Brown Frandsen 37

6. Effects of Metformin on Glycaemic Control and Cardiovascular Risk in Type 2 Diabetes
   G. Perriello 47

7. Dyslipidemia and Cardiovascular Risk in Diabetes
   R. Carmena, J.F. Ascaso 53

8. Hypertension in Type 2 Diabetes Mellitus
   M. Serrano Rios, M.T. Martinez Larad 63

9. Microalbuminuria and Cardiovascular Disease in Type 2 Diabetes
   M. Massi Benedetti, M. Orsini Federici 85

10. Cardiovascular Risk in Obese Type 2 Diabetes Mellitus Patients
    G. Roman, X. Formiguera, N. Hâncu 98

11. The Hypertriglyceridemic Waist Concept: Implication for Evaluation and Management of Cardiovascular Disease Risk in Type 2 Diabetes
    I. Lemieux, J.-P. Després 118

12. Oxidative Stress and Cardiovascular Risk in Type 2 Diabetes
    A. Ceriello 140

13 Lifestyle and Cardiovascular Risk in Type 2 Diabetes
   M.W. Conard, W.S. Carlos Poston 150

14 The Prothrombotic Syndrome in Type 2 Diabetes: Assessment
   and Control
   M. Cucuianu, M. Coca 159

15 Hyperhomocysteinemia as Cardiovascular Risk Factor
   in Type 2 Diabetes Mellitus
   A. de Leiva 173

16 Cardiac Autonomic Neuropathy: Is it a Cardiovascular Risk Factor
   in Type 2 Diabetes?
   P. Kempler 181

17 Thiazolidinediones in Cardiovascular Risk in Type 2 Diabetes
   Mellitus
   M. Khamaisi, L. Symmer, I. Raz 193

18 Hyperglycemia and Cardiovascular Disease in Type 2 Diabetes
   Mellitus: Evidence-based Approach to Primary and Secondary
   Prevention
   Z. Milicevic, N. Hâncu, I. Raz 204

19 Cardiac Exploration of Diabetic Patients
   R. Căpâlneanu 212

20 Assessment of Peripheral Vascular Disease
   I.A. Veresiu 227

21 Global Approach to Cardiovascular Risk in Type 2 Diabetic Persons
   N. Hâncu, A. Cerghizan 240

Subject Index 277

Contributors

Ascaso, J.F.
Department of Medicine, University of Valencia, Avda Blasco Ibanez 15, 46010 Valencia, Spain

Brown Frandsen, K.
Novo Nordisk A/S, Building 9 RS,28, Bagsvaerd, Denmark

Brunetti, P.
DiMISEM, Via E Dal Pozzo, 06126 Perugia, Italy

Căpâlneanu, R.
Heart Institute "Niculae Stancioiu", 19 – 21 Motilor St., 3400 Cluj-Napoca, Romania

Carlos Poston, W.S.
4825 Troost, Suite 124, University of Missouri-Kansas City, Kansas City, MO 64110, USA

Carmena, R.
Department of Medicine, University of Valencia, Avda Blasco Ibanez 15, 46010 Valencia, Spain

Cerghizan, A.
Diabetes Center and Clinic, 2 – 4 Clinicilor St., 3400 Cluj-Napoca, Romania

Ceriello, A.
Internal Medicine, University of Udine, P. le S. Maria della Misericordia, 33100 Udine, Italy

Coca, M.
Diabetes Center and Clinic, 2 – 4 Clinicilor st., 3400 Cluj-Napoca, Romania

Conard, M.W.
4825 Troost, Suite 124, University of Missouri-Kansas City, Kansas City, MO 64110, USA

Cucuianu, M.
Diabetes Center and Clinic, 2-4 Clinicilor St., 3400 Cluj-Napoca, Romania

Dabelea, D.
Preventive Medicine and Biometrics, University of Colorado, Health Sciences Center, 4200 East 9th Ave, Box C245, Denver, CO 80262, USA

Després, J.-P.
Lipid Research Center, CHUL Research Center, 2705 Laurier Blvd, Room TR-93, Ste-Foy(Quebec), Canada, G1V 4G2

Formiguera, X.
Institut Catala de la Salud, Hospital Universitario Germans Triasi Pujol, Ctra de Canet, Sin, 08916 Badalona, Spain

Hâncu, N.
Diabetes Center and Clinic, Iuliu Hatieganu University of Medicine and Pharmacy, 2-4 Clinicilor St., 3400 Cluj-Napoca, Romania

Kempler, P.
Internal Department of Medicine, Semmelweis University, Koranyi S.u.2/a, 1083 Budapest, Hungary

Khamaisi, M.
Center of Diabetes, Hadassah University Hospital, Kiryat Hadassah, P.O. Box 12000, Jerusalem 91120, Israel

Laakso, M.
Department of Medicine, University of Medicine, 702110 Kuopio, Finland

de Leiva, A.
Department of Endocrinology, Diabetes and Nutrition, Hospital de la Santa Creu i Sant Pau, Universitat Autonoma de Barcelona, Avda. Sant Antoni M. Claret, 167, 08025 Barcelona, Spain

Lemieux, I.
Lipid Research Center, CHUL Research Center, 2705 Laurier Blvd, Room TR-93, Ste-Foy (Quebec), Canada, G1V 4G2

Martinez Larrad, M.T.
Hospital Clinico San Carlos, Department of Internal Medicine II, Plaza Cristo Rey S/N, 28040 Madrid, Spain

Massi Benedetti, M.
Department of Internal Medicine and Endocrine and Metabolic Sciences, University of Perugia, Perugia, Italy

Milicevic, Z.
Eli Lilly regional Operations Ges.m.b.H., Area Medical Center Vienna, Barichgasse 40-42, 1030 Vienna, Austria

Orsini Federici, M.
Department of Internal Medicine and Endocrine and Metabolic
Sciences, University of Perugia, Perugia, Italy

Perriello, G.
DiMISEM, Via E Dal Pozzo, 06126 Perugia, Italy

Raz, I.
Center of Diabetes, Hadassah University Hospital, Kiryat Hadassah,
P.O. Box 12000, Jerusalem 91120, Israel

Roman, G.
Diabetes Center and Clinic, Iuliu Hatieganu University of Medicine
and Pharmacy, 2 - 4 Clinicilor St., 3400 Cluj-Napoca, Romania

Serrano Rios, M.
Hospital Clinico San Carlos, Department of Internal Medicine II,
Plaza Cristo Rey S/N, 28040 Madrid, Spain

Symmer, L.
Center of Diabetes, Hadassah University Hospital, Kiryat Hadassah,
P.O. Box 12000, Jerusalem 91120, Israel

Veresiu, I.A.
Diabetes Center and Clinic, 2 - 4 Clinicilor St., 3400 Cluj-Napoca,
Romania

Weekes, A.J.
Servier International, 31 Rue de Pont, 92200, Neuilly-sur-Seine, France

CHAPTER 1

The Heavy Burden of Cardiovascular Disease in Type 2 Diabetes

M. Laakso

Abstract. All manifestations of macrovascular disease, coronary heart disease, cerebrovascular disease, and peripheral vascular disease are significantly more common in diabetic patients than in nondiabetic subjects. Although several cardiovascular risk factors are abnormal in patients with type 2 diabetes we can not explain the excess of cardiovascular disease among these patients. The most important risk factors for cardiovascular disease in type 2 diabetic patients are dyslipidemia (elevation of total and low-density lipoprotein cholesterol, decrease in high-density lipoprotein cholesterol and elevation of total triglycerides), elevated blood pressure, smoking and poor glycemic control. Several recent clinical trials have given evidence that the normalization of total and low-density lipoprotein cholesterol and elevated blood pressure reduces the risk of cardiovascular disease similarly in type 2 diabetic patients and nondiabetic individuals. The correction of poor glycemic control reduces microvascular complications but its effect on the prevention of cardiovascular disease is more limited. Drug treatment of established cardiovascular disease in patients with type 2 diabetes should follow the recommendations given for nondiabetic subjects.

Introduction

Several studies have indicated that all manifestations of macrovascular disease, coronary heart disease (CHD), cerebrovascular disease, and peripheral vascular disease, are significantly more common in diabetic patients than in nondiabetic individuals (Laakso and Lehto 1997). The risk for cardiovascular disease (CVD) events is relatively higher among female type 2 diabetic patients than among male type 2 diabetic patients, and it is largely independent of age. Although we can identify several risk factors for macrovascular disease we can not explain the excess of cardiovascular complications among diabetic patients. Both micro- and macrovascular complications are tightly linked with poor metabolic control in patients with type 1 diabetes, but this association in patients with type 2 diabetes is more complex. Because type 2 diabetic patients are > 80 % of all cases of diabetes I will concentrate in this review only on type 2 diabetic subjects.

One of the paradoxes of CVD in type 2 diabetes is that macrovascular disease starts even before the diagnosis of frank hyperglycemia, a sharp contrast to microvascular complications which are mainly depending on glycemic control. In order to understand why type 2 diabetic patients have so high prevalence of macrovascular complications already at diagnosis we have to try to dissect out factors responsible for accelerated atherothrombosis in the prediabetic state, particularly in impaired glucose tolerance (IGT).

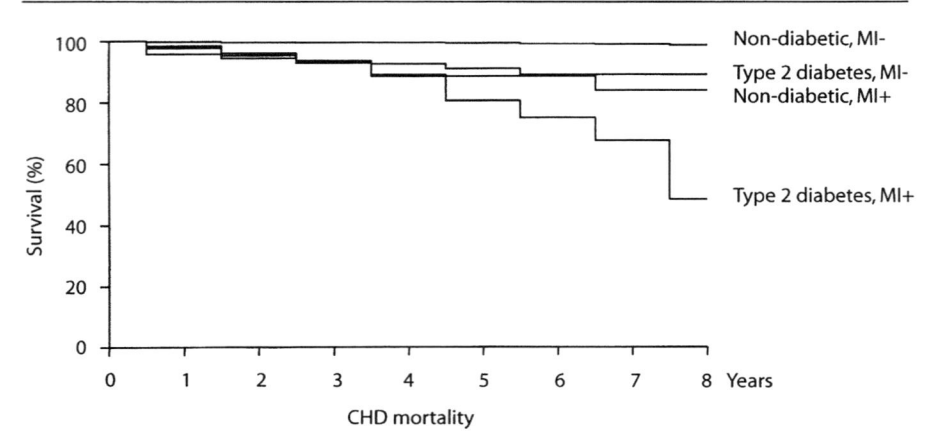

Fig. 1.1. Kaplan-Meier estimates of the probability of death from coronary heart disease in 1,059 subjects with type 2 diabetes and 1,378 nondiabetic subjects with and without prior myocardial infarction. *MI,* myocardial infarction. (Haffner et al. 1998)

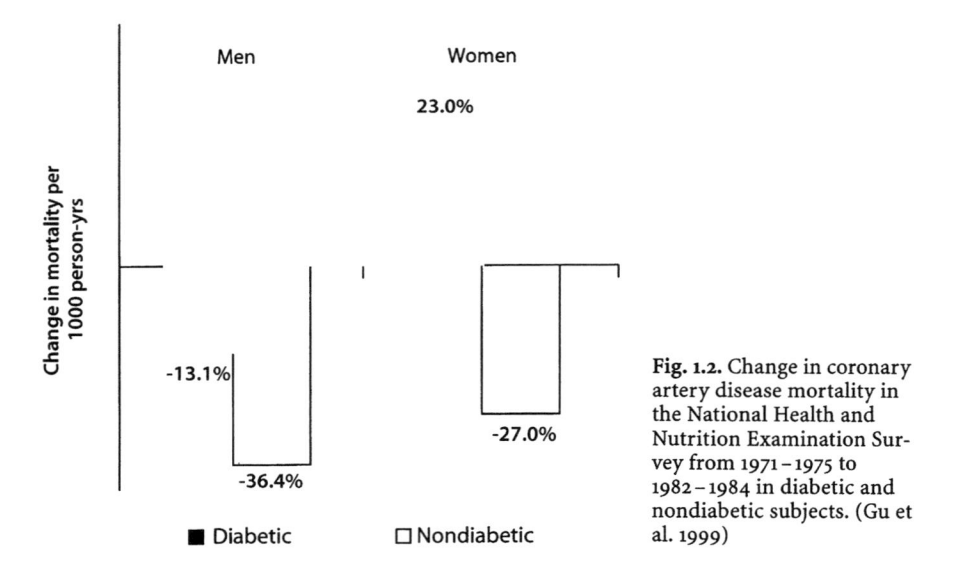

Fig. 1.2. Change in coronary artery disease mortality in the National Health and Nutrition Examination Survey from 1971–1975 to 1982–1984 in diabetic and nondiabetic subjects. (Gu et al. 1999)

The prognosis of type 2 diabetic patients is heavily dependent on the presence of CHD. Our study based on 7-year follow-up of 1059 type 2 diabetic subjects suggested that type 2 diabetic patients without prior myocardial infarction (MI) have as high risk of a new MI as nondiabetic patients with prior MI (Fig. 1.1; Haffner et al. 1998). These findings imply that probably type 2 diabetic patients should be treated as aggressively as nondiabetic patients with MI.

Not only is the incidence and prevalence of type 2 diabetes increasing but also the occurrence of diabetes-related CVD. Furthermore, the time trends in mortality from all causes and CVD based on data from the US show that when nondiabetic subjects have had a decline in coronary artery disease mortality over the years the corresponding decline among diabetic subjects has been considerably less (Gu et al. 1999). In fact, age-adjusted heart disease mortality has even increased in diabetic women (Fig. 1.2). This offers us an important challenge to reduce the risk of CVD events in patients with type 2 diabetes in the future.

Hyperglycemia-Independent Increase in Cardiovascular Disease in the Prediabetic State – Does It Exist?

Two recent studies have indicated that even a slight increase in glucose level is associated with mortality. A meta-regression analysis performed by Coutinho et al. (1999) included 95783 non-diabetic individuals followed for 12.4 years. The study showed that fasting glucose >6.1 mmol/l increased the relative risk of cardiovascular events by 33% (hazard ratio and its 95% confidence intervals 1.33 (1.06–1.17)) compared with a fasting glucose of 4.2 mmol/l or less. Two-hour glucose >7.8 mmol/l and <11.0 mmol/l increased the risk even more, by 58% (1.58[1.19–2.10]). The DECODE Study (1999) included 18048 men and 7316 women from 12 European cohort studies and showed that in men with IGT hazard ratio of death was 1.51 (1.32–1.72) and in women with IGT 1.60 (1.22–2.10) compared to corresponding subjects with fasting glucose <6.1 mmol/l. Thus, in subjects with IGT the risk for CHD and mortality is considerably increased.

What could be the explanation why even a slight increase of glucose is associated with an elevated risk of cardiovascular disease? Of classic risk factors elevated blood pressure is a common finding in subjects with IGT. Furthermore, these subjects are often obese, centrally obese, have high levels of triglycerides and low high-density-lipoprotein (HDL) cholesterol. Although total and low-density lipoprotein (LDL) cholesterol levels are often unchanged these subjects have small dense LDL particles. IGT subjects have also increased thrombosis formation and impaired fibrinolysis. It is important to note that cardiovascular risk factors do not change much into more atherogenic direction when these subjects develop diabetes.

What is the evidence that the clustering of risk factors in the prediabetic state really predicts CHD? We have recently followed elderly nondiabetic subjects for 7 years. By applying statistical technique, factors analysis, we could find a clustering of risk factors with hyperinsulinemia and named this clustering as the insulin resistance syndrome(IRS) factor having the highest loading for insulin and also significant loadings for obesity, high triglycerides, and high glucose (Fig. 1.3; Lempiäinen et al. 1999). Because glucose clustered with other cardiovascular risk factors we can conclude that glucose was not an independent contributor of cardiovascular disease but rather an essential component of the IRS. With logistic regression model we could demonstrate that the IRS factor predicted CHD among these individuals. Therefore, it is likely that in subjects with a slight elevation of glucose an increase in CVD risk is independent of glucose level. Furthermore, it is likely that general cardiovascular risk factors operate similarly in subjects with IGT or other mild abnormalities in glucose metabolism as in normoglycemic subjects although we do not have prospective cohort studies to substantiate this conclusion.

Nondiabetic men　　*Type 2 diabetic subjects*

IRS
- Body mass index ↑
- Insulin ↑
- Triglycerides ↑
- Glucose ↑

⇓

CHD ↑

IRS
- HDL cholesterol ↓
- Insulin ↑
- Triglycerides ↑
- Body mass index ↑

⇓

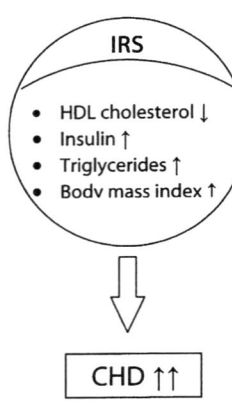

CHD ↑↑

Fig. 1.3. Insulin resistance syndrome (*IRS*) factor (↑ positive loading, ↓ negative loading) in nondiabetic men (Lempiäinen et al. 1999) and in type 2 diabetic subjects (Lehto et al. 2000). *CHD*, coronary heart disease

Type 2 Diabetes and Elevated Risk for Cardiovascular Disease

Type 2 diabetes is associated with multiple adverse changes in cardiovascular risk factors, obesity, central obesity, elevation of blood pressure, elevation of small dense LDL particles and total and very-low-density lipoprotein (VLDL) triglycerides, decrease in HDL cholesterol, enhanced thrombus formation and impaired fibrinolysis (Laakso 1995; Table 1.1).

Several explanations can be offered why type 2 diabetes increases the risk of all manifestations of CVD: (1) Abnormalities in cardiovascular risk factors are more common among type 2 diabetic patients than in nondiabetic subjects and they have a more deleterious effect on the risk of CVD among type 2 diabetic patients than among nondiabetic subjects; (2) Hyperglycemia has a deleterious effect on cardiovascular risk factors leading indirectly to CVD; (3) Hyperglycemia and cardiovascular risk factors have an interaction to increase the risk for CVD; (4) Hyperglycemia itself directly explains an excess risk for CVD in type 2 diabetic patients; and (5) There are unknown risk factors in type 2 diabetic patients leading to increased risk for CVD.

Table 1.1. Summary of risk factors for cardiovascular disease in patients with type 2 diabetes

Risk factor	Abnormality	Independent risk factor	Positive treatment effect
Total cholesterol	±	Yes	Yes
HDL cholesterol	↓	Yes	Yes
Total triglycerides	↑	Yes	Yes
Blood pressure	↑	Yes	Yes
Smoking	±	Yes	NA
Hyperglycaemia	↑	Yes	Yes
Insulin resistance/hyperinsulinemia	↑	?	NA
Obesity/central obesity	↑	No	NA

NA, data not available; ±, no change; ↓, decrease; ↑, increase.

No evidence is available to show that abnormalities in established cardiovascular risk factors have a more deleterious effect on CVD risk in type 2 diabetic patients than in nondiabetic subjects. In fact, several studies have indicated that classic risk factors, elevated total and LDL cholesterol, smoking and elevated blood pressure, operate in a similar way in diabetic and nondiabetic subjects (Laakso and Lehto 1997, Stamler et al. 1993). However, it is possible that low HDL cholesterol is a stronger risk factor for CHD in type 2 diabetic patients than in nondiabetic individuals (Lehto et al. 1997, Turner et al. 1998). Because type 2 diabetic patients are at high risk for CVD these results imply that absolute risk induced by abnormalities in cardiovascular risk factors among type 2 diabetic patients is considerably elevated compared to that among normoglycemic subjects.

Several studies have indicated that hyperglycemia contributes to abnormalities in cardiovascular risk factors. Poor metabolic control leads to high total and LDL cholesterol, high total and VLDL triglycerides and elevation of blood pressure (Laakso and Lehto 1997). The effect of hyperglycemia on HDL cholesterol is more limited. Hyperglycemia favors thrombus formation and impaired fibrinolysis. Furthermore, hyperglycemia is likely to have an interaction with other cardiovascular risk factors, particularly with elevated blood pressure leading to an excess risk for CVD events.

Is hyperglycemia among patients with type 2 diabetes an independent risk factor for CVD? This is certainly the case according to several prospective population-based studies from Caucasian and non-Caucasian populations (Laakso 1999, Laakso 2000). However, the relative predictive power of poor glycemic control for CVD events is likely to be less than that of classic cardiovascular risk factors (total and LDL cholesterol, elevated blood pressure and smoking) on the basis of the United Kingdom Prospective Diabetes Study (UKPDS) (Turner et al. 1998) and our own study (Lehto et al. 1997). The mechanisms via which hyperglicemia could directly exert its harmful effects on the vascular wall are largely unknown. Furthermore, there might be yet unidentified environmental and genetic risk factors which contribute to accelerated atherothrombosis.

Insulin resistance is a characteristic finding in patients with type 2 diabetes. Our study has shown that a clustering of cardiovascular risk factors around hyperinsulinemia also occurred in type 2 diabetic patients (Lehto et al. 2000). Interestingly, and in contrast to nondiabetic subjects (Lempiäinen et al. 1999), hyperglycemia was not significantly loaded on the insulin resistance syndrome factor (Fig. 1.3). Because insulin resistance syndrome factor predicted CHD events independently of hyperglycemia in patients with type 2 diabetes our study indicates that in frank hyperglycemia glucose level is not a part of the IRS, but rather an independent risk factor for CVD events.

How to Treat Cardiovascular Risk Factors Among Type 2 Diabetic Patients

Because several modifiable risk factors in patients with type 2 diabetes predict CVD complications there is a great potential to reduce the burden of atherothrombotic complications in type 2 diabetic patients by intensive treatment (Table 1.1).

Dyslipidemia

Although based on subgroup analyses of larger trials several studies have given a convincing evidence that the treatment of dyslipidemia is of benefit also for type 2 diabetic patients. Statin treatment has been shown to be effective in the primary and secondary prevention of CHD in patients with type 2 diabetes. The reduction of CHD risk by lovastatin treatment was 33% (p=NS) in the Air Force/ Texas Coronary Atherosclerosis Prevention Study (Downs et al. 1998), 55% (p=0.002) by simvastatin treatment in the Scandinavian Simvastatin Survival Study (Pyörälä et al. 1997), 25% (p=0.05) by pravastatin treatment in the Cholesterol And Recurrent Events Trial (Goldberg et al. 1998), and 19% (p=NS) in the Long-term Intervention with Pravastatin in Ischemic Disease trial (1998).

Two studies have indicated that triglyceride lowering and HDL cholesterol elevation are also effective in the prevention of CVD events. In the Helsinki Heart Study (Koskinen et al. 1992) gemfibrozil treatment reduced CHD events by 60% in patients with type 2 diabetes but because only 125 patients were randomized into the trial the reduction was not statistically significant. In the Veterans Affairs High-density Lipoprotein Cholesterol Intervention Trial (Rubins et al. 1999) gemfibrozil reduced the risk of CHD by 24% in diabetic patients (p=0.05).

Elevated Blood Pressure

Two sub-group analyses of larger trials have indicated that drug treatment of isolated systolic hypertension is effective in the prevention of CVD events. The Systolic Hypertension in the Elderly Program showed that in diabetic patients (Curb et al. 1996), most of them having type 2 diabetes, chlorthalidone reduced CVD mortality more effectively than did placebo. Similarly, according to the results of the Systolic Hypertension in Europe Trial (Tuomilehto et al. 1999) nitrendipine reduced CVD events more effectively than did placebo in nondiabetic and diabetic individuals. The lowering of blood pressure levels down to 80 mm Hg by felodipine-based drug treatment in diabetic patients reduced CVD events significantly more than blood pressure level of 90 mm Hg according to the Hypertension Optimal Treatment Study (Hansson et al. 1998). The UKPDS (1998a) included type 2 diabetic patients only and compared tight and less tight control of elevated blood pressure. Intensive treatment with atenolol or captopril reduced diabetes-related deaths by 32%, stroke by 44%, and microvascular complications by 37%. Atenolol and captopril reduced end-points similarly. In contrast, in the Captopril Prevention Project (Hansson et al. 1999) captopril reduced CVD events by 41% more than did the conventional treatment by beta-blockers or diuretics.

Hyperglycemia

The University Group Diabetes Program was the first study aiming to investigate the treatment of hyperglycemia in patients with type 2 diabetes but it did not solve the problem whether or not intensive glycemic control is beneficial in the reduction of CVD in type 2 diabetic patients (Knatterud et al. 1978). The UKPDS (1998b) based on 10-year follow-up of 3867 newly diagnosed patients with type 2 diabetes showed that intensively treated group had 0.9% lower hemoglobin A1c than did the conventionally treated group (7.0 vs. 7.9%). Intensive treatment reduced any diabetes-related end-points by 12% ($p=0.029$), myocardial infarction by 16% ($p=0.052$), and microvascular complications by 25% ($p=0.0099$). Chlorpropamide, glibenclamide and insulin similarly reduced diabetic complications. The Swedish Diabetes Mellitus and Insulin Glucose Infusion in Acute Myocardial Infarction study demonstrated that the institution of intensive insulin treatment during an acute myocardial infarction reduced mortality significantly during the mean follow-up of 3.4 years (Malmberg et al. 1999).

Other Risk Factors

A majority of type 2 diabetic patients are obese and centrally obese, and obesity has a profound effect on all cardiovascular risk factors. Unfortunately, although weight loss and execise still remain the cornerstones of the treatment of type 2 diabetic patients we do not have trials showing that the treatment of obesity has beneficial effects on the reduction of CVD events. Insulin resistance is a central metabolic disturbance in type 2 diabetes. Similarly, no trials have been published whether or not CVD events can be reduced by improving insulin sensitivity by non-pharmacological (weight loss, exercise) or pharmacological treatment.

Drug Treatment of Established Cardiovascular Disease in Patients with Type 2 Diabetes

Patients with type 2 diabetes have not only a greater incidence and prevalence of CVD, but clinical outcomes, such as MI and sudden death, are more frequent than in nondiabetic subjects. The number of diabetic patients who die outside the hospital is particularly high (Miettinen et al. 1998). Therefore, the question how to treat established CVD in diabetic patients is of crucial importance.

In general the trials published so far including a considerable number of diabetic patients have indicated in the treatment of an acute MI, stable CHD, and cardiac failure diabetic patients benefit similarly or more of drug therapy as do nondiabetic individuals. Beta-blocking agents have been shown to be effective also in diabetic patients acutely and chronically after MI and in stable CHD (Malmberg et al. 1989, Jonas et al. 1996). Thrombolytic therapy in acute MI (Fibrinolytic Therapy Trialists' Collaborative Group 1994) and aspirin treatment (Antiplatelet Trialists' Collaborative Group 1994) in chronic CHD are also beneficial in diabetic patients. Similarly, angiotensin-converting enzyme inhibitors reduce mortality after MI (Zuanetti et al. 1997). Particularly interesting is the recently published HOPE study showing that ramipril effectively reduced CVD events in diabetic patients (Heart Outcomes Prevention Evaluation Study Investigators 2000). The blood pressure reduction was only 3 mm Hg, and therefore the reduction of CVD events was more than expected by blood pressure reduction alone. Furthermore, in nondiabetic subjects ramipril prevented at least partly the incidence of type 2 diabetes.

Conclusions

Diabetes is a major risk factor for all manifestation of CVD in addition to elevated cholesterol and blood pressure, smoking, low HDL cholesterol and aging (Grundy et al. 1999). In patients with CVD the prevalence of known diabetes seems to be about 20% (EUROASPIRE Study Group 1997) indicating that diabetes-related atherothrombosis forms a significant health problem.

Intensive treatment of all modifiable risk factors is indicated on the basis of recently published trials. If we assume that type 2 diabetic patients are at the same risk for CVD as are nondiabetic subjects who have suffered from MI the level of LDL cholesterol should be lowered to < 2.6 mmol/l acccording to the National Cholesterol Education Expert Panel recommendations (1988). Elevated blood pressure should be lowered to < 140/80 mm Hg, and smoking should be stopped. Because glycated hemoglobin A1c level is linearly associated with the risk of CVD (Stratton et al. 2000) normoglycemia should be the goal in the treatment of hyperglycemia. Although trial evidence is missing normal weight is highly desirable because obesity and central obesity worsen all cardiovascular risk factors. Lowering of total triglycerides and raising HDL cholesterol seems to be beneficial in the prevention of CVD events but for definite treatment goals more data from ongoing trials are needed. Trials aiming to investigate the effect of the improvement of insulin sensitivity on the reduction of CVD risk are urgently needed.

Finally, several recent trials have indicated that drug treatment of established CVD in type 2 diabetic patients, if needed, should follow the recommendations for nondiabetic subjects.

Acknowledgements. Our research projects refered to in this review have been financially supported by grants from the Academy of Finland, and the Kuopio University Hospital (EVO grants no 5019 and 5123).

References

Antiplatelet Trialist' Collaboration (1994) Collaborative overview of randomised trials of antiplatelet therapy – I: Prevention of death, myocardial infarction, and stroke by prolonged antiplatelet therapy in various categories of patients. BMJ 308; 81–106

Coutinho M, Gerstein HC, Wang Y, Yusuf S (1999) The relationship between glucose and incident cardiovascular events: a metaregression analysis of published data from 20 studies of 95783 individuals followed for 12.4 years. Diabetes Care 22:233–240

Curb DJ, Pressel SL, Cutler JA, Savage PJ, Applegate WB, Black H, Camel G, Davis BR, Frost PH, Gonzales N, Guthrie G, Oberman A, Rutan GH, Stamler (1996) Effect of diuretic-based antihypertensive treatment on cardiovascular disease risk in older diabetic patients with isolated systolic hypertension. Systolic Hypertension in the Elderly Program Cooperative Research Group. JAMA 276, 1886–1892

Downs JR, Clearfield M, Weis S, Whitney E, Shapiro DR, Beere PA, Langerdorfer A, Stein EA, Kruyer W, Gotto AM Jr for the AFCAPS/TexCAPS Research Group (1998) Primary prevention of acute coronary events with lovastatin in men and women with average cholesterol levels: results of AFCAPS/TexCAPS. Air Force/Texas Coronary Atherosclerosis Prevention Study. JAMA 279:1615–1622

EUROASPIRE (1997) A European Society of Cardiology survey of secondary prevention of coronary heart disease: principal results. EUROASPIRE Study Group. European Action on Secondary Prevention through Intervention to Reduce Events. Eur Heart J 18:1569–1589

Fibrinolytic Therapy Trialists' Collaborative Group (1994) Indications for fibrinolytic therapy in suspected acute myocardial infarction: collaborative overview of early mortality and major morbidity results from all randomised trials of more than 1000 patients. Lancet 343:311–322

Goldberg RB, Mellies MJ, Sacks FM, Moye LA, Howard BV, Howard WJ, Davis BR, Cole TG, Pfeffer MA, Braunwald E for the CARE Investigators (1998) Cardiovascular events and their reduction with pravastatin in diabetic and glucose-intolerant myocardial infarction survivors with average cholesterol levels: subgroup analyses in the Cholesterol And Recurrent Events (CARE) Trial. Circulation 98:2513–2519

Grundy SM, Benjamin IJ, Burke GL, Chait A, Eckel RH, Howard BV, Mitch W, Smith SC Jr, Sovers JR (1999) Diabetes and cardiovascular disease: a statement for healthcare professionals from the American Heart Association. Circulation 100:1134-1146

Gu K, Cowie CC, Harris MI (1999) Diabetes and decline in heart disease motality in US adults. JAMA 281:1291–1297

Haffner SM, Lehto S, Rönnemaa T, Pyörälä K, Laakso M (1998) Mortality from coronary heart disease in subjects with type 2 diabetes and in nondiabetic subjects with and without prior myocardial. N Engl J Med 339:229–234

Hansson L, Zanchetti A, Carruthers SG, Dahlöf B, Elmfeldt D, Julius S, Menard J, Rahn KH, Wedel H, Westerling S (1998) Effects of intensive blood-pressure lowering and low-dose aspirin in patients with hypertension: principal results of the Hypertension Optimal Treatment (HOT) randomised trial. HOT Study Group. Lancet 351:1755–1762

Hansson L, Lindholm LH, Niskanen L, Lanke J, Hedner T, Niklason A, Loumanmäki K, Dahlöf B, de Faire U, Morlin C, Karlberg BE, Wester PO, Björck JE (1999) Effect of angiotensin-converting-enzyme inhibition compared with conventional therapy on cardiovascular morbidity and mortality in hypertension: the Captopril Prevention Project (CAPPP) randomised trial. Lancet 353:611–616

Heart Outcomes Prevention Evaluation study investigators (2000) Effects of ramipril on cardiovascular and microvascular outcomes in people with diabetes mellitus: results of the HOPE study and MICRO-HOPE substudy. Lancet 355:253–259

Jonas M, Reicher-Reiss L, Boyko V, Shotan A, Mandelzweig L, Goldbourt U, Behar S, for the Bezafibrate Infarction Prevention (BIP) Study Group (1996) Usefulness of beta-blocker therapy in patients with non-insulin-dependent diabetes mellitus and coronary artery disease . Am J Cardiol 77:1273–1277

Knatterud GL, Klimt CR, Levin ME, Jacobson ME, Goldner MG (1978) Effects of hypoglycemic agents on vascular complications in patients with adult-onset diabetes. VII. Mortality and selected nonfatal events with insulin treatment. JAMA 240:37–42

Koskinen P, Mänttäri M, Manninen V, Huttunen JK, Heinonen OP, Frick MH (1992) Coronary heart disease incidence in NIDDM patients in the Helsinki Heart Study. Diabetes Care 15:820–825

Laakso M (1995) Epidemiology of diabetic dyslipidemia. Diabetes Rev. 3:408–422

Laakso M (1999) Hyperglycemia and cardiovascular disease in type 2 diabetes. Diabetes 48:937–942

Laakso M (2000) Hyperglycemia as a cardiovascular risk factor. International Diabetes Monitor 12:1–5, 2000

Laakso M, Lehto S (1997) Epidemiology of macrovascular disease in diabetes. Diabetes Rev 5:294–315

Lehto S, Rönnemaa T, Haffner SM, Pyörälä K, Kallio V, Laakso M (1997) Dyslipidemia and hyperglycemia predict coronary heart disease events in middle-aged patients with NIDDM. Diabetes 48:1354–1359

Lehto S, Rönnemaa T, Pyörälä K, Laakso M (2000) Cardiovascular risk factors clustering with endogenous hyperinsulinaemia predict death from coronary heart disease in patients with type 2 diabetes. Diabetologia 43:148–155

Lempiäinen P, Mykkänen L, Pyörälä K, Laakso M, Kuusisto J (1999) Insulin resistance syndrome predicts coronary heart disease events in elderly nondiabetic men. Circulation 100:123–128

Malmberg K, Herlitz J, Hjalmarson Å, Ryden L (1989) Effects of metoprolol on mortality and late infarction in diabetics with suspected acute myocardial infarction: retrospective data from two large studies. Eur Heart J 10:423–428

Malmberg K, Norhammar A, Wedel H, Ryden L (1999) Glycometabolic state at admission: important risk marker of mortality in conventionally treated patients with diabetes mellitus and acute myocardial infarction: long term results form the Diabetes and Insulin-Glucose Infusion in Acute Myocardial Infarction (DIGAMI) study. Circulation 99:2626–2632

Miettinen H, Lehto S, Salomaa V, Mähönen V, Niemelä M, Haffner SM, Pyörälä K, Tuomilehto J (1998) Impact of diabetes on mortality after the first myocardial infarction. The FINMONICA Myocardial Infarction Register Study Group. Diabetes Care 21:69–75

National Cholesterol Education Program Expert Panel, National Heart, Lung, and Blood Institute (1988) Report of the National Cholesterol Education Expert Panel on detection, evaluation, and treatment of high blood cholesterol in adults. Arch Intern Med 148:36–69

Pyörälä K, Pedersen TR, Kjekshus J, Faergeman O, Olsson AG, Thorgeirsson G for the Scandinavian Simvastatin Survival Study (4 S) Group (1997) Cholesterol lowering with simvastatin improves prognosis of diabetic patients with coronary heart disease: a subgroup analysis of the Scandinavian Simvastatin Survival Study (4 S). Diabetes Care 0:614–620

Rubins HB, Robins SJ, Collins D, Fye CL, Anderson JW, Elam MB, Faas FH, Linares E, Schaefer EJ, Schectman G, Wilt TJ, Wittes J (1999) Gemfibrozil for the secondary prevention of coronary heart disease in men with low levels of high-density lipoprotein cholesterol. Veterans Affairs High-density Lipoprotein Cholesterol Intervention Trial Study Group. N Engl J Med 341:410–418

Stamler J, Vaccaro O, Neaton JD, Wentworth D for the Multiple Risk Factor Intervention Trial Research Group (1993) Diabetes, other risk factors, and 12-yr cardiovascular mortality for men screened in the multiple risk factor intervention trial. Diabetes Care 16:434–444

Stratton IM, Adler AI, Neil AW, Matthews DR, Manley SE, Cull CA, Hadden D, Turner RC, Holman RR on behalf of the UK Prospective Diabetes Study Group (2000) Association of Glycaemia with macrovascular and microvascular complications of type 2 diabetes (UKPDS 35): prospective observational study. BMJ 321:405–412

The DECODE Study Group on behalf of the European Diabetes Epidemiology Group (1999) Glucose tolerance and mortality: comparison of WHO and American Diabetes Association diagnostic criteria. Lancet 354:617–621

The Long-term Intervention with Pravastatin in Ischaemic Disease (LIPID) Study Group (1998) Prevention of cardiovascular events and death with pravastatin in patients with coronary heart disease and a broad range of initial cholesterol levels. N Engl J Med 339:1349–1357

Tuomilehto J, Rastenyte D, Birkenhäger WH, Thijs L, Antikainen R, Bulpitt CJ, Fletcher AE, Forette F, Goldhaber A, Palatini P, Sarti C, Fagard R (1999) Effects of calcium-channel blockade in older patients with diabetes and systolic hypertension. Systolic Hypertension in Europe Trial Investigators. N Engl J Med 340:677–684

Turner RC, Millns H, Neil HA, Stratton IM, Manley SE, Matthews DR, Holman RR for the United Kingdom Prospective Diabetes Study Group (1998) Risk factors for coronary artery disease in non-insulin dependent diabetes mellitus: United Kingdom Prospective Diabetes Study (UKPDS:23). BMJ 316:823–828

UK Prospective Diabetes Study Group (1998a) Tight blood pressure control and risk of macrovascular and microvascular complications in type 2 diabetes: UKPDS 38. BMJ 317:703-713

UK Prospective Diabetes Study Group (1998b) Intensive blood-glucose control with sulphonylureas or insulin compared with conventional treatment and risk of complications in patients with type 2 diabetes. UKPDS 33. Lancet 352:837–853

Zuanetti G, Latini R, Maggioni AP, Franzosi MG, Santoro L, Tognoni G, on behalf of GISSI-3 Investigators (1997) Effect of the ACE-inhibitors lisinopril on mortality in diabetic patients with acute myocardial infarction: the data from the GISSI-3 Study. Circulation 96:4239–4245

CHAPTER 2

Atherogenesis in Diabetes

D. Dabelea

Abstract. The association between diabetes mellitus and an increased risk for cardiovascular disease (CVD) has been well documented. Among diabetic patients, morbidity and mortality rates from myocardial infarction are increased, as are the risks for recurrent infarction, congestive heart failure, stroke, and peripheral vascular disease. Many efforts have been made in elucidating the relation between the metabolic derangements of diabetes and the increased risk for the development of macrovascular disease Most of the known risk factors that predict large vessel disease in the general population, including dyslipidemia, cigarette smoking, and hypertension have been shown to apply equally in the presence of diabetes and, in general, they can be treated in the same ways, but more aggressively. Overall, about 50 percent of excess heart disease in diabetes can be attributed to associated abnormalities in other known CVD risk factors. However, diabetic status appears to confer risk such that even after correction of other risk factors, the diabetic remains at high risk for macrovascular disease. The excess risk is so high that being diabetic is considered to place a patient in the same risk category as having established coronary and other atherosclerotic disease. The degree of risk is, at least in part, influenced by the degree of glycaemic control. Thus, diabetes may increase CVD risk by both direct and indirect effects.

This chapter reviews current concepts of atherogenesis and highlights some of the ways in which diabetes mellitus is thought to accelerate the progress.

Lesions of Atherosclerosis

The term "atherosclerosis" comes from the Greek words athere (gruel or porridge) and sclerosis (hardening) and was first used in 1904. Albrecht von Haller introduced the term "atheroma" in 1755 (Wolf 1999). Morphologically, atherosclerosis (ATS) is characterized by focal lesions confined to the large elastic and muscular arteries (i.e. aorta, the epicardial coronary arteries, femoral and carotid arteries). These lesions form the base for occurrence of some well-recognized clinical syndromes. When the increase in volume of such a lesion on coronary arteries is sufficiently severe to reduce the cross-sectional area of the lumen by at least 75 percent or the diameter by 50 percent or more, the patient may develop *stable angina*. A lesions with certain morphologic characteristics, an advanced lesion, is more likely to develop intimal injury, which can lead to intraplaque or intraluminal thrombosis, situation that may lead to *unstable angina, acute myocardial infarction* and *sudden death*.

First Lesion: The Fatty Streak

The earliest detectable lesion of ATS is the fatty streak. It is a slightly elevated above the intima, lipid-rich lesion made up of foam cells. The foam cells are mostly derived from circulating monocytes; a smaller number are derived from smooth muscle cells. The main processes involved in the genesis of fatty streak are (Wolf 1999):

- The accumulation within the intima of excess amounts of blood derived LDL cholesterol
- The migration of monocytes, T lymphocytes, and smooth muscle cells into these areas, followed by differentiation of monocytes into macrophages and their uptake of large quantities of modified LDL

First step of fatty streak formation is the adhesion of monocytes and T lymphocytes to an *intact endothelial surface*. Endothelial cells then express all sorts of *cytokines* and *growth factors*: adhesion molecules of the immunoglobulin gene family, selectins, integrins, and vascular cell adhesion molecule-1 (VCAM-1) (Li et al. 1993). These cells then migrate into the subendothelial space, where they differentiate into macrophages and fill-up with large amounts of lipids (*foam cells*) (Seddon et al. 1987, Fagiotto et al. 1994).

Macrophages do not bind LDL via the LDL receptor described by Glodstein and Brown (Brown, Goldstein 1986), but instead they recognize and bind LDL via a family of receptors that only can bind *chemically modified LDL*. They presumably do not down-regulate, and modified LDL can be taken up via these receptors fast enough to progressively build up the foam cells (Steinberg 1997). The first such receptor, which was cloned and characterized by Kodama and colleagues (Kodama et al. 1990), was the *acetyl LDL receptor*. They called it the "*scavenger receptor*". It now appears that there are several families of scavenger receptors, and the acetyl LDL receptor is now referred to as a class A scavenger receptor. However, there is no evidence that LDL acetylation occurs in vivo. In 1981, Henriksen and colleagues described that an *oxidative modification of LDL* might account for the foam cell formation in vivo (Henriksen et al. 1981). Oxidized LDL seems to be taken up quite fast both via the acetyl LDL receptor and via another different scavenger receptor. Moreover, oxidized LDL has biologic properties that enhance its atherogenicity (Steinberg 1997). Oxidative modification of the LDL particle starts to some degree before its recognition by scavenger receptors. At this stage, the LDL is *minimally oxidized*. The minimally oxidized LDL is capable to stimulate the release from endothelial cells chemical signals such as macrophage, granulocyte-macrophage, and granulocyte colony-stimulating factors (M-CSF, GM-CSF, G-CSF), all of which are potent stimulators of leucopoiesis. In addition, minimally oxidized LDL is able to stimulate the secretion of monocyte chemotactic protein-1 (MCP-1), and may influence arterial functions through impairing the nitric-oxide mediated vasodilatation that occurs in response to acethylcoline, bradikinin, and thrombin, and through increasing the release of plasminogen activator inhibitor-1 (PAI-1) (Wolf 1999). To what extent these in vitro properties are important in atherogenesis remains to be ascertained. Conversion of LDL to its oxidized form is associated with more atherogenic features; therefore, any metabolic abnormality that increases the rate of LDL oxidation could accelerate ATS.

Fibrolipid Plaques or Advanced Lesions

Fatty streak progression to fibrous plaque or advanced lesion is a process that shares many features with chronic inflammation. All the main cells involved – endothelial, macrophages, T lymphocytes, and smooth muscle cells – can generate and release chemotactic, vasoactive, mitogenic and growth factors, cytokines and leukotrienes. The result is the a recruitment of smooth cell muscle from the media into the intima, where they proliferate and secrete proteoglycans, collagen, elastin, and other connective tissue proteins, which form a fibrous cap over the top of the lesion. The result is the formation of a large fibrolipid plaque rich in both connective tissue and lipids (Wolf 1999). The fibrolipid plaque represents the substrate on which thrombosis can occur and its extent in the arterial wall predicts the development of CVD in any population (Deupree 1973). The relative proportion of the cap and core in a fibrolipid plaque correlate with the future acute event: a large lipid core and a thin fibrous cap are associated with a higher risk of plaque injury and subsequent thrombosis than a thick cap with a small lipid pool.

Exactly what triggers the progression from fatty streak to fibrolipid plaque is still uncertain. However, progression is by no means inevitable and it would be of utmost importance to identify the trigger(s). One hypothesis is that the endothelial layer that covers the fatty streak loses its integrity, exposing the underlying lesion to the blood stream *(the response to injury hypothesis)*. This could be followed by platelet aggregation and release of cytokines such as platelet-derived growth factors (PDGF), which can modulate recruitment and proliferation of smooth muscle cells, in a way that would represent a reparatory process (Wolf 1999).

Plaque Injury and Thrombosis

The fibrolipid plaque can probably build up over several years until it matures enough to become an *advanced lesion*. The morphological correlate of potential life-threatening events is the *unstable plaque*, which has undergone injury and thrombosis. Plaque injury can be superficial and deep. Superficial injury is a denudation of the surface endothelium. In such large areas of denudation mural and sometimes occlusive thrombi may form. Plaques in which superficial injury occurs are those in which the collagen strands are separated by large numbers of foam cells (Davies et al, 1988; Davies 1990). Deep injury is a plaque split or rupture from the luminal surface down to the soft lipid pool. Blood from the lumen enters the plaque and thrombus formation takes place within the plaque itself. Both mural and occlusive thrombi can develop this way (Falk 1985; Fuster et al. 1992). Plaques in which such fissuring occurs are those with a large lipid-rich core (Richardson et al. 1989).

Atherosclerosis in Diabetes

It is now widely accepted that ATS in diabetic patients is qualitatively identical to ATS in non-diabetic individuals, since the histological appearance of the lesions, the chemical composition, and the sites of predilection are almost exactly the same. The

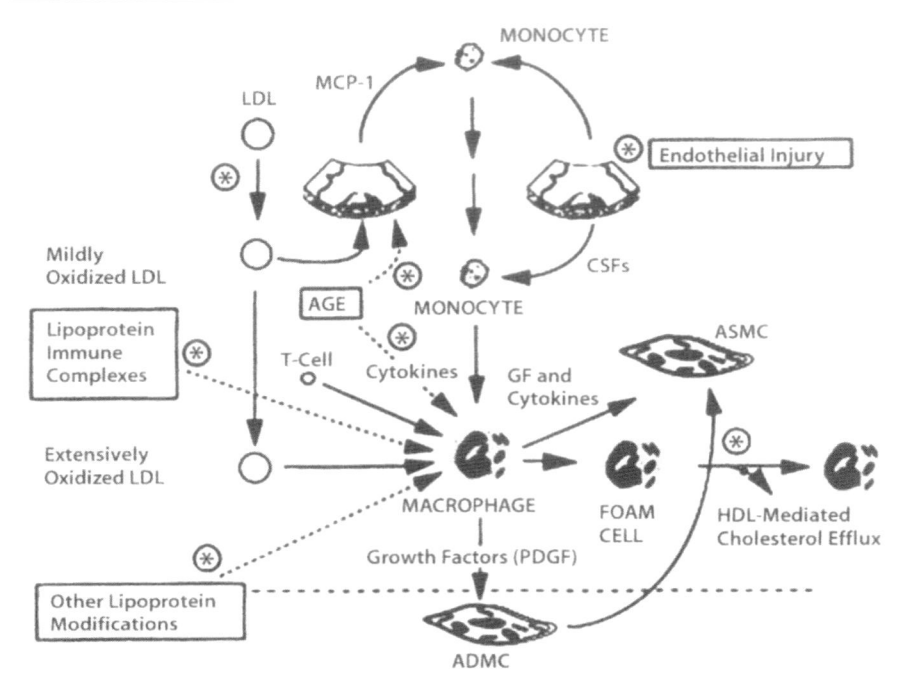

Fig. 2.1. Sites at which DM is thought to influence atherogenesis. *CSFs*, colony-stimulating factors; *GF,* growth factors; *ASMC*, arterial smooth muscle cell; *PDGF,* platelet-derived growth factor; *MCP-1*, monocyte chemotactic protein-1. [Reprinted from Bierman EL (1992) Atherogenesis in diabetes. Arteriosclerosis and thrombosis 12)]

only – significant – difference is the excess and premature morbidity from ATS in diabetic subjects of both sexes. Why this is the case it is not clear, but several possibilities are thought to account for this observation. One is the higher prevalence of all known CVD risk factors in diabetes, another is the presence of diabetic dyslipidemia, which has unique features shown to be atherogenic, but there are also other mechanisms through which diabetes "per se" is thought to contribute to premature ATS (Fig. 2.1). The next part of this chapter summarizes some of the current knowledge.

Diabetic Dyslipidemia

Disturbances in lipoprotein patterns in diabetes are both quantitative and qualitative. Thus, dyslipidemia may be a contributing factor to the premature ATS in diabetic subjects, but there are also many diabetic patients who do not have dyslipidemia but in whom premature ATS is present.

Type 1 Diabetes Mellitus

In general the lipoprotein pattern is anti-atherogenic in individuals with type 1 diabetes mellitus (DM) who are insulin treated and have optimal glycemic control (Taskinen 1992). The lack of abnormalities of lipoprotein levels does not exclude the possibility that there are compositional changes that may be atherogenic. James and Pometta (James, Pometta 1990) found that in poorly controlled type 1 diabetic patients both VLDL and LDL sub-fractions showed multiple abnormalities. First, all three VLDL subclasses were increased and contained excess of non-apo B apolipoproteins (apo Cs and Es). Second, LDL subclasses distribution demonstrated a shift to relative excess of small dense LDL. Third, LDL particles were more triglyceride rich but depleted in esterified cholesterol as compared to normal subjects. Importantly, intensive insulin therapy was associated with a marked fall of VLDL particles and also corrected the distribution of LDL subclasses.

Type 2 Diabetes Mellitus

The major lipid abnormalities found in type 2 diabetic patients are *elevation of serum VLDL triglycerides associated with a low concentration of HDL cholesterol* (Taskinen 1992). Usually, the elevation of serum triglycerides is mild or moderate and the triglyceride values are 1.5 to 3.0 fold compared with those of non-diabetic cohorts matched for age, sex, and BMI. The HDL cholesterol is on average reduced by 10–20%. The sex difference for HDL is less in type 2 diabetic patients than in nondiabetic cohorts. The recognition that hypertriglyceridemia is associated with multiple alterations of other lipoproteins that are potentially atherogenic has expanded the picture of diabetic dyslipidemia (Jonasson et al. 1986). Type 2 diabetic patients commonly have increased production of VLDL particles and this defect is the principal cause for the raised levels of plasma triglycerides (Syvänne, Taskinen 1997). In addition, impaired clearance of triglyceride rich particles contributes to the elevation of plasma triglycerides. The traditional concept is that hyperinsulinemia, compensatory to insulin resistance, stimulates the VLDL production in the liver in the presence of enhanced free fatty acid (FFA) flux (Reaven 1988). There is convincing evidence that the substrate flux of FFA into liver is increased in type 2 DM, and in insulin resistant states (Lewis 1997). Malmström and colleagues (Malmström et al. 1997) reported that type 2 diabetic patients in contrast to normal men failed to suppress large VLDL particles (VLDL1) release from the liver in response to acute hyperinsulinemia. This failure of insulin to suppress large VLDL particles production in type 2 diabetes results in *inappropriate production of large buoyant VLDL1* in the postprandial phase and most likely contributes *to postprandial lipemia* and to the raised triglyceride levels seen with type 2 DM (Knudsen et al. 1995). In type 2 DM, the delipidation rate of triglyceride rich particles is delayed. Another key feature of diabetic dislipidemia is the *excess formation of small dense LDL particles*. They are the product of large VLDL (triglyceride enriched VLDL1 particles) delipidation, the principal component of VLDL subclasses in type 2 DM. The delayed passage of triglyceride-rich lipoproteins (TRL) through the lipolytic cascade favors enhanced core lipid exchange between TRL and LDL, mediated by cholesterol-ester-transfer-protein (CETP). Large lipid rich LDL particles which result are a good substrate for hepatic lipase and its action leads to formation of smaller dense LDL particles, thought to be *the most atherogenic LDL subclass, since they are most susceptible to glycation and oxidation*. There seem to be symmetry of mechanism for the lowering of HDL cholesterol to the formation of small dense LDL. The long residence time of TRLs in circulation also results in enhanced exchanges of core lipids between TRLs and HDL particles. This process leads to formation of triglyceride rich HDL particles, which are good substrate for hepatic lipase. The end-result of this process is a *reduced number of small size HDL particles* (HDL3), the principal HDL subclass in type 2 DM (Frénais et al. 1997). HDL is the particle involved in cholesterol efflux from the arterial wall cells. *DM is associated with a decreased removal of cholesterol from arterial wall*. Several modifications of HDL, which alter its functions, have also been described in diabetes. Extensively glycated HDL as well as HDL that has been oxidized with copper bind poorly to cell-surface proteins and does not facilitate cholesterol efflux to the same extent as unmodified HDL.

Hyperglycemia and Insulin Resistance

DM is characterized by major abnormalities in glucose metabolism and insulin action, which can lead to a whole range of vascular changes in the area of leukocyte adhesions, smooth muscle cell proliferation, contractility and coagulation (Caprio et al. 1997).

The molecular mechanisms through which hyperglycemia may cause vascular dysfunction are at least four: *non-enzymatic glycation of proteins, lipid oxidation, polyol-myoinositol pathway*, and *activation of diacylglycerol (DAG) and protein kinase C (PKC)* (Chait, Heinecke 1999).

Non-enzymatic Glycation

Glucose reacts non-enzymatically with amino groups from all of the plasma proteins and probably all of the cell surface membrane proteins to form Schiff bases. The rate of this process is proportional to glucose concentration. The early steps in glycation are reversible but if the process continues, and this happens often with diabetic patients when their glycemic control is poor, the protein-glucose adducts spontaneously suffer an Amadori rearrangement, giving rise to *advanced glycosylation end products (AGE)*. There is accumulating evidence that AGEs have several interactions with the atherosclerotic process, and contribute to the pathogenesis of macrovascular disease at least as much as they are involved in the pathogenesis of microvascular complications of diabetes.

- Reactive oxygen species generated from glycation increase cross-linking of extracellular matrix, quench nitric oxide, and may damage DNA (Brownlee 1993).
- Several cell-surface receptors for AGEs-modified proteins have been described; these findings support the theory that there are receptor-mediated signaling processes that alter vascular functions (Vlassara 1992; Khoo et al. 1992).
- Glycation of connective tissue matrix proteins increases the probability that LDL is trapped in the vessel wall where it undergoes more extensive oxidation and fur-

ther glycation (Brownlee et al. 1984). LDL binds easily to all the matrix proteins, but it binds even stronger when these proteins carry AGEs.
- LDL could undergo non-enzymatic glycation, and this decreases its affinity for the native LDL receptor, prolonging its plasmatic lifetime, and increasing the probability of its undergoing oxidation (Witzum et al. 1981). Oxidative modifications as well as non-enzymatic glycation of trapped LDL increase its uptake by scavenger receptors on macrophages in the subendothelial space.
- Autoantibodies against glycated LDL (Witzum et al. 1981) and against oxidized LDL (Palinski 1994) have been demonstrated in both normal subjects and, at high titers, in diabetic patients. Immune complexes of oxidized LDL have been found in atherosclerotic lesions in receptor-deficient rabbits (Palinski et al. 1989). They can be recognized by the Fc receptor and provide an additional pathway for rapid uptake and built-up of foam cells (Khoo et al. 1988). Immune complexes are also cytotoxic and could thus favor the progression of the lesions. It has been shown that T-lymphocytes are almost universally present in atherosclerotic lesions (Jonasson et al. 1986), although the precise role of these cells in atherogenesis in not known.
- AGEs are chemotactic for monocytes and activate them. They selectively induce monocyte migration across an intact endothelium. When monocytes interact with the AGEs in the matrix, they increase their production of PDGF, IGF-I, IL-I, and TNF, which are all implicated in the pathogenesis of the atherosclerotic lesion (Steinberg 1997).

Lipid Oxidation

Hyperglycemia has been reported to be associated with an increase in oxidants, both extracellular and intracellular (Feener, King 1997). However, decreased serum antioxidant activity has not been a consistent finding (Wells-Knecht et al. 1995). Free oxygen radicals can arise from either glycation or increased oxidase activity that occurs with activation of protein kinase C. Moreover, DM seems to be associated with an increased lipoprotein oxidation (Sato et al. 1979; Nishigaki et al. 1981). Studies in streptozotocin-diabetic animals showed that there is increased lipid oxidation in the plasma lipoproteins and red cell membranes, and this increase can be prevented by treating the animal with antioxidants (Chisolm et al. 1992).

Glycation and lipid oxidation may be interactive and synergistic. Glycosylated proteins may be more susceptible to oxidative modifications and oxidized lipoproteins are more susceptible to glycation. The connection between diabetes and oxidation seems to work in both ways: oxidation of LDL is enhanced in the presence of hyperglycemia and the rate of generation of glycosylated proteins is accelerated under pro-oxidant conditions (Hickes et al. 1988; Hunt et al. 1990). In atherosclerotic lesions one can find both oxidized LDL and advanced AGEs, compatible with an interaction between the two mechanisms (Haberland et al. 1988; Nakamura et al. 1993).

Polyol-myoinositol Pathway

Hyperglycemia with increased glucose metabolism can lead to the accumulation of sorbitol via aldose reductase. Sorbitol can be subsequently converted to fructose by sorbitol dehydrogenase. Increased sorbitol concentrations in tissues increase osmotic pressure, decrease myoinositol concentrations, and, in combination with glycolisis, alter the intracellular redox balance. However, to what extent this pathway is important in the pathogenesis of vascular complications of diabetes is still not clear (Sorbinil Retinopathy Trial Research Group 1993).

Diacylglycerol and Protein Kinase C Pathways

Glycolisis is the major pathway of glucose metabolism and hyperglycemia increases diacylglycerol (DAG) concentrations in several types of vascular cells and tissues. This increase is the result of accelerated DAG synthesis through the stepwise acylation of triose intermediates generated from glycolisis, which leads to fatty-acid synthesis and the subsequent acylation of glycerol (Feener, King 1997). DAG is a rate-limiting co-factor for protein kinase C (PKC). Recent studies have shown an increase in DAG levels and activation of PKC activities in vascular cells exposed to hyperglycemia, both in culture and in diabetic patients (Ishii et al. 1996). PKC is a family of 12 isoforms of serine and threonine kinases (Feener, King 1997). The βI and II isoforms are predominantly increased in the vascular cells of diabetic subjects. This specific activation of PKCβ isoforms has been related to several biochemical, cellular and physiological changes in the vasculature. The changes are associated with a higher transcription of transforming growth factor β (TGFβ), which in turn leads to an increase synthesis of extra-cellular matrix proteins such as type IV and VI collagen and fibronectin, resulting in capillary membrane thickening (Sharma et al. 1996). This thickening can lead to vascular dysfunction and to acceleration of ATS.

A new theory is suggesting that insulin has both atherogenic and anti-atherogenic effects on the vasculature (Kinball et al. 1994). The *anti-atherogenic actions* include vasodilatation through nitric oxide release, inhibition of tumor necrosis factor and angiotensin II activities, amino acid transport, and conversion of glucose into glycogen (Caprio 1997). The *atherogenic functions* include smooth muscle cell growth, and increased basement matrix synthesis and PAI-I expression. Given these totally opposite effects of insulin on the vasculature, information about the balance between them in insulin resistant states is important. Insulin action is thought to be increased in the vascular tissues under these conditions, but the ability of insulin to induce vasodilatation is low in insulin resistance and diabetes (Khoo et al. 1992). This might be due to inactivation of nitric oxide or to a general impairment in the ability of the endothelium to produce nitric oxide (Steinberg et al. 1996). Al these findings suggest a *vascular insulin resistance in diabetes*. Thus, at physiological concentrations, insulin has anti-atherogenic properties that can be lost in diseases characterized by insulin resistance or insulin deficiency.

Several epidemiological studies have demonstrated an association between insulin resistance, hypertension and CVD. Angiotensin II has been implicated in ATS through its effects on smooth muscle cell growth and migration, and on expression of putative atherogenic and thrombogenic genes such as PAI-I (Hamdan et al. 1996). Similarly, the vasopressor peptide endothelin 1, whose expression in endothelial cells in also increased by angiotensin II and insulin, is believed to be involved in the pathogenesis of CVD. The *increased activity of vasopressor peptides, combined with diminished action of nitric oxide*, may partially account for the excess hypertension in insulin resistant states and diabetes (Feener, King 1997).

Diabetes and Thrombosis

Diabetes may influence the latter stages of ATS, the terminal fatal thrombosis. DM has long time thought to be a pro-coagulant state. Plasma concentrations of plasminogen activator inhibitor I (PAI-I) are increased in insulin resistant states and type 2 DM, and may account for the decrease in fibrinolysis. Several factors, such as hyperinsulinemia, insulin precursors, and tumor necrosis factor α (TNF α) *increase PAI-I concentrations*. In addition, *endothelial dysfunction*, described both in insulin resistant states and DM, may reduce the anticoagulant properties of the endothelium. A decrease in the synthesis of prostaglandin I2 and in nitric oxide action may reduce the endothelium's protective effects against platelet adhesion (Wolf 1999). Thrombosis is often triggered by erosion of the fibrous cap, exposing blood to thrombogenic factors in the lipid core of the lesion. The rupture generally happens at the margin of the lesion, where there are higher densities of macrophages. It might be possible that macrophages are less robust and more prone to lyse and spill their content or to release lytic enzymes in lesions from diabetic than in those from non-diabetic patients. Because there is evidence that conversion from a fatty streak to a fibrous plaque is associated with *loss of endothelial integrity*, this may be another way in which the lesions in diabetic patients advance faster that in non-diabetic individuals.

Conclusions

The macrovascular complications associated with DM are a result of combination of metabolic and hormonal imbalances. The past decade has seen some outstanding progress in understanding the vascular pathobiology so that sequential important events leading to ATS can now be described. Moreover, explicit ways through which DM may lead to accelerated atherogenesis can now be recognized. Intensive glycemic control seems to delay the onset and slow the progression of vascular dysfunction and diseases, as demonstrated by DCCT and UKPDS, but does not eradicate them (Feener, King 1997). Of utmost importance, management of all of the conventional risk factors for ATS in diabetic patients should rank as high as control of hyperglycemia.

References

1. Brown MS, Goldstein JL (1986). A receptor-mediated pathway for cholesterol homeostasis. Science 232: 34–47
2. Brownlee M (1994). Lilly Lecture 1993. Diabetes 43: 836–841
3. Brownlee M, Vlassara H, Cerami A (1984). Nonenzymatic glycosylation products of collagen covalently trap low-density lipoprotein. Diabetes 34: 938–941
4. Caprio S, Wong S, Alberti KGMM, King G (1997). Cardiovascular complications of diabetes. Diabetologia 40: B78-B82
5. Chait A, Heinecke JW (1999). Lipoproteins, modified lipoproteins and atherosclerotic vascular disease. In: In: Betteridge DJ, Illingworth DR, Sheperd J (eds). Lipoproteins in health and disease. Arnold, pp 597–611
6. Chisolm GM, Irwin KC, Penn MS (1992). Lipoprotein oxidation and lipoprotein-induced cell injury in diabetes. Diabetes 41 (suppl 2): 61–66

7. Davies MJ (1990) A macro and micro view of coronary vascular insult in ischemic heat disease. Circulation 82: 1138–1146
8. Davies MJ, Wolf N, Rowles O, Pepper J (1988). Morphology of the endothelium over atherosclerotic plaques in human coronary arteries. British Heart Journal 60: 459–464
9. Deupree R, Fields R, McMahan C, and Strong JP (1973). Laboratory Investigation 28: 252–262
10. Faggiotto A, Ross R, Harker L (1984). Studies of hypercholesterolemia in the nonhuman primate. I Changes that lead to fatty streak formation. Arteriosclerosis 4: 232–240
11. Falk E (1985) Unstable angina with fatal outcome: dynamic coronary thrombosis leading to infarction and/or sudden death. Autopsy evidence of recurrent mural thrombosis with peripheral embolization culminating in total vascular occlusion. Circulation 71: 699–708
12. Feener EP, King GL (1997). Vascular dysfunction in diabetes mellitus. Lancet 350 (suppl I): 9–13
13. Frénais R, Ouguerranm K, Maugeais C, Mahot P, Maugère P, Krenpf M, Magot T (1997). High-density lipoprotein apolipoprotein AI kinetics in NIDDM: a stable isotope study. Diabetologia 40: 578–583
14. Fuster V, Badimon L, Badimon JJ, and Chesebro JH (1992). The pathogenesis of coronary artery disease and the acute coronary syndromes (2). New England Journal of Medicine 326: 310–318
15. Haberland ME, Fong D, Cheng L (1988). Malondialdehyde-altered protein occurs in atheroma of Watanabe heritable hyperlipidemic rabbits. Science 241: 215–218
16. Hamdan AD, Quist WC, Gagne JB, Feener EP (1996). Angiotensin-converting enzyme inhibition suppresses plasminogen activator inhibitor-1 expression in the neointima of balloon-injured rat aorta. Circulation 93: 1073–1078
17. Henriksen T, Mahoney EM, Steinberg D (1981). Enhanced macrophage degradation of low-density lipoprotein previously incubated with cultured endothelial cells: recognition by receptors for acetylated low density lipoproteins. Proc Natl Acad Sci USA 78: 6499–6503
18. Hickes M, Delbridge L, Yue DK, Reeve TS (1988). Catalysis of lipid peroxidation by glucose and glycosylated collagen. Biochem Biophys Res Comm 151: 629–655
19. Hunt JV, Smith CCT, Wolff SP (1990). Autoxidative glycosylation and possible involvement of peroxides and free radicals in LDL modification by glucose. Diabetes 39: 1420–1424
20. Ishii H, Jirousek M, Ballas L, et al (1996). Prevention of diabetes-induced vascular dysfunctions by oral PKC isoenzyme-selective inhibitor. Science 272: 728–731
21. James RW, Pometta D (1990). Differences in lipoprotein subfraction composition and distribution between type 1 diabetic men and control subjects. Diabetes 39: 1158–1164
22. Jonasson L, Holm J, Shalli O, et al (1986). Regional accumulations of T cells, macrophages, and smooth muscle cells in the human atherosclerotic plaque. Arteriosclerosis 6: 131–138
23. Kahri J, Groop P-H, Viberti GC, Elliott T, Taskinen M-R (1993). Regulation of apolipoprotein A-I containing lipoproteins in IDDM. Diabetes 42: 1281–1288
24. Khoo JC, Miller E Pio F, et al (1992). Monoclonal antibodies against LDL further enhance macrophage uptake of LDL aggregates. Arterioscler Thromb 12: 1258–1266
25. Khoo JC, Miller E, McLoughlin P, Steinberg D (1988). Enhanced macrophage uptake of low-density lipoprotein after self-aggregation. Arteriosclerosis 8: 348–358
26. Kinball TR, Daniels SR, Khoury PR, Magnotti RA, Turn AM, Dolan LM (1994) Cardiovascular status in young patients with insulin-dependent diabetes mellitus. Circulation 90: 357–361
27. Knudsen P, Eriksson J, Lahdenperä S, Kahri J, Groop L, Taskinen M-R (1995). Changes of lipolytic enzymes cluster with insulin resistance syndrome. Diabetologia 38: 344–350
28. Kodama T, Freeman M, Rohrer L, et al (1990). Type I macrophage scavenger receptor contains α-helical and collagen-like coiled coils. Nature 343: 531–535
29. Lewis GF (1997). Fatty acid regulation of very low-density lipoprotein production. Curr Opin Lipidol 8: 146–153
30. Li H, Cybulsky MI, Gimbrone MA Jr, Libby P (1993). An atherogenic diet rapidly induces VCAM-1, a cytokine-regulatable mononuclear leukocyte adhesion molecule in rabbit aortic endothelium. Arterioscler Thromb 13: 197–204
31. Malmström R, Packard C, Caslake M, Bedford D, Steward P, Yki-Järvinen H, Sheperd T, Taskinen M-R (1997). Defective regulation of triglyceride metabolism by insulin in the liver in NIDDM. Diabetologia 40: 454–462
32. Nakamura Y, Horii Y, Nishino T, et al (1993). Immunocytochemical localization of advanced glycosylation end products in coronary atheroma and cardiac tissue in diabetes mellitus. Am J Pathol 143: 1649–1656

33. Nishigaki I, Haghihara M, Tsunekava HT, et al (1981). Lipid peroxides and atherosclerosis. Biochem Med 25: 373–378
34. Palinski W, Ord V, Plump AS, et al (1994). Apoprotein A-deficient mice are a model of lipoprotein oxidation in atherogenesis: Demonstration of oxidative-specific epitopes in lesions and high titers of autoantibodies to malondialdehidehydelsine in serum. Arterioscler Thromb 14: 605–616
35. Palinski W, Rosenfeld ME, Ylä-Herttuala S, et al (1989). Low density lipoproteins undergoes oxidative modification in vivo. Proc Natl Acad Sci USA 86: 1372–1376
36. Reaven GM (1988) Role of insulin resistance in human disease. Diabetes 37: 1595–1607
37. Richardson P, Davies MJ, and Born G (1989) Influence of plaque configuration and stress distribution on fissuring of coronary atherosclerotic plaques. Lancet ii: 941–944
38. Sato Y, Hotta N, Sakamoto N, et al (1979). Lipid peroxide level in plasma of diabetic patients. Biochem Med 21: 104–107
39. Seddon AM, Wolf N, LaVille A, et al. (1987). Hereditary hyperlipidemia and atherosclerosis in the rabbit due to overproduction of lipoproteins. II Preliminary report of arterial pathology. Arteriosclerosis 7: 113–124
40. Sharma K, Jin Y, Guo J, Ziyadeh FN (1996). Neutralization of TGF-beta antibody attenuates kidney hypertrophy and the enhanced extra cellular matrix gene expression in STZ-induced diabetic mice. Diabetes 45: 522–530
41. Sorbinil Retinopathy Trial Research Group (1993). The sorbinil retinopathy trial: neuropathy results. Neurology 43: 1141–1149
42. Steinberg D (1997) Diabetes and atherosclerosis. In: Ellenberg & Rifkin's Diabetes Mellitus, 5th Edition, Appeton & Lange, pp 193–207
43. Steinberg HO, Chaker H, Leaming R, Johnson A, Brechtel G, Baron AD. Obesity/insulin resistance is associated with endothelial dysfunction. J Clin Invest 1996; 97: 2601–2610
44. Syvänne M, Taskinen M-R (1997). Lipids and lipoproteins as coronary risk factors in non-insulin-dependent diabetes mellitus. Lancet 350: 20–23
45. Taskinen M-R (1992). Quantitative and qualitative lipoprotein abnormalities in diabetes mellitus. Diabetes 41: 12–17
46. Taskinen M-R Lahdenperä S, Syvänne M (1996). New insights into lipid metabolism in non-insulin-dependent diabetes mellitus. Ann Med 28: 335–340
47. Vlassara H (1992). Receptor-mediated interactions of advanced glycosylation endproducts with cellular components within diabetic tissues. Diabetes 41 (suppl2): 52–56
48. Wells-Knecht MC, Thorpe SR, Baynes JW (1995). Pathways of formation of glycoxidation products during glycation of collagen. Biochemistry 34: 15134–15141
49. Withzum JL, Steinbrecher UP, Kesaniemi YA, Fisher M (1984). Autoantibodies to glucosylated proteins in the plasma of patients with diabetes mellitus. Proc Natl Acad Sci USA 81: 3204–3208
50. Witzum JL, Mahoney EM, Branks MJ, et al (1981). Nonenzymatic glycosilation of low-density lipoproteins alters its biological activity. Diabetes 31: 283–291
51. Wolf N (1999) Pathology of atherosclerosis. In: Betteridge DJ, Illingworth DR, Sheperd J (eds). Lipoproteins in health and disease. Arnold, pp 533–541

CHAPTER 3

Hyperglycaemia as Cardiovascular Risk in Type 2 Diabetes

P. Brunetti, G. Perriello

Cardiovascular disease is responsible for approximately 70 % of all causes of death in type 2 diabetes (Laakso and Lehto 1997). Among cardiovascular diseases ischemic cardiopathy represents the primary cause of death, since mortality rates for coronary artery disease (CHD) are 2 – 4 times greater in diabetics than in non diabetic individuals (Haffner et al. 1998). Cerebrovascular events are the second cause of death in patients with type 2 diabetes.

Morbidity rates are substantially superimposed to mortality rates. In Framingham study, CHD incidence was 2 – 4 times greater in diabetics than in general population (Garcia et al. 1983). These results are consistent with those of other studies, which confirm that CHD, stroke and peripheral vascular disease are more frequent in patients with type 2 diabetes (Pyorala et al. 1987).

In epidemiological studies looking at the importance of conventional risk factors in causing vascular disease in diabetics, the levels of these factors (smoking, hypertension, hypercolesterolemia, etc.) often resulted to be increased, but not enough to explain the exaggerated risk for macrovascular complications in diabetic population (Stamler et al. 1993). Therefore, diabetes itself, and perhaps hyperglycaemia, should be involved in determining the excess risk in patients with type 2 diabetes.

Although the excess risk of CHD in diabetics has been recognised from several decades, the role of hyperglycaemia has been ignored until the late 80s. In fact, an old metaanalysis of some prospective studies did not provide clear evidence that hyperglycemia is a risk factor for CHD, because of small number of subjects and inconsistent findings (International Collaborative Group 1979).

In the last decade, several prospective studies including larger number of patients have shown that hyperglycemia is clearly involved in determining cardiovascular complications. One of these studies showed that in more than 100 newly diagnosed type 2 diabetics, the cardiovascular mortality increased three times according to tertiles of glycaemic control in a 10-year follow-up (Uusitupa et al. 1993). The same finding was confirmed in older diabetic patients (Fig. 3.1), in whom HbA1c and diabetes duration were related to CHD (Kuusisto et al. 1994) and cerebrovascular (Kuusisto et al. 1994a) events. Other European studies have confirmed these findings. In 411 patients with type 2 diabetes, aged 23 – 94 years and followed for 7 years, CHD mortality and morbidity were related to glycaemic control (Andersson and Svardsudd 1995). Similar results were obtained in another study from Northern Europe (Gall et al. 1995), in which a relationship between glycaemic control and cardiovascular mortality was shown in 328 patients with type 2 diabetes, aged 20 – 65 years and followed for

3 Hyperglycaemia as Cardiovascular Risk in Type 2 Diabetes

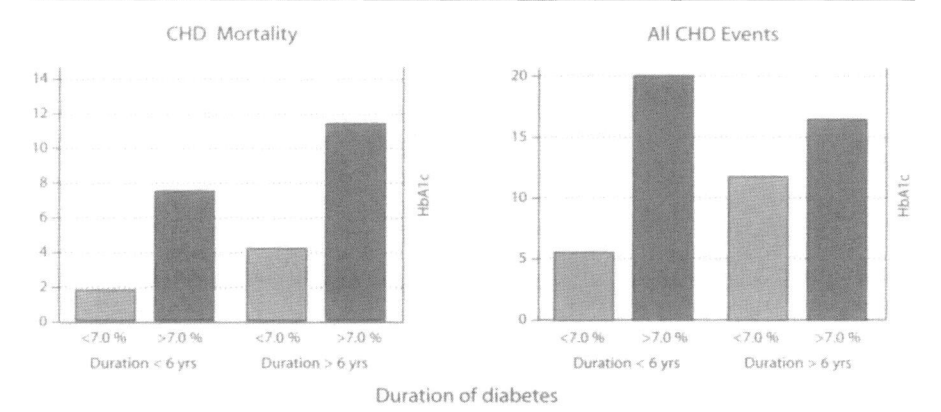

Fig. 3.1. 3.5-year incidence (%) of CHD deaths and all CHD events with respect to median of HbA1c and duration of diabetes. (Kuusisto et al 1994)

5 years. These results were confirmed by another study performed in 190 diabetic patients, who were followed for 10 years (Standl et al. 1996).

In more recent studies it has been appeared that also other risk factors are important contributors to macrovascular complications in patients with type 2 diabetes. In 2693 newly diagnosed patients included in the UKPDS, multivariate analysis showed that the high LDL level is the most powerful risk factor for CHD, followed by low HDL and high HbA1c (Turner et al. 1998). Similar results were accomplished in other two Finnish studies, in which approximately 1000 patients were followed for 7 years and high fasting plasma glucose predicted CHD (Lehto et al. 1997) and cerebrovascular (Lehto et al. 1996) events. Other studies reported similar data (Klein et al. 1995), indicating that hyperglycaemia is a risk factor not only in Caucasians but also in other ethnic groups (Wei et al. 1998).

More recently the incidence of myocardial infarction and CHD mortality have found to be correlated to postprandial hyperglycaemia but not to fasting hyperglycaemia (Hanefeld et al 1996), raising the possibility that not only fasting but also postprandial hyperglycaemia is related to cardiovascular disease in type 2 diabetes. This finding has been confirmed by the DECODE study (Fig. 3.2), in which high 2-hour

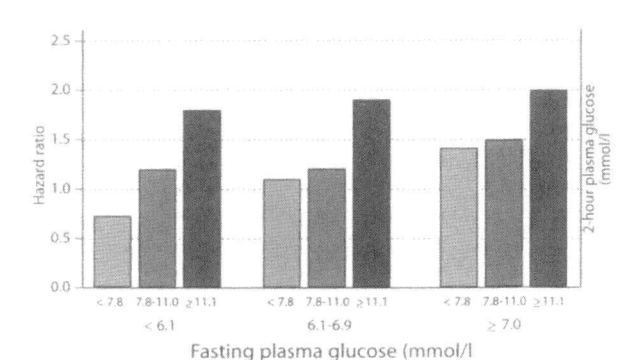

Fig. 3.2. Relative risk for all-cause mortality in subjects not known as diabetic. (DECODE 1999)

post-load blood glucose was found to be associated with increased relative risk of all-cause mortality (DECODE 1999).

In the last decade a number of evidence has been accumulated and collected in a recent metaanalysis (Coutinho et al. 1999) of twenty studies including approximately 100000 individuals without known diabetes, followed for more than 10 years. In this review, fasting, 1-h and 2-h after load glucose values correlated with the risk of cardiovascular events. Moreover, fasting as well as 2-h glucose levels of 6.1 and 7.8 mmol/L, respectively, increased the risk of cardiovascular events, thus suggesting that not only glycaemic value diagnostic for diabetes (>7 mmol/L) are harmful and strongly indicating that glycemia is a continuous cardiovascular risk factor, such as cholesterol or blood pressure.

These results were confirmed by a twofold increase in the risk of CHD observed in subjects with impaired glucose tolerance (IGT), a prediabetic state (Pyorala et al. 1987). IGT, identified using OGTT (75 g), was found in 16% of the US subjects aged 40-74 years (Harris et al. 1998), in 13% of the DECODE (DECODE 1998) and in 15% of the DECODA subjects (Qiao and Tuomilehto 2001). Interestingly, 58% of individuals with IGT had normal fasting glucose levels in the DECODE and 73% in the DECODA study. In addition, other conditions, such as hypertension, dyslipidemia, often are present together in the Metabolic Syndrome and are associated with high risk of CHD.

Fasting and postprandial hyperglycaemia can determine macrovascular complications in type 2 diabetes, through several pathogenetic mechanisms (Fig. 3.3). Non enzymatic glycosylation, or glycation, of structural and functional proteins is very important, because of the strict link with the degree of glycaemic control (Brownlee 1994). Protein glycation induces AGE (Advanced Glycosylation End-Products) formation through a complete and irreversible process of re-arrangement of intermediate glycosylation products. AGEs tend to self-associate and form cross-links which alter the structure and function of tissues and cells.

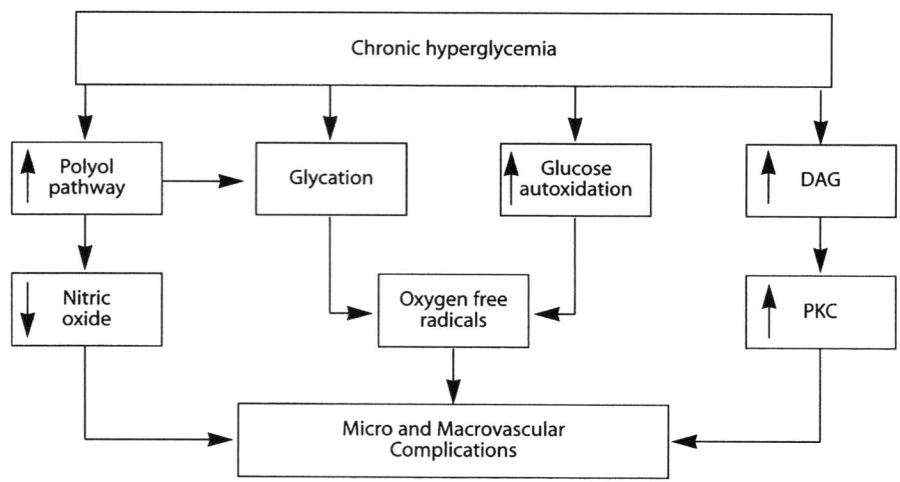

Fig. 3.3. Pathogenetic mechanisms of microvascular and macrovascular complications in diabetes

3 Hyperglycaemia as Cardiovascular Risk in Type 2 Diabetes

Moreover, AGEs may determine auto-oxidation and free-radical formation (Ceriello et al. 1997). These events cause a damage of both microvasculature through an increase in permeability of capillary wall and thickness of basal membrane, but also of macrovasculature promoting the migration and accumulation of LDL in vascular wall. Particularly, glycated ApoB and LDL are captured by macrophages with formation of foam cells, associated to increased susceptibility to oxidation with consequent enhancement of atherogenecity and stimulation of platelet aggregation.

The conclusive answer to the question on the existence of cause-effect relationship between hyperglycaemia and CHD derives from intervention studies (Fig. 3.4). The UKPDS has clearly demonstrated that chronic complications, mainly microvascular, can be prevented in T2DM through intensive therapy leading to optimise glycemic levels (UKPDS 1998). However, the risk of myocardial infarction reduces slightly but not significantly of about 15%, and less than treatment of hypertension (21%) or hyper-colesterolemia (30%) does. Since in UKPDS the reduction of hyperglycaemia has not been too pronounced, it appears to be an underestimation of the role of hyperglycemia in preventing cardiovascular complications. Nevertheless, the targets of management of type 2 diabetes have to be multifactorial in order to reduce cardiovascular mortality and morbidity. The optimal approach should comprise behaviour, diagnostic and therapeutic measures to control the whole spectrum of metabolic and vascular risk factors. This is possible through the adoption of protocols of primary prevention for early diagnosis in patients with family history, obese, anamnestic hyperglycemia, hypertriglyceridemia, hypertension and smokers. Protocols of secondary interventions should be finalised to correct all risk factors through a rational treatment of hyperglycaemia with diet and physical activity and eventually oral hypoglycaemic drugs or insulin. In this regard we need new drugs and therapeutic strategies for treatment of hyperglycemia, which remains the most difficult target to be reached in patients with type 2 diabetes.

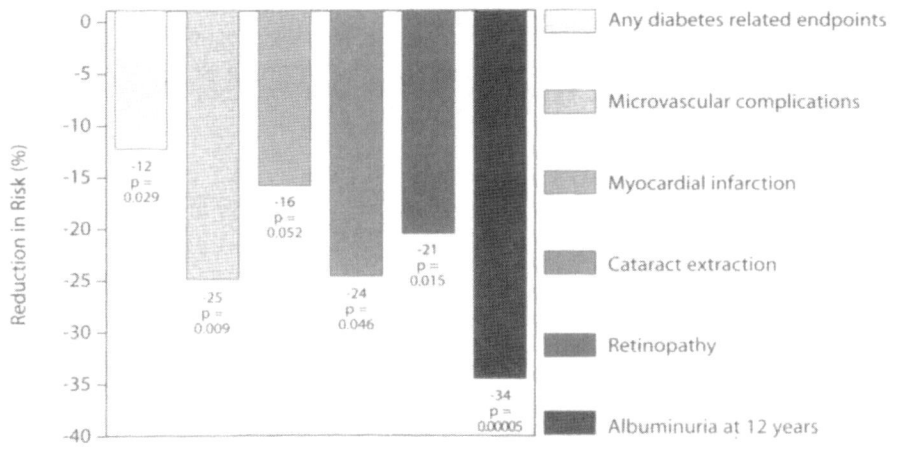

Fig. 3.4. Effects of lowering HbA1c on microvascular and macrovascular complications in patients with type 2 diabetes. (UKPDS 1998)

References

Andersson DKG, Svardsudd K (1995) Long-term glycemic control relates to mortality in type II diabetes. Diabetes Care 18:1534–43

Brownlee M (1994) Glycation and diabetic complications. Diabetes 43:836–41

Ceriello A (1997) Acute hyperglycaemia and oxidative stress generation. Diabet Med. 14 Suppl 3:S45–9

Coutinho M, Gerstein HC, Wang Y, Yusuf S (1999) The relationship between glucose and incident cardiovascular events. A metaregression analysis of published data from 20 studies of 95,783 individuals followed for 12.4 years. Diabetes Care 22:233–40

Will new diagnostic criteria for diabetes mellitus change phenotype of patients with diabetes? Reanalysis of European epidemiological data. DECODE Study Group on behalf of the European Diabetes Epidemiology Study Group (1998) BMJ 317:371–5

Glucose tolerance and mortality: comparison of WHO and American Diabetes Association diagnostic criteria. The DECODE study group. European Diabetes Epidemiology Group. Diabetes Epidemiology: Collaborative analysis Of Diagnostic criteria in Europe (1999) Lancet 354:617–21

Qiao Q, Tuomilehto J (2001) Diagnostic criteria of glucose intolerance and mortality. Minerva Med. 92:113–9

Gall MA, Borch-Johnsen K, Hougaard P, Nielsen FS, Parving HH (1995) Albuminuria and poor glycemic control predict mortality in NIDDM. Diabetes 44:1303–9

Garcia MJ, McManara PM, Gordon T, Kannel WB (1983) Morbidity and mortality in diabetics in the Framingham population. Diabetes 23: 336–341

Hanefeld M, Fischer S, Julius U, Schulze J, Schwanebeck U, Schmechel H, Ziegelasch HJ, Lindner J (1996) Risk factors for myocardial infarction and death in newly detected NIDDM: the Diabetes Intervention Study, 11-year follow-up. Diabetologia 39:1577–83

Haffner SM, Lehto S, Ronnemaa T, Pyorala K, Laakso M (1998) Mortality from coronary heart disease in subjects with type 2 diabetes and in nondiabetic subjects with and without prior myocardial infarction. N Engl J Med. 339:229–34

Harris MI (1998) Diabetes in America: epidemiology and scope of the problem. Diabetes Care 21 Suppl 3:C11–4

Klein R (1995) Hyperglycemia and microvascular and macrovascular disease in diabetes. Diabetes Care18:258–68

Kuusisto J, Mykkanen L, Pyorala K, Laakso M (1994) NIDDM and its metabolic control predict coronary heart disease in elderly subjects. Diabetes 43:960–7

Kuusisto J, Mykkanen L, Pyorala K, Laakso M (1994) Non-insulin-dependent diabetes and its metabolic control are important predictors of stroke in elderly subjects. Stroke 25:1157–64

International Collaborative Group (1979) Asymptomatic hyperglycemia and coronary artery disease: a series of papers by the International Collaborative Group based on studies in fifteen populations. J Chronic Dis 32:829–837

Laakso M and Lehto S (1997) Epidemiology of macrovascular disease in diabetes. Diabetes Rev 5:294–315

Lehto S, Ronnemaa T, Pyorala K, Laakso M (1996) Predictors of stroke in middle-aged patients with non-insulin-dependent diabetes. Stroke 27:63–8

Lehto S, Ronnemaa T, Haffner SM, Pyorala K, Kallio V, Laakso M (1997) Dyslipidemia and hyperglycemia predict coronary heart disease events in middle-aged patients with NIDDM. Diabetes 46:1354–9

Pyorala K, Laakso M, Uusitupa M (1987) Diabetes and atherosclerosis: an epidemiologic view. Diabetes Metab Rev 3:463–524

Stamler J, Vaccaro O, Neaton JD, Wentworth D (1993) Diabetes, other risk factors, and 12-yr cardiovascular mortality for men screened in the Multiple Risk Factor Intervention Trial. Diabetes Care 16:434–44

Intensive blood-glucose control with sulphonylureas or insulin compared with conventional treatment and risk of complications in patients with type 2 diabetes (UKPDS 33). UK Prospective Diabetes Study (UKPDS) Group (1998). Lancet 352:837–53

Uusitupa MI, Niskanen LK, Siitonen O, Voutilainen E, Pyorala K Ten-year cardiovascular mortality in relation to risk factors and abnormalities in lipoprotein composition in type 2 (non-insulin-dependent) diabetic and non-diabetic subjects. Diabetologia 36:1175–84

Standl E, Balletshofer B, Dahl B, Weichenhain B, Stiegler H, Hormann A, Holle R (1996) Predictors of 10-year macrovascular and overall mortality in patients with NIDDM: the Munich General Practitioner Project. Diabetologia 39(12):1540–5

Turner RC, Millns H, Neil HA, Stratton IM, Manley SE, Matthews DR, Holman RR (1998) Risk factors for coronary artery disease in non-insulin dependent diabetes mellitus: United Kingdom Prospective Diabetes Study (UKPDS: 23) BMJ 316:823–8

Wei M, Gaskill SP, Haffner SM, Stern MP (1998) Effects of diabetes and level of glycemia on all-cause and cardiovascular mortality. The San Antonio Heart Study. Diabetes Care 21:1167–72

CHAPTER 4

Gliclazide and Diabetic Angiopathy

A.J. Weekes

Abstract. Vascular disease remains the major contributor to morbidity and mortality in the diabetic population. Conventional classification into micro- and macrovascular disease is a useful distinction for the purposes of research and debate, although several risk factors and mechanisms appear to be implicated in both patterns of disease. The results of recent intervention trials, including the Kumamoto, UKPDS 33, and Steno 2 studies, concur that tight glycemic control benefits vascular prognosis in type 2 diabetes.

Hypercoagulability, oxidative stress, and endothelial dysfunction are common in diabetic patients, and an increasing body of evidence points to their role in both micro- and macrovascular disease. Research into the hemovascular properties of gliclazide has paralleled this progress in the understanding of pathophysiology, with interest focusing on the potential for this molecule to provide glycemia-independent vascular protection in the management of type 2 diabetic patients.

The Impact and Pathophysiology of Vascular Complications in Type 2 Diabetes

Despite modern therapeutic strategies, vascular disease remains the major contributor to morbidity and mortality in the type 2 diabetic population. The socioeconomic impact of these conditions makes elucidation of their pathogenesis, and hence of strategies for prevention and treatment, a priority. Conventional classification into microvascular and macrovascular disease is a useful distinction for the purpose of research and debate, although several risk factors and mechanisms appear to be implicated in both patterns of disease.

In the United Kingdom, microvascular pathology has an estimated lifetime incidence of about 9%, and the estimated prevalence of macrovascular complications in type 2 diabetic patients is around 20% (UKPDS Group 1998).

Conclusions from animal, epidemiological, and intervention studies coincide to implicate hyperglycemia and hypertension in the pathogenesis of microvascular disease. Hyperglycemia is equally acknowledged as an independent marker of cardiovascular risk, commonly associated features like obesity and dyslipidemia being additive in impact. The presence of hypercoagulability, oxidative stress, and endothelial dysfunction have been relatively recently identified in type 2 diabetes, and their pathophysiological role in vascular disease considered. Hypercoagulability, which may be accounted for by elevated levels of fibrinogen, factor VII, and plasminogen activator inhibitor-1 (PAI-1), leads to excess formation and impaired degradation of fibrin. Prospective clinical follow-up implicates increased blood viscosity and coagulability in microvascular disease (Barnes et al. 1987) and, similarly, several studies have associated these abnormalities with increased coronary morbidity and mortality (Thompson et al. 1995). Furthermore, increased free-radical production from glucose oxidation and reduced antioxidant defenses promotes LDL oxidation in diabetic patients, a primordial step in the atherosclerotic process, making this a widely hypothesized mechanism for accelerated vascular disease. Additionally, oxidative stress and advanced glycation end-product (AGE) deposition have been linked to diabetic endothelial dysfunction, which leads to arterial narrowing and susceptibility to atheroma deposition; in microvascular disease this has been described as the "choreographer" of the pathological process (Tooke 1996) due to the widespread microcirculatory changes it causes. These are manifested clinically in vulnerable structures by pathologies such as retinopathy, nephropathy, and neuropathy.

Hence, aside from hyperglycemia, hypertension, and associated "classic" vascular risk factors, hypercoagulability, oxidative stress, and endothelial dysfunction are common and interlinked abnormalities in diabetic patients. Laboratory and epidemiological evidence points to a role for these abnormalities in both micro- and macrovascular disease.

Gliclazide: Structure–Function Relationships

The second-generation sulfonylurea, gliclazide, is differentiated from the other members of the class mainly by its hemovascular properties. The unique feature of the gliclazide molecule is its amino azabicyclo [3.3.0] octane ring, grafted to a sulfonylurea group.

Recent observations of free-radical scavenging and interference with lipid oxidation reactions by hydrazine (H_2N-NH_2) (Zhou et al. 1998), suggest a molecular mechanism for the ability of gliclazide to reduce oxidative stress at therapeutic concentrations (Scott et al. 1991) (O'Brien and Luo 2000). The azabicyclo octane moiety has also recently been credited with the strong selectivity and high affinity of gliclazide for β-cell sulfonylurea receptors (Gribble and Ashcroft 1999) which may contribute to the very good tolerability and safety of this molecule observed in clinical studies and in daily practice.

Gliclazide and Glycemic Control

Glycemic control is an unquestionable component of the necessarily multifactorial approach to vascular risk reduction, as has recently been underlined by the Kumamoto and UKPDS results.

The Kumamoto study (Ohkubo et al. 1995) showed that tight glycemic control, to a mean HbA_{1c} of 7.1%, was effective in both primary and secondary prevention of retinopathy and nephropathy. Furthermore, although based on a small number of events, a trend in favor of tight glycemic control was observed on macrovascular end points. These results to some extent anticipated those of UKPDS 33 (UKPDS Group 1998), where intensive glycemic control to a mean HbA_{1c} of 7.0% over 10 years was associated with a 25% reduction in microvascular end points, including the need for retinal photocoagulation. An apparent risk reduction of 16% in myocardial infarction was of borderline significance ($P=0.052$). Hence, these data from prospective follow-up studies lend strong support to the current HbA_{1c} criterion of 7% for good glycemic control (American Diabetes Association 2000). Glycemic control on gliclazide has been studied in a large number of complementary studies in different populations. In obese, diet-resistant diabetics with a mean time from diagnosis of 8.3 years, gliclazide treatment was associated with a reduction in HbA_{1c} of 30% over 1 year, to a final mean value of 7.02% (Kilo et al. 1991). These results reflect those seen in longer-term studies, where maintenance of control (to a mean HbA_1 of 7.3%) was observed over 5 years of treatment (Guillausseau 1991).

The recent Steno 2 study (Gaede et al. 1999) chose gliclazide as the reference sulfonylurea. Microalbuminuric type 2 diabetic patients were randomized to standard or intensive multifactorial management. A period of 3.8 years of intensive management was associated with a significant reduction in risk of progression to nephropathy, of progression of retinopathy, of progression of autonomic neuropathy, and, interestingly, of progression of peripheral arterial disease.

Gliclazide and the Thrombotic Process

From some of the earliest studies in the development of gliclazide, inhibition of platelet adhesion and aggregation has been observed and identified as a potential benefit in terms of vascular risk reduction More recently, these observations have been confirmed and the likely mechanism elucidated in a series of studies. Reduced platelet aggregation to collagen was observed in gliclazide-treated, but not in glibenclamide-treated patients in a randomized study of type 2 diabetic patients with microvascular disease (Jennings et al. 1992). These results were significant at 3 months, and were maintained at 6 months' treatment. Glycemic control was not significantly different between the groups, and concomitant improvements in markers of oxidative stress reduced plasma thiols and lipid peroxides, and increased superoxide dismutase activity were observed on gliclazide treatment. Additional data of interest come from an uncontrolled study showing significantly decreased thromboxane B_2, lipid peroxides, and protein oxidation products over 36 weeks' treatment of 17 type 2 diabetic patients (Florkowski et al. 1988). Therefore, an attractive hypothesis to explain these observations is reduction in oxidative stress by gliclazide, leading to a reduction in lipid peroxide levels, hence improving the balance between prostacyclin and thromboxane A_2 production, and reducing excessive platelet activity. This idea is supported by the observation of a markedly improved thromboxane:prostacyclin ratio, calculated from assays of the metabolites 6-keto-PGF_1 and thromboxane B_2, in another study of type 2 diabetics switched from glibenclamide to an equipotent dose of gliclazide (Fu et al. 1992).

Other effects of gliclazide on the thrombotic process include alterations in fibrin structure and fibrinolysis seen during treatment. Ex vivo studies were performed in platelet-free plasma from diabetic subjects and age, sex-matched controls (Nair et al. 1991). In plasma from uncontrolled diabetics, using turbidity and permeability measures, reduced fibrin fiber thickness and permeability of fibrin networks were found, this being attributed to inhibition of lateral polymerization, and probably related to glycation of plasma proteins including fibrinogen. This altered fibrin network structure is associated with resistance to lysis (Nair et al. 1989). Pretreatment with a therapeutic concentration of gliclazide was found to significantly increase fibrin fiber thickness, diminish tensile strength, and reduce permeability. These effects were attributed to enhanced lateral polymerization and enhanced crosslinking within the network, and were not reproduced by metformin, glibenclamide, or insulin pretreatment. Gliclazide was also associated with some enhancement of fibrinolysis in this model, this fitting in with previous results from several studies specifically dedicated to fibrinolytic activity in diabetes and the effect of gliclazide treatment.

Tolbutamide-treated type 2 diabetic patients were switched from their previous treatment to gliclazide for 12 months (Gram et al. 1989). Sustained increases in tissue-type plasminogen activator (t-PA) activity were seen in those with no detectable t-PA activity at baseline. Interestingly, no changes in this variable were observed in a subgroup of patients with marked t-PA activity at baseline. As plasminogen activator inhibitor (PA-I) remained constant throughout the study, increased endothelial cell production or release of t-PA was thought likely, this theory being supported by a significant increase in t-PA antigen following venous occlusion. As metabolic control was unchanged during the study, this effect seems to be glycemia-independent, further evidence for this coming from another study showing increased activity of both t-PA and prekallikrein during 6 months of treatment of male type 1 diabetics with gliclazide (Gram et al. 1988).

Another study included chlorpropamide-treated type 2 diabetic patients with low plasminogen activator activity. These patients showed normalization of this variable after switching to an equipotent dose of gliclazide for 6 months, this change being sustained at 24 and 48 months of follow-up despite the fact that these was no difference in glycemic control (Almer 1984). Concomitant normalization of plasminogen activator levels was observed, along with a significant fall in fibrinogen level during gliclazide therapy. The various investigators of these studies of gliclazide, platelets, and fibrin have hypothesized positive implications for the reduction of occlusive vascular events during gliclazide treatment.

Gliclazide, Oxidative Stress, and the Atherosclerotic Process

General free-radical scavenging activity with gliclazide at therapeutic concentrations was demonstrated by the inhibition of photooxidation of o-dianisidine (Scott et al. 1991) and has been confirmed in other models and conditions (Noda et al. 1997). These effects of gliclazide in reducing oxidative stress contrast with those of glibenclamide, which shows no effect even in concentrations well above the therapeutic range.

The potential implications of reduced oxidative stress on gliclazide for the atherosclerotic process have been explored in ex-vivo studies of LDL from type 2 diabetic subjects and controls (O'Brien and Luo 2000). Gliclazide, at therapeutic concentrations, highly significantly increased the lag-time between exposure of LDL to a prooxidant (copper), and the commencement of oxidation. This effect was more marked than that of equimolar vitamin C, and was not reproduced by the other sulfonylureas tested – glibenclamide, glimepiride, tolbutamide, and glipizide (Fig. 4.1).

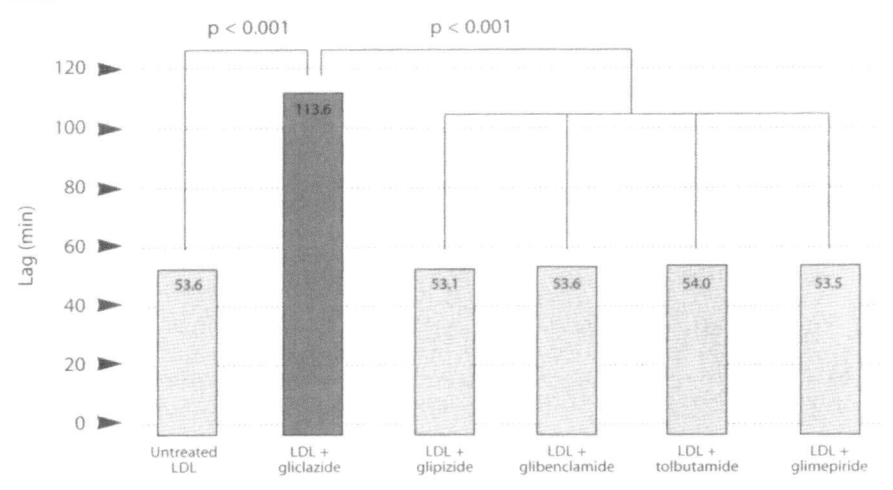

Fig. 4.1. Effect on LDL oxidation (lag-time) of sulfonylureas

The effect of gliclazide on circulating lipid peroxides (the in-vivo correlates of LDL oxidation) has also been demonstrated (Jennings et al. 1992). In this study, type 2 diabetics with retinopathy and/or incipient nephropathy were selected, and randomized to treatment with either gliclazide or an equipotent dose of glibenclamide. A significant reduction in lipid peroxides was observed by 3 months in the gliclazide, but not the glibenclamide, group, this effect being maintained at 6 months. Associated improvements in oxidative status were seen in gliclazide-treated patients, and as glycemic control was similar in the 2 groups, the authors were led to conclude that the gliclazide effect was glycemia-independent.

These results may be of particular interest in the light of a study correlating susceptibility of LDL to oxidation with the extent of coronary atherosclerosis (Regnstrom et al. 1992). Oxidized LDL is thought to play several roles in atherogenesis, including foam-cell formation via unregulated uptake into macrophages, enhanced adherence to the vascular endothelium via increased expression of cell adhesion molecules, and enhanced production of proatherogenic factors including growth factors and cytokines. The effects of gliclazide on these processes have been elucidated in a series of studies. Type 2 diabetic patients previously poorly controlled on glibenclamide, that is with HbA_{1c} levels greater than 9%, were switched to an equipotent dose of gliclazide for 3 months' treatment. All patients were also taking metformin throughout this study before and after the exchange of therapy. Lipid peroxide levels, serum cytokine levels, monocyte cytokine production, and monocyte adhesion to endothelial cells were assessed and compared with results from healthy nonsmoking control subjects matched for sex and body mass index. Both high lipid peroxide levels and monocyte adhesion to endothelial cells were completely reversed by gliclazide treatment, and an associated reduction in production of the proatherogenic tumor necrosis factor-α was observed (Desfaits et al. 1998). Subsequently, an in vitro study employing human monocytes and cultured human endothelial cells extended these findings (Desfaits et al. 1999). Incubation of these cells in the presence of glycated albumin was associated with a time-dependent increase in monocyte adhesion, which could be significantly reduced by preincubation with gliclazide in therapeutic concentration. A probable molecular mechanism for inhibition of monocyte adhesion by gliclazide was suggested by demonstration of marked reductions in induction of both soluble and cell-associated adhesion molecules; ELAM-1, ICAM-1, and VCAM-1. Inhibition of expression of these adhesion molecules by gliclazide appeared to be exerted at the transcriptional level, as a concurrent suppressive effect on the activation of the transcriptional factor NF-κB was observed.

Gliclazide and Vascular Function

An expanding body of research has examined the effects of gliclazide on vascular function, specifically vascular permeability and endothelium-dependent relaxation. Gliclazide's effects on capillary macromolecular permeability and reactivity were studied in a hamster cheek-pouch preparation (Bouskela et al. 1997). Gliclazide, applied topically, dose-dependently inhibited increases in vascular permeability induced both by histamine in nondiabetic hamsters, and by ischemia/ reperfusion in streptozotocin-treated hamsters with no residual pancreatic function. No changes in glycemia were observed in either model, and in the postischemic model the effect of gliclazide was comparable with that of equimolar vitamin C, supporting the hypothesis that reduced vascular permeability is a glycemia-independent effect mediated via reduction in oxidative stress.

Another similar animal model of diabetes (Pagano et al. 1998), the alloxan-treated rabbit was employed to further study the effects of gliclazide on the vasculature. Again, gliclazide has no effect on glycemia or insulinemia in this model, so any effect identified can be considered glycemia-independent. Relaxation responses of sections of precontracted aorta were recorded in a number of experimental conditions, before and after 6 weeks treatment with gliclazide at 10 mg/kg/day. Diabetes was associated with significant impairment of acetylcholine-induced endothelium-dependent relaxation of the abdominal aorta, these responses being restored to a level which was not different from nondiabetic controls during gliclazide treatment. Similarly, augmented aortic contractions to acetylcholine in the presence of the NO synthase inhibitor, L-NAME, were significantly reduced by gliclazide to a level which was not different from that of normal rabbits. This effect of gliclazide appears to be specific to the abnormality arising in diabetes, as 6 weeks' gliclazide treatment of nondiabetic rabbits did not affect vessel responses.

Dose-dependent improvement of diabetic endothelial dysfunction by gliclazide has also been observed in human microvessels (Vallejo et al. 1999). Omental microvessels were obtained from nondiabetic, normotensive nonsmokers undergoing surgical intervention. Glycated oxyhemoglobin at 10% or more was found to inhibit relaxation responses of precontracted vessels to bradykinin, this effect appearing to be NO-mediated, as it mirrored the effects seen with L-NAME, but not with indomethacin, in the same model. The impaired relaxation induced by glycated oxyhemoglobin could be dose-dependently inhibited by gliclazide in concentrations within the therapeutic range, or by either equimolar vitamin C or superoxide dismutase at 100 U/l (Fig. 4.2).

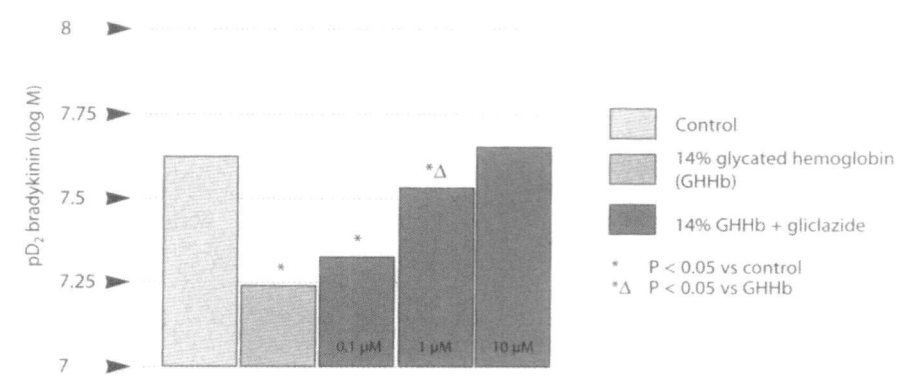

Fig. 4.2. Endothelial dysfunction (expressed as pD_2 values for bradykinin) – effect of gliclazide

Neither glibenclamide nor indomethacin alone showed any effect on impaired relaxation responses. Besides showing, for the first time, a deleterious effect of glycated hemoglobin on endothelial function in human vessels, these data support the view that gliclazide has its protective effect on the endothelium via reduction in oxidative stress, thus preserving NO-mediated vessel relaxation responses.

Gliclazide and Clinical Vascular Complications

This review has presented evidence that gliclazide provides effective, long-term glycemic control and additional properties with vasculoprotective potential; namely, reduction in excessive platelet activity; improved fibrinolysis; reduced oxidative stress, lipid peroxidation, and monocyte adhesion; and preservation of endothelial function. There are some existing clinical data to support the view that gliclazide may improve type 2 diabetic patients' vascular prognosis to a greater degree than other sulfonylureas, this data coming primarily from studies in retinopathy.

A per-protocol analysis after a mean of 39 months' follow-up of a randomized, single-blind comparative study of gliclazide vs glibenclamide revealed significantly fewer capillary occlusions and microaneurysms in the gliclazide-treated than in the glibenclamide-treated patients (Régnault 1980). Retinal photographs were rated for overall severity by a blinded observer on a 5-grade scale, and the percentage of patients considered to have stabilized or improved in each treatment group analyzed. A difference, significant at the 5% level, was found between gliclazide-treated (65%) and glibenclamide-treated (35%) patients. Gliclazide's apparent benefit in this study was attributed to a glycemia-independent mechanism on the basis of the difference with glibenclamide, and the interesting observation that these findings were mirrored in a small study subpopulation of type 1 diabetics. A per-protocol analysis of a second study was published at 5 years of follow-up of 60 type 2 diabetics with no or simple retinopathy at inclusion (Akanuma et al. 1991). Twenty-one of these patients had been randomized to gliclazide 160 to 240 mg, 19 to continue on their previous sulfonylurea, and a third group of 20 patients had been allocated a diet-only regime. Retinopathy was scored from funduscopy and fluorescein angiography on a 5-grade adaptation of the Scott scale. In this study, progression to proliferative retinopathy was significantly less frequent in the gliclazide group than the other sulfonylurea group, again despite the absence of difference in glycemic control.

Conclusion

There is an emerging body of evidence indicating that, in addition to effective long-term glycemic control, gliclazide, in contrast to other sulfonylureas, has a direct action on the pathophysiological processes of diabetic micro- and macrovascular disease. The main results of interest concern reduced thrombotic tendency, reduction in oxidized LDL and monocyte/endothelium interactions, and preservation of endothelial function during gliclazide administration. The results of ongoing and planned studies will further elucidate the potential for glycemia-independent vascular protection with gliclazide.

References

Akanuma Y, Kosaka K, Kanazawa Y, Kasuga M, Fukuda M, Aoki S (1991) Diabetic retinopathy in non-insulin-dependent diabetes mellitus patients: the role of gliclazide. Am J Med 90(6A): 6–74

Almer LO (1984) Effect of gliclazide on plasminogen activator activity in vascular walls in patients with maturity onset diabetes. Thromb Res 35:19–25

American Diabetes Association (2000) Standards of medical care for patients with diabetes mellitus (Position statement). Diabetes Care 23(Suppl 1):S32-S42

Barnes AJ, Oughton J, Kohner EM (1987) Blood rheology and the progression of diabetic retinopathy: a prospective study. Clin Hemorheol 7:460

Bouskela E, Cyrino F, Conde C, Garcia A (1997) Microvascular permeability with sulfonylureas in normal and diabetic hamsters. Metabolism 46:26–30

Desfaits A-C, Serri O, Renier G (1998) Normalization of plasma lipid peroxides, monocyte adhesion and tumor necrosis factor-α production in NIDDM patients after gliclazide treatment. Diabetes Care 21:487–493

Desfaits A-C, Serri O, Renier G (1999) Gliclazide reduces the induction of human monocyte adhesion to endothelial cells by glycated albumin. Diabet Obes Metab 1:113–120

Florkowski CM, Richardson MR, Le Guen C, Jennings PE, Jones AF, Lunec J (1988) Effect of gliclazide on thromboxane B_2 parameters of haemostasis, lipid peroxides and fluorescent IgG in type 2 (non-insulin-dependent) diabetes mellitus. Diabetologia 31:490 A

Fu ZZ, Yan T, Chen Y-J, Quang Sang J (1992) Thromboxane/prostacyclin balance in type II diabetes: gliclazide effects. Metabolism 41:33–35

Gæde P, Vedel P, Parving H-H, Pedersen O (1999) Intensified multifactorial intervention in patients with type 2 diabetes mellitus and microalbuminuria: the Steno type 2 diabetes study. Lancet 353:617–622

Gram J, Jespersen J, Kold A (1988) Effects of an oral antidiabetic drug on the fibrinolytic system of blood in insulin-treated diabetic patients. Metabolism 37:937–943

Gram J, Kold A, Jespersen J (1989) Rise of plasma t-PA fibrinolytic activity in a group of maturity onset diabetic patients shifted from a first generation (tolbutamide) to a second generation sulphonylurea (gliclazide). J Int Med 225:241–247

Gribble FM, Ashcroft FM (1999) Differential sensitivity of beta-cell and extrapancreatic K_{ATP} channels to gliclazide. Diabetologia 42:845–848

Guillausseau P-J (1991) An evaluation of long-term glycemic control in non-insulin-dependent diabetes mellitus: the relevance of glycated hemoglobin. Am J Med 90(6A):46–49

Jennings PE, Scott NA, Saniabadi AR, Belch JJF (1992) Effects of gliclazide on platelet reactivity and free radicals in type 2 diabetic patients: clinical assessment. Metabolism 41:36-39

Kilo C, Dudley J, Kalb B (1991). Evaluation of the efficacy and safety of Diamicron in non-insulin-dependent diabetic patients. Diabetes Res Clin Pract 14:S79-S82

Nair CH, Sullivan JR, Singh D, Azhar A, Van Gelder J, Dhall DP (1989) Fibrin network structure as a determinant of fibrinolysis. Thromb Haemos 62:86

Nair CH, Azhar A, Wilson JD, Dhall DP (1991) Studies in fibrin network structure in human plasma. Part II - clinical application: diabetes and antidiabetic drugs. Thromb Res 64:447-485

Noda Y, Mori A, Packer L (1997) Gliclazide scavenges hydroxyl, superoxide and nitric oxide radicals: an ESR study. Res Comm Mol Path Pharm 96;115-124

O'Brien RC, Luo M, Balazs N, Mercuri J (2000) In-vitro and in-vivo antioxidant properties of gliclazide. J Diabetes Complications 14;201-206

Ohkubo Y, Kishikawa H, Araki E, et al (1995) Intensive insulin therapy prevents the progression of diabetic microvascular complications in Japanese patients with non-insulin-dependent diabetes mellitus: a randomized prospective 6 year study. Diab Res Clin Prac 28:103-119

Pagano PJ, Griswold MC, Ravel D, Cohen RA (1998) Vascular action of the hypoglycemic agent gliclazide in diabetic rabbits. Diabetologia 41:9-15

Régnault AF (1980) Prognosis of non-proliferative diabetic retinopathy during treatment with gliclazide. Roy Soc Med Int Congr Symp Ser 20:249-257

Regnstrom J, Nilsson J, Tornvall P, et al (1992) Susceptibility to low density lipoprotein oxidation and coronary atherosclerosis in man. Lancet 339:1183-1186

Scott NA, Jennings PE, Brown J, Belch JJF. (1991) Gliclazide: a general free radical scavenger. Eur J Pharmacol 208:175-177

Thompson FG, Kienast J, Pyke SDM, Havarkate F, Van De Loo JCW, for the European concerted action on thrombosis and disabilities angina pectoris study group (1995) Haemostatic factors and the risk of myocardial infarction or sudden death in patients with angina pectoris. N Engl J Med 332:635-641

Tooke JE (1996) Endothelium: the main actor or choreographer in the remodeling of the microvasculature in diabetes? Diabetologia 39:745-746

UKPDS Group (1998) Intensive blood-glucose control with sulfonylureas or insulin compared with conventional treatment and risk of complications in patients with type 2 diabetes (UKPDS 33). Lancet 352:837-853

Vallejo S, Angulo J, Peiró C, et al (1999) Highly glycosylated oxyhaemoglobin impairs nitric oxide relaxations in human mesenteric microvessels. Diabetologia 43:83-90

Zhou S, Dickinson LC, Yang Li, Decker EA (1998) Identification of hydrazine in commercial preparations of carnosine and its influence on carnosine's antioxidative properties. Analyt Biochem 261:79-86

CHAPTER 5

Clinical Experience with Repaglinide, the First Prandial Glucose Regulator in Type 2 Diabetes

K. Brown Frandsen

Abstract. Repaglinide is a novel prandial glucose regulator developed for the treatment of Type 2 diabetes mellitus. Its pharmacokinetic profile – rapid onset and short duration of action – is able to limit postprandial blood glucose excursions, and allows convenient administration in a flexible schedule at meal times. Placebo-controlled and comparative studies have demonstrated that prandial repaglinide achieves a high level of overall glycaemic control by synchronising insulin secretion to insulin need. Glycaemic control can be further improved in drug-resistant patients when repaglinide is combined with insulin-sensitising agents, such as metformin or troglitazone.

The major limitation of the traditional insulin secretagogues, the sulphonylureas, has been the risk of hypoglycaemia. This stems from the relatively prolonged action of these agents, whereby inappropriate stimulation of beta-cells may take place during periods of low blood glucose. Data from comparative studies show that repaglinide reduces the risk of major hypoglycaemia by more than 50%, compared with sulphonylureas. This advantage may be even more marked when the patient is free to adopt a flexible/normal meal pattern. To reduce the risk of hypoglycaemia, the sulphonylurea-treated patient must consume meals at regular intervals, and take snacks between meals. However, assuming compliance, this approach restricts the patient's routine and ability to implement lifestyle measures such as caloric restriction. Advising patients to snack between meals and achieve weight loss at the same time may also seem illogical.

Compelling reasons for considering a prandial approach to glycaemic management include risk reductions for late diabetic complications and hypoglycaemia, and greater flexibility for the patient. Available data concerning repaglinide suggest that many theoretical benefits of prandial glucose regulation may be achievable in clinical practice.

Introduction: The Need for Refined Antidiabetic Therapies

Type 2 diabetes mellitus is a major and increasing cause of global mortality, morbidity and healthcare expenditure (Amos et al. 1997). Consequently, the need for effective antidiabetic therapies has never been greater. There are encouraging data to show that when strict targets for glycaemic control are met with drug treatment, the pay-off is a significant risk reduction for adverse diabetic outcomes (Ohkubo et al. 1995; UKPDS group, 1998). Thus, an intensified use of antidiabetic therapies can be anticipated. However, traditional drug treatment methods have limitations that can place burdens on the patient.

The most widely used agents, the sulphonylureas, are effective antidiabetic drugs, but have pharmacokinetic profiles that result in continuous stimulation of beta-cells across dosing intervals, regardless of the patient's plasma glucose concentration (Melander et al. 1998). Consequently, hypoglycaemia is an inevitable risk. This risk can be minimised if the patient takes care to consume meals at regular intervals and supplement caloric intake through additional snacks. However, compliance to such regimens may be poor. Symptomatic hypoglycaemia is the most common side effect associated with sulphonylurea therapy; irregular or missed meals are a major contributory factor, and have been identified as the precipitating event in about one third of sulphonylurea-related hospital admissions for severe hypoglycaemia (Asplund et al. 1983; Gill and Huddle 1993; Robertson and Home 1993; Teo and Ee 1997; Stahl and Berger 1999). Accumulation of sulphonylureas that require renal elimination may be another cause of hypoglycaemic events, especially in the elderly (Robertson and Home 1993; Melander et al. 1998). Despite these risks being well known, surveys show that the majority of patients prescribed sulphonylureas have predisposing risks for hypoglycaemia, including compromised renal function (Paterson et al. 1989; Yap et al. 1998).

Alternative antidiabetic agents such as the thiazolidinediones and the biguanide metformin, are not associated with hypoglycaemia, but have other limitations. The insulin-sensitising thiazolidinediones require the presence of adequate insulin levels as a prerequisite for drug efficacy (Sparano and Seaton 1998; Emilien et al. 1999), and may be ineffective in 25 – 55 % of patients unless sufficient insulin is provided via supplementation or the concomitant use of an insulin secretagogue (Sparano and Seaton 1998). Troglitazone has been withdrawn due to hepatotoxicity, raising concerns about these agents.

Metformin inhibits hepatic glucose output, and may also increase peripheral insulin sensitivity (Feinglos and Bethel 1998). Tolerability is the major clinical limitation of this agent; it is associated with a high incidence of adverse gastrointestinal side effects, occurring in 20 – 30 % of patients (Feinglos and Bethel 1998). Metformin is excreted unchanged via the kidneys, so should not be used in patients with any degree of renal impairment. This and further contraindications preclude its use in many patients with Type 2 diabetes.

Prandial Glucose Regulation: The Modern Approach to Diabetic Risk Management

Given that Type 2 diabetes is characterised by abnormal beta-cell function with a relative or absolute deficiency of insulin secretion (Polonsky 1999), the most logical approach to initial therapy may be to address this fundamental defect, either through the use of exogenous insulin, or the more physiological method of insulin secretagogue therapy. In either case, avoidance of hypoglycaemia requires that insulin availability be synchronised with need. Traditional regimens have attempted to do this by compelling the patient to adhere to regular mealtimes supplemented by snacks. This way, patients attempt to optimise glucose intake to the pharmacokinetic properties of their treatment, but this approach is restrictive and the risk of nocturnal hypoglycaemia may remain. Poor compliance with either the treatment or mealtime regimen may jeopardise glycaemic control or risk hypoglycaemia.

A more recent approach to the problem has been to reverse this situation by attempting to optimise treatments to patients' glucose intake. This results in flexible regimens, with interventions taken on an 'as-needed' basis. This is the logic that underlies basal-bolus regimens with exogenous insulins. It is also the logic that led to repaglinide, the first insulin secretagogue specifically developed for prandial glucose regulation (PGR). Repaglinide is taken before meals, whenever they are eaten, and only when they are eaten.

An effective prandial glucose regulator must have pharmacokinetic properties that induce prandial insulin responses close to normal physiology. In health, the prandial insulin response is biphasic; an early burst of secretion reduces hepatic gluconeogenesis and glycogenolysis, and increases splanchnic glucose sequestration (Mitrakou et al. 1990; Crepaldi and Del Prato 1995; Bruttomesso et al. 1999). Subsequently, a more sustained phase of insulin secretion increases peripheral glucose disposal until intestinal glucose absorption declines. In Type 2 diabetes, the early phase of insulin secretion is delayed and blunted, so endogenous glucose production continues in spite of prandial intake, resulting in postprandial hyperglycaemia (Polonsky et al. 1988; Mitrakou et al. 1990; Crepaldi and Del Prato 1995; Coates et al. 1994; Owens et al. 1996). Therefore, optimal kinetic properties of a prandial glucose regulator include a sufficiently rapid onset and intensity of action to curtail endogenous glucose production, and a duration of action sufficient to dispose of the exogenous glucose load, but which does not continue into the postprandial phase to the point of risking hypoglycaemia. By stimulating insulin secretion when most appropriate, and limiting postprandial hyperglycaemia, good overall glycaemic control can be achieved with PGR, as it is in health.

As well as reducing the relative risk of hypoglycaemia, PGR provides mealtime flexibility for patients and releases them from dependencies on snacks. Thus, a spin-off benefit for patients may be the opportunity to implement caloric restriction and avoid weight-gain (Home 1999). Indeed, patients may be confused by the apparently conflicting advice to consume regular snacks between meals, and yet attempt to lose weight.

Another theoretical benefit of PGR is that blood glucose levels are selectively decreased at times when hyperglycaemia may pose the greatest long-term risk. In Type 2 diabetes, the greatest imbalances between insulin supply and metabolic demands are detected at mealtimes. Postprandial blood glucose peaks may be 3-fold higher than in healthy controls, and the duration of elevated blood glucose, greatly prolonged (Polonsky et al. 1988; Coates et al. 1994; Owens et al. 1996; Home 1999). There is increasing evidence that many vascular morbidities associated with diabetes have aetiologies that are accelerated during these periods (Ceriello 1998; Haller 1998; Haffner 1998; Lefebvre and Scheen 1998). Furthermore, epidemiological data suggest that postprandial hyperglycaemia is associated with a greater risk of vascular morbidity and mortality than is fasting hyperglycaemia (Hanefeld et al. 1996; Tominaga et al. 1999; DECODE study group, 1999).

Fortunately, these risks are modifiable, and outcome benefits have been demonstrated when rigorous glycaemic control is achieved through pharmacological intervention (Ohkubo et al. 1995; UKPDS group, 1998). Thus, good glycaemic control achieved by PGR may represent both a physiological and beneficial strategy for improving long-term prognosis in Type 2 diabetes.

Repaglinide – Pharmacology

Repaglinide, a carbamoylmethyl benzoic acid (CMBA) derivative, increases the secretion of endogenous insulin from pancreatic beta-cells by blocking ATP-gated potassium channels (Owens 1998). In this respect, it has a similar action to the sulphonylureas, although it binds with markedly different affinities compared with glibenclamide to two receptor sites in the beta-cell membrane (Fuhlendorff et al. 1998). Repaglinide also differs from the sulphonylureas in that it does not stimulate insulin release independently of its effects on beta-cell potassium channels (Fuhlendorff et al. 1998; Bokvist et al. 1998), and does not inhibit insulin biosynthesis (Vinambres et al. 1996; Louchami et al. 1998). Furthermore, *in vitro*, repaglinide uniquely augments insulin release from pancreatic islets only in the presence of glucose (Bakkali-Nadi et al. 1994; Fuhlendorff et al. 1998). Thus, repaglinide appears to enhance *glucose-mediated* insulin release, a property suited to PGR.

The most important characteristics of repaglinide, from the point of view of PGR, are its rapid onset and appropriate duration of action. Maximum plasma concentrations are reached 50 minutes after oral dosing, and the terminal elimination half-life is just 32 minutes (Oliver and Ahmad 1997). These properties ensure that, with preprandial dosing, it is just the prandial insulin response that is selectively enhanced. Sulphonylureas have much more prolonged secretagogue activities, so may enhance fasting insulin secretion (Melander et al. 1998).

Repaglinide's elimination profile also reduces the risk of hypoglycaemia when compared to sulphonylureas such as glibenclamide, as repaglinide is not dependent on renal elimination and does not have active metabolites. It is extensively metabolised in the liver and its inactive metabolites are excreted in bile (Owens 1998). Repaglinide does not accumulate and is not contraindicated, in patients with mild–moderate renal dysfunction (Hatorp et al. 1999), although it should be avoided in patients with severe renal impairment (Ruckle and Hatorp 1998).

Interactions with drugs that inhibit, induce or act as substrates for the cytochrome CYP3A4 enzyme could be anticipated with repaglinide, but unpublished interaction studies involving ketoconazole, rifampicin, nifedipine and simvastatin have not identified clinically significant interactions. Further studies have shown repaglinide to have no clinically relevant effect on the pharmacokinetics of digoxin, warfarin or theophylline, while co-administration of cimetidine does not affect the kinetics of repaglinide (Owens 1998).

Prandial Repaglinide and Glycaemic Control

The antidiabetic efficacy of PGR with repaglinide has been demonstrated in a number of placebo-controlled and comparative studies. For example, a 16-week, placebo-controlled study randomised 408 patients with Type 2 diabetes who were naïve to antidiabetic pharmacotherapy, but poorly controlled by diet (Brown Frandsen et al. 1999). Repaglinide was associated with a significant improvement in HbA_{1c} from 7.8% at baseline to 6.6% at endpoint ($p < 0.001$), whereas no significant change in HbA_{1c} occurred with placebo (7.6% and 7.4% at baseline and endpoint, respectively). The reduction in HbA_{1c} associated with repaglinide occurred regardless of whether patients ate two, three or four meals per day, confirming the feasibility of the PGR strategy. Repaglinide was associated with a reduction in HbA_{1c} in all patient categories regardless of age or body mass index, and there was no indication of weight gain with repaglinide. Furthermore, there was no increased risk of hypoglycaemia observed with repaglinide, whichever meal pattern was followed.

Comparative studies have shown repaglinide to provide a level of glycaemic control at least equivalent to that obtained with sulphonylureas or metformin and superior to troglitazone. For example, a 1-year study randomised 576 patients with Type 2 diabetes to repaglinide or glibenclamide (Marbury et al. 1999). The overall level of glycaemic control was similar with either drug, but it was noted that pharmacotherapy-naïve patients gained less weight when treated with repaglinide than glibenclamide. Both repaglinide and glibenclamide lowered HbA_{1c} rapidly in pharmacotherapy-naïve patients; from 9.4% to 7.6%, and from 9.6% to 8.0%, respectively, over 3 months.

Another study randomised 195 patients with Type 2 diabetes to receive either preprandial repaglinide or once or twice daily glibenclamide for 14 weeks (Landgraf et al. 1999). This study also showed equivalent levels of glycaemic control in terms of HbA_{1c}, fasting glucose, C-peptide, insulin and proinsulin, but a between-group difference in 2-hour postprandial blood glucose level was reported that approached statistical significance (repaglinide, 8.1 mmol/l versus glibenclamide, 9.1 mmol/l, $p = 0.07$). A long-term trial that compared repaglinide with glipizide, showed repaglinide to have superior efficacy in terms of reducing HbA_{1c} and fasting glucose (Dejgaard et al. 1998). Thus, the level of glycaemic control achievable with repaglinide is at least equivalent to that with sulphonylurea treatment, but repaglinide treatment is associated with significantly less hypoglycaemia, as discussed below.

Glycaemic Control with Repaglinide Combination Regimens

As Type 2 diabetes is a progressive disease, many patients will ultimately require combination drug therapy to maintain glycaemic control (Turner et al. 1999). Such regimens are likely to be used increasingly given that strict glycaemic control, often only achievable with combination treatment, can significantly improve prognosis (UKPDS group 1998; Matthews 1998). The suitability of repaglinide for use in combination regimens involving metformin and troglitazone has therefore been investigated.

A study of 83 patients with Type 2 diabetes, no longer adequately controlled by metformin after treatment for 4 years, showed repaglinide to provide a level of glycaemic control at least equivalent to that of metformin when used as monotherapy, but to provide a synergistic effect when used in combination with metformin (Fig. 5.1) (Moses et al. 1999). Patients continuing metformin monotherapy did not show any significant changes in parameters of glycaemic control over the 3-month study period, but patients given additional preprandial repaglinide had significant decreases in HbA_{1c} (from 8.3% to 6.9%, $p = 0.0016$) and fasting plasma glucose level (from 10.22 mmol/l to 8.04 mmol/l, $p = 0.0003$). Of the patients receiving combination therapy, 59% achieved an HbA_{1c} of less than 7.1%.

Repaglinide has also been studied in combination with, and in comparison to, troglitazone. In a 22-week study involving 256 patients with Type 2 diabetes, HbA_{1c}

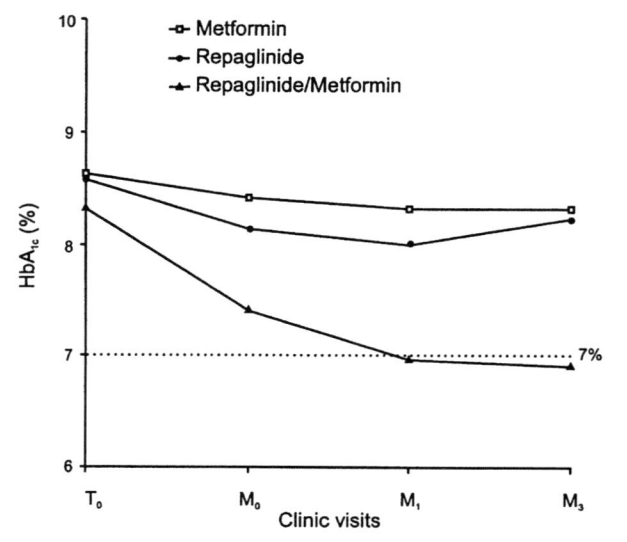

Fig. 5.1. HbA$_{1c}$ at baseline (first titration visit, T_o) and at clinic visits at 0 (M_o), 1, (M_1) and 3 (M_3) months in patients with Type 2 diabetes treated with metformin, repaglinide, or a combination of repaglinide and metformin. (Reproduced from Moses at al. 1999)

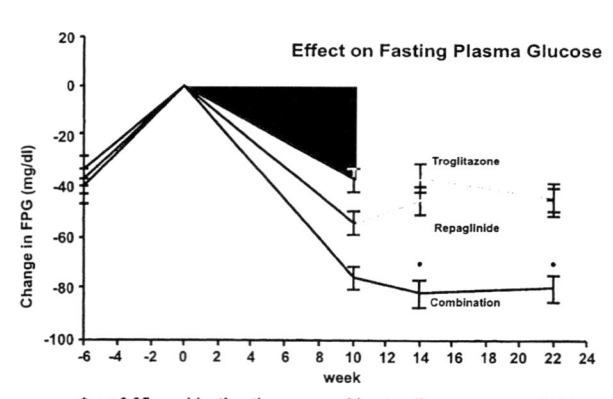

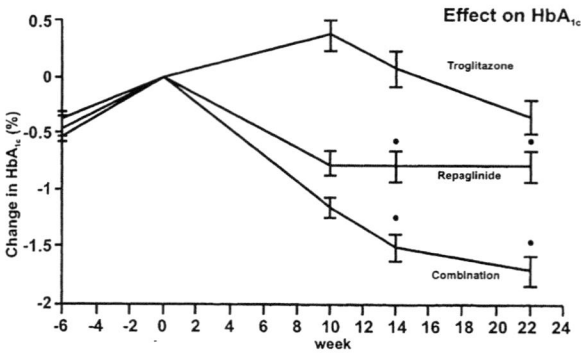

Fig. 5.2. Change in fasting glucose and HbA$_{1c}$ over time in patients with Type 2 diabetes treated with repaglinide, troglitazone or the combination of these two drugs. (Reproduced from Raskin et al. 1999)

decreased from 8.8% to 8.0% in repaglinide-treated patients, from 8.5% to 8.1% in troglitazone-treated patients, and from 8.7% to 7.0% in patients receiving a repaglinide–troglitazone combination (Raskin et al. 1999). Repaglinide was significantly more effective than troglitazone, while combination therapy was significantly more effective than monotherapy in terms of glycaemic control (Fig. 5.2).

Prandial Repaglinide and Hypoglycaemia

An important predicted advantage of the PGR strategy is that it will reduce the incidence and severity of hypoglycaemia relative to traditional regimens involving sulphonylureas. As discussed above, this is a particular concern when meals are taken at irregular intervals or missed altogether, as it is on such occasions that severe hypoglycaemia may be precipitated.

The ability of PGR with repaglinide to minimise the risk of hypoglycaemia in such situations was demonstrated in a randomised study of 43 patients with well-controlled Type 2 diabetes who received either repaglinide taken only with meals or glibenclamide given as per label recommendations (Damsbo et al. 1999). These patients were assessed with and without omission of lunch. The mean minimum blood glucose level remained unchanged at 4.3 mmol/l in repaglinide-treated patients when lunch was omitted, whereas omission of lunch in glibenclamide-treated patients led to a fall from 4.3 to 3.4 mmol/l (between-group difference, $p = 0.014$). Six episodes of hypoglycaemia, four requiring treatment, occurred, all of them in glibenclamide-treated patients and in association with omission of lunch.

This has been the only study designed to assess the impact of repaglinide in the context of poor compliance to mealtime regimens. In long-term comparative studies, ethical considerations demand that dosing and food consumption are tightly controlled in line with the requirements of sulphonylurea therapy. Nevertheless, a meta-analysis from comparative studies involving glibenclamide, gliclazide and glipizide show that repaglinide incurs a significantly lower risk of major hypoglycaemia, even under tightly controlled circumstances (Fig. 5.3); the relative risk for major hypoglycaemia being 2.8 for sulphonylurea-treated patients compared with repaglinide-treated patients (Smedegaard Kristensen et al. 1999). Furthermore, this difference was manifest despite identical levels of metabolic control with all treatments. Objec-

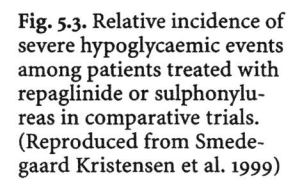

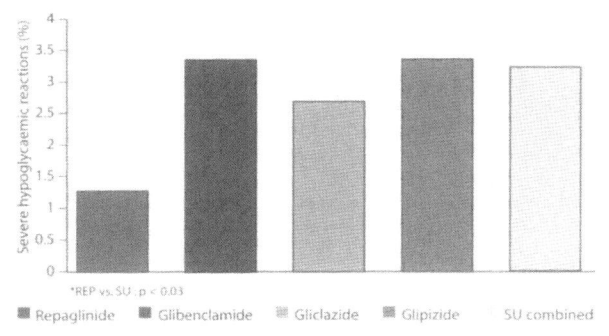

Fig. 5.3. Relative incidence of severe hypoglycaemic events among patients treated with repaglinide or sulphonylureas in comparative trials. (Reproduced from Smedegaard Kristensen et al. 1999)

tive evidence from those patients in whom blood glucose measurements were made show the relative risk of hypoglycaemia (blood glucose < 2.5 mmol/l) to be two-fold higher with glibenclamide and glipizide, and four-fold higher with gliclazide, in comparison to repaglinide (Owens 1998).

This finding was underlined by a comparative study of repaglinide and glibenclamide (Marbury et al. 1999). In this study, 15% and 19% of patients receiving repaglinide and glibenclamide, respectively, reported symptoms of hypoglycaemia. This difference was not significant, but the study also provided data concerning the objective parameter of self-assessed blood glucose level measured at the time of hypoglycaemic symptoms. Blood glucose levels were found to be significantly lower at these times in patients receiving glibenclamide than in those receiving repaglinide ($p = 0.004$). This finding raises the possibility that the threshold for awareness of hypoglycaemia may be higher in association with repaglinide than with sulphonylureas. The incidence of patient-reported, symptomatic hypoglycaemia associated with repaglinide in clinical trials has been 16%, with severe hypoglycaemia occurring only rarely – in just 1.3% of patients.

The overall conclusion to be drawn from these studies is that while prandial repaglinide does not eliminate the risk of hypoglycaemia, it does reduce the incidence and severity of hypoglycaemic events in comparison to traditional regimens of sulphonylureas, even under well-controlled conditions. In the context of poor compliance to mealtime regimens, the advantage of repaglinide in this respect may be great.

Conclusion

A treatment strategy based upon prandial blood glucose regulation is logical, given the deficiency of the prandial insulin response characteristic of Type 2 diabetes, the association between postprandial hyperglycaemia and vascular disease, and the risks of hypoglycaemia inherent in traditional methods of increasing blood insulin levels. This strategy is also highly effective: prandial repaglinide has been shown to provide control of all measures of glycaemia, as well as offering greater flexibility for the patient and the potential for improved compliance. Thus, PGR with repaglinide can be regarded as an advance compared to traditional sulphonylurea-based regimens. It is a treatment strategy that improves prognosis through maximal metabolic control, yet minimises the risk of treatment-induced hypoglycaemia.

References

Amos AF, McCarty DJ, Zimmet P (1997) The rising global burden of diabetes and its complications: estimates and projections to the year 2010. Diabet Med 14:1–85

Asplund K, Wiholm B-E, Lithner F (1983) Glibenclamide-associated hypoglycaemia: a report on 57 cases. Diabetologia 24:412–417

Bakkali-Nadi A, Mailaisse-Lagae F, Malaisse WJ (1994) Insulinotropic action of meglitinide analogues; concentration–reponse relationship and nutrient dependency. Diabetes Res 27:81–87

Bokvist M, Høy M, Poulsen CR, Buschard K, Gromada J (1998) A4166 but not repaglinide stimulate Ca^{2+}-evoked, K_{ATP} channel independent, secretion in rat pancreatic α- and β-cells. Diabetologia 41 (Suppl 1):Abstract 543

5 Clinical Experience with Repaglinide

Brown Frandsen K, Moses RG, Gomis R, Clauson P, Schlienger J-L, Dedov I (1999) The efficacy and safety of repaglinide used as a flexible prandial glucose regulator in patients with type 2 diabetes: a multi-center, randomized, placebo-controlled, double-blind study. Diabetes 48 (Suppl 1): Abstract 112

Bruttomesso D, Pianta A, Mari A, Valerio A, Marescotti MC, Avogaro A, Tiengo A, Del Prato S (1999) Restoration of early rise in plasma insulin levels improves the glucose tolerance of type 2 diabetic patients. Diabetes 48:99–105

Ceriello A (1998) The emerging role of post-prandial hyperglycaemic spikes in the pathogenesis of diabetic complications. Diabet Med 15:188–193

Coates PA, Ollerton RL, Luzio SD, Ismail I, Owens DR (1994) A glimpse of the 'natural history' of established type 2 (non-insulin dependent) diabetes mellitus from the spectrum of metabolic and hormonal responses to a mixed meal at the time of diagnosis. Diabetes Res Clin Pract 26:177–187

Crepaldi G, Del Prato (1995) What therapy do our NIDDM patients need? Insulin releasers. Diabetes Res Clin Pract 28 Suppl: 159–165

Damsbo P, Clauson P, Marbury TC, Windfeld K (1999) A double-blind randomized comparison of meal-related glycemic control by repaglinide and glibenclamide in well-controlled type 2 diabetic patients. Diabetes Care 22:789–794

DECODE study group, European Diabetes Epidemiology group (1999) Glucose tolerance and mortality: comparison of WHO and American Diabetes Association diagnostic criteria. Lancet 354:617–621

Dejgaard A, Madsbad S, Kilhovd B, Lager I, Mustajoki P (1998) Repaglinide compared to glipizide in the treatment of type 2 diabetic patients. Diabetologia 41 (Suppl 1):Abstract 236.

Emilien G, Maloteaux J-M, Ponchon M (1999) Pharmacological management of diabetes: recent progress and future perspective in daily drug treatment. Pharmacol Ther 81:37–51

Feinglos MN, Bethel MA (1998) Treatment of Type 2 diabetes mellitus. Med Clin North America 82:757–790

Fuhlendorff J, Rorsman P, Kofod H, Brand CL, Rolin B, MacKay P, Shymko R, Carr RD (1998) Stimulation of insulin release by repaglinide and glibenclamide involves both common and distinct processes. Diabetes 47:345–351

Gill GV, Huddle KR (1993) Hypoglycaemic admissions among diabetic patients in Soweto, South Africa. Diabetic Med 10:181–183

Haffner SM (1998) The importance of hyperglycaemia in the nonfasting state to the development of cardiovascular disease. Endocrine Rev 1998;19:583–92

Haller H. The clinical importance of postprandial glucose. Diabet Res Clin Pract 40:43–49

Hanefeld M, Fischer S, Julius U, Schulze J, Schwanebeck U, Schmechel H, Ziegelasch HJ, Lindner J (1996) Risk factors for myocardial infarction and death in newly detected NIDDM: the Diabetes Intervention Study, 11-year follow-up. Diabetologia 39:1577–1583

Hatorp V, Hasslacher C, Clauson P (1999) Pharmacokinetics of repaglinide in Type 2 diabetes patients with and without renal impairment. Diabetologia 42 (Suppl 1):Abstarct 242

Home PD (1999) Rapid-acting insulin secretagogues: a clinical need? Exp Clin Endocrinol Diabetes 107:115–119

Landgraf R, Bilo HJ, Muller PG (1999) A comparison of repaglinide and glibenclamide in the treatment of type 2 diabetic patients previously treated with sulphonylureas. Eur J Clin Pharmacol 55:165–171

Lefèbvre PJ, Scheen AJ (1998) The postprandial state and risk of cardiovascular disease. Diabet Med 15(Suppl 4):63–68

Louchami K, Jijakli H, Sener A, Malaisse WJ (1998) Effect of repaglinide upon nutrient metabolism, biosynthetic activity, cationic fluxes and insulin release in rat pancreatic islets. Res Commun Mol Pathol Pharmacol 99:155–168

Marbury T, Huang WC, Strange P, Lebovitz H (1999) Repaglinide versus glibenclamide: a one-year comparison trial. Diabetes Res Clin Pract 43:155–166

Matthews DR, Cull CA, Stratton IM, Holman RR, Turner RC (1998) UKPDS 26: Sulphonylurea failure in non-insulin-dependent diabetic patients over six years. UK Prospective Diabetes Study (UKPDS) Group. Diabet Med 15:297–303

Melander A, Donnelly R, Rydberg T (1998) Is there a concentration-effect relationship for sulphonylureas? Clin Pharmacokinet 34:181–188

Mitrakou A, Kelley D, Veneman T, Jenssen T, Pangburn T, Reilly J, Gerich J (1990) Contribution of abnormal muscle and liver glucose metabolism to postprandial hyperglycaemia in NIDDM. Diabetes 39:1381–1390

Moses R, Slobodniuk R, Boyages S, Colagiuri S, Kidson W, Carter J, Donnelly T, Moffitt P, Hopkins H (1999) Effect of repaglinide addition to metformin monotherapy on glycemic control in patients with type 2 diabetes. Diabetes Care 22:119

Ohkubo Y, Kishikawa H, Araki E, Miyata T, Isami S, Motoyoshi S, Kojima Y, Furuyoshi N, Shichiri M (1995) Intensive insulin therapy prevents the progression of diabetic microvascular complications in Japanese patients with non-insulin-dependent diabetes mellitus: a randomized prospective 6-year study. Diabetes Res Clin Pract 28:103–117

Oliver S, Ahmad S (1997). Pharmacokinetics and bioavailability of repaglinide, a new oral antidiabetic agent for patients with Type 2 diabetes (NIDDM). Diabetologia 40(Suppl 1):Abstract320

Owens DR (1998) Repaglinide – prandial glucose regulator: a new class of oral antidiabetic drug. Diabet Med 15(Suppl 4):28–36

Owens DR, Luzio SD, Coates PA (1996). Insulin secretion and sensitivity in newly diagnosed NIDDM Caucasians in the UK. Diabet Med 13(Suppl 6):19–24

Paterson JR, Orrell JM, Neithercut WD et al. (1989) Drug therapy in patients with diabetes mellitus: an audit. Diabetes Research 12:169–171

Polonsky KS (1999) Evolution of β-cell dysfunction in impaired glucose tolerance and diabetes. Exp Clin Endocrinol Diabetes 107:124–127

Polonsky KS, Given BD, Hirsch LJ, Tillil H, Shapiro ET, Beebe C, Frank BH, Galloway JA, Van Cauter E (1988) Abnormal patterns of insulin secretion in non-insulin-dependent diabetes mellitus. N Engl J Med 318:1231–1239

Raskin P, Kennedy F, Woo V, Jain R, Mueller PG (1999) A multicenter, randomized study of the therapeautic effect of repaglinide combined with troglitazone in subjects with Type 2 diabetes. Diabetes 48(Suppl 1):Abstract107, Abstract 0463

Robertson DA, Home PD (1993) Problems and pitfalls of sulphonylurea therapy in older patients. Drugs Aging 3:510–524

Ruckle JL, Hatorp V (1998) Repaglinide pharmacokinetics in patients with renal impairment versus healthy volunteers. Diabetologia 41 (Suppl 1):Abstract235

Smedegaard Kristensen J, Clauson P, Bayer T, Brown Frandsen K The frequency of severe hypoglycaemia is reduced with repaglinide treatment compared with sulphonylurea treatment. Presented at Scandinavian Society for the Study of Diabetes, Turku, Finland

Sparano N, Seaton TL (1998) Troglitazone in type II diabetes mellitus. Pharmacotherapy 18:539–548

Stahl M, Berger W (1999). Higher incidence of severe hypoglycaemia leading to hosptial admission in Type 2 diabetic patients treated with long-acting versus short-acting sulphonylureas. Diabetic Med 16:586–590

Teo SK, Ee CH (1997) Hypoglycaemia in the elderly. Singapore Med J 38:432–434

Tominaga M, Eguchi H, Manaka H, Igarashi K, Kato T, Sekikawa A (1999) Impaired glucose tolerance is a risk factor for cardiovascular disease, but not impaired fasting glucose. Diabetes Care 22:920–924

Turner RC, Cull CA, Frighi V, Holman RR for the UKPDS group (1999) Glycemic control with diet, sulfonylurea, metformin, or insulin in patients with Type 2 diabetes mellitus. J Am Med Assoc 281:2005–2012

UK Prospective Diabetes Study (UKPDS) Group 91998) Intensive blood-glucose control with sulphonylureas or insulin compared with conventional treatment and risk of complications in patients with type 2 diabetes (UKPDS 33). Lancet 352:837–853

Vinambres C, Villanueva-Penacarrillo ML, Valverde I, Malaisse WJ (1996) Repaglinide preserves nutrient-stimulated biosynthetic activity in rat pancreatic islets. Pharmacol Res 34:83–85

Yap WS, Peterson GM, Vial JH, Randall CTC, Greenaway TM (1998) Review of management of type 2 diabetes mellitus. J Clin Pharmacol Therapeutics 23:457–465

CHAPTER 6

Effects of Metformin on Glycaemic Control and Cardiovascular Risk in Type 2 Diabetes

G. Perriello

Cardiovascular disease is the major cause of death in patients with type 2 diabetes (Pyorala et al 1987). The excess cardiovascular risk of patients with type 2 diabetes may be explained by detrimental action of hyperglycaemia and deleterious effects of other metabolic abnormalities, such as visceral obesity, dyslipidemia and hypertension, associated to type 2 diabetes and related to insulin resistance (Reaven and Laws 1994).

Management of patients with type 2 diabetes should reduce cardiovascular mortality, which is associated to diabetes, as well as prevent or minimise micro-vascular complications (Klein 1995). Intervention trials have shown that decreasing hyperglycaemia can effectively reduce micro-vascular but at a lesser extent macro-vascular complications in type 2 diabetes (UKPDS 1998).

Several longitudinal studies have demonstrated a relationship between glycaemic control and development of cardiovascular disease (Coutinho et al. 1999). Other cardiovascular risk factors, such as dyslipidemia, hypertension and obesity, are very common in patients with type 2 diabetes and contribute to development of cardiovascular complications (Turner et al. 1998). Reducing macro-vascular complications requires concomitant management of all cardiovascular risk factors.

In type 2 diabetes insulin resistance is a fundamental defect, which impairs insulin-dependent production of nitric oxide, without affecting insulin-dependent vascular smooth muscle cell growth and migration. These changes contribute to determine a pro-atherogenic state in type 2 diabetes (Tooke and Hannemann 2000). Therefore, insulin resistance, rather than hyperglycaemia, appears to be the primary factor in determining endothelial dysfunction, which in turn initiates and largely contributes to development and progression of cardiovascular disease.

Insulin resistance often leads to hyperinsulinaemia, which is associated with hypertension, atherogenic dyslipidemia, left ventricular hypertrophy, impaired fibrinolysis and visceral obesity (Fagan et al. 1998). Although all these conditions are associated with atherosclerosis and adverse cardiovascular events, the therapeutic efforts in patients with type 2 diabetes have focussed predominantly on normalising blood glucose. Improvement of insulin sensitivity should lower both insulin and glucose levels as well as diminish hypertension and dyslipidemia (Henry 1998).

These observations indicate that the treatment of type 2 diabetes requires therapeutic agents which do more than simply lower hyperglycaemia. Pharmacological agents with anti-hyperglycaemic effects and also beneficial effects on dyslipidemia, hypertension, obesity, hyperinsulinaemia and insulin resistance should be preferred

Table 6.1. Metabolic effects of Metformin

↓ Plasma insulin levels
↓ Body weight
↓ Free fatty acid levels and oxidation
↓ TG and LDL cholesterol levels
↓ Post-prandial hyperlipidemia
↑ HDL cholesterol
↓ Plasma levels of PAI-1

(Bailey 1999). In this respect metformin has an important and established role: this drug has been shown to lower blood glucose and triglyceride levels, and to assist with weight reduction and to reduce hyperinsulinaemia and insulin resistance (DeFronzo 1999). Moreover, metformin treatment may improve endothelial function and insulin resistance, with a strong relationship between relative changes of these parameters, in patients with type 2 diabetes (Mather et al. 2001).

Metformin is an oral biguanide which ameliorates hyperglycaemia by improving insulin sensitivity. It does not stimulate insulin secretion and aggravate hyperinsulinaemia or cause hypoglycaemia or weight gain. It also has beneficial effects on serum lipid profiles (Table 6.1). Typically it reduces basal and post-prandial hyperglycaemia by about 25% in more than 90% of patients with type 2 diabetes (Zimmet and Collier 1999).

Metformin is rapidly and completely absorbed from the small intestine reaching a plasma concentration peak in 2 h after oral administration. It is not bound to plasma proteins, is not transformed in active metabolites and is eliminated only by kidney with a half-life of 2–5 h. Metformin should be administered three times a day to reach a total daily dose of 2–2.5 g (Bailey and Turner 1996).

The effect on fasting, rather than on post-prandial hyperglycaemia, is more pronounced because metformin acts predominantly on the liver to suppress gluconeogenesis, mainly potentiating insulin action, reducing hepatic extraction of certain substrates, such as lactate, diminishing the energy supply by suppressing fatty acid oxidation and opposing the effects of glucagon (Wiernsperger and Bailey 1999).

A recent study has shown that metformin could reduce gluconeogenesis through short-term (metabolic) and long-term (genic) effects, which involves a reduction of about 30–60% of fatty acid oxidation, ketogenesis and gluconeogenesis and a 250% increase in glycolisis (Fulgencio et al. 2001).

The most serious complication associated with metformin is lactic acidosis which has an incidence of about 0.03 cases per 1000 patients years of treatment and a mortality risk of about 0.015 per 1000 patient-years. Most cases occur in patients who are wrongly prescribed the drug, particularly patients with impaired renal function, i.e. serum creatinine level >1.5 g/L. Other major contraindications include congestive heart failure, hypoxic states and advanced liver disease. Serious adverse events with metformin are predictable rather than spontaneous and are potentially preventable if the prescribing guidelines are respected. Gastrointestinal adverse effects, notably diarrhoea, occur in less than 20% of patients and remit when the dosage is reduced. The life-threatening risks associated with metformin are rare and could mostly be avoided by strict adherence to the prescribing guidelines (Howlett and Bailey 1999).

Metformin decreases blood glucose concentrations in patients with type 2 diabetes at a similar extent of sulfonylureas (Davidson and Peters 1997). In the US Multicenter Metformin Study obese patients with type 2 diabetes, not controlled with diet, were randomised to either metformin (2.5 g/d) or placebo for about 30 weeks. At the end of observation period, fasting blood glucose concentration was 55 mg/dl lower in metformin group compared to placebo (189 vs 244 mg/dl). In the same study metformin added to glyburide determined a substantial improvement in fasting blood glucose (187 vs 261 mg/dl) in patients not controlled with glyburide alone (DeFronzo and Goodman 1995).

Metformin consistently is not associated with weight gain, even though it lowers glycosuria significantly and at a similar extent of other hypoglycaemic agents (Lebovitz 1999). In the 9-year follow up of the obese type 2 diabetic group of the UKPDS, the change in mean weight in the metformin group compared with the diet treated controls resulted in a 2 kg less weight gain (UKPDS 1998). In the US metformin trial patients who were switched from glyburide to metformin lost 4.1 kg of weight compared with those who continued to use glyburide (DeFronzo and Goodman 1995). A 4 kg weight difference was observed in nine randomised trials between metformin and sulfonylurea treatment despite comparable improvements in glycaemic control (Campbell and Howlett 1995). The BIGPRO study which examined the effect of 1-year of treatment in non-diabetic subjects with an increased waist-to-hip ratio with metformin versus placebo, showed a mean weight loss with metformin of 2.0 kg compared with 0.8 kg in the placebo treated group (Fontbonne et al. 1996).

The mechanism underlying the beneficial effect of metformin on body weight is uncertain, but may be related to a decrease in energy intake. In a short-term study, hunger rating and snacks eaten were found to be decreased after only 3 days of metformin therapy (Lee et al. 1998). In 10 obese type 2 diabetes subjects it was found that metformin decreased mildly appetite and largely fat mass but not lean body mass, thus indicating a prominent effect of the drug on lipid deposits independent with the reduced energy intake (Stumvoll et al. 1995). In contrast, metformin reduced body weight by decreasing energy intake which counterbalanced the reduction in BMR and glycosuria due to the improvement of blood glucose (Makimattila et al. 1999).

Metformin has a prominent lipid lowering effect, producing a significant reduction in serum triglyceride and free fatty acid concentrations, a small reduction in serum LDL, and an elevation in HDL (Schneider et al. 1990). The effects on triglycerides and LDL cholesterol are in a range of 4–5%, as it has been demonstrated in patients poorly controlled with glyburide and switched to metformin, even though the glycaemic control was unchanged (DeFronzo and Goodman 1995). In another study a better improvement in plasma LDL and HDL cholesterol was obtained with metformin compared to insulin independently from plasma glucose control (Fanghanel et al. 1996). Metformin added to sulfonylurea-treated patients decreased postprandial triglyceride-rich particles of intestinal origin (Abbasi et al. 1997). Regarding the mechanism by which metformin improve plasma lipid profile, some recent studies have focussed the attention on the effect of metformin on decreasing lipolysis and lowering plasma free fatty acid concentration. This effect is strictly related to the reduction in fatty acid oxidation, which may decrease energy in hepatic cell for gluconeogenesis and contribute to the anti-hyperglycaemic action of metformin (Perriello et al 1994).

A few studies suggested that metformin treatment decreases blood pressure (Giugliano et al 1993). Other studies (Dorella et al 1996, Snorgaard et al 1997) as well as the UKPDS trial failed to show any blood pressure lowering effect of metformin. A more detailed analysis of blood pressure responses to angiotensin II or norepinephrine infusions have shown no effect of metformin treatment.

Metformin treatment does modify the procoagulant state in type 2 diabetes. It has a specific effect in decreasing plasminogen activator inhibitor I (PAI-1) levels in type 2 diabetic patients. Metformin decreased PAI-1 levels in the centrally obese nondiabetic patients in the BIGPRO trial (Fontbonne et al 1996).

Recently, it has been demonstrated that metformin may reduce dicarbonil compounds, such as methylglyoxal and glyoxal, which are extremely reactive glycating agents involved in the formation of advanced glycation end products (AGEs), which in turn are associated with diabetic vascular complications (Beisswenger et al 1999). These results suggest that besides its known anti-hyperglycaemic effect, metformin could reduce also AGE formation by reacting with alpha-dicarbonyl compounds. This is relevant to a potential clinical use of metformin in the prevention of diabetic complications by inhibition of carbonyl stress.

In UKPDS, overweight patients who received metformin gained less weight and had fewer hypoglycemic episodes than those treated with either insulin or sulfonylureas (Table 6.2). Patients who received metformin also had a more favorable outcome with respect to development of diabetes-related end points, all cause mortality and stroke (UKPDS 34).

The choice of therapeutic agents to treat hyperglycemia or indeed any other abnormality in type 2 diabetes should take into acconunt the effects of those agents on other metabolic abnormalities. Improved glycemic control reduces glycosuria, decreases calorie loss and improves anabolic state. These changes can determine weight gain, a decrease in VLDL concentration, triglycerides and cholesterol and blood pressure. Therefore, managament of type 2 diabetes should consider not only the magnitude of effect on glycemic control and its specific mechanism but also the profile of effects on other components of the insulin resistance syndrome.

Table 6.2. Metformin vs other treatments (from UKPDS 1998)

Aggregate endpoint	P
Any diabetes related endpoint	0.0034
Diabetes related deaths	0.11
All cause mortality	0.021
Myocardial infarction	0.12
Stroke	0.032
Peripheral vascular disease	0.62
Microvascular	0.39

References

Abbasi F, Kamath V, Rizvi AA, Carantoni M, Chen YD, Reaven GM (1997) Results of a placebo-controlled study of the metabolic effects of the addition of metformin to sulfonylurea-treated patients. Evidence for a central role of adipose tissue. Diabetes Care 20:1863-69
Bailey CJ (1999) Insulin resistance and antidiabetic drugs. Biochem Pharmacol 58:1511-20
Bailey CJ, Turner RC (1996) Metformin N Engl J Med 334:574-9
Beisswenger PJ, Howell SK, Touchette AD, Lal S, Szwergold BS (1999) Metformin reduces systemic methylglyoxal levels in type 2 diabetes. Diabetes 48:198-202
Campbell IW and Howlett HC (1995) Worldwide experience of metformin as an effective glucose-lowering agent: a meta-analysis. Diabetes Metab Rev 11 Suppl 1:S57-62
Coutinho M, Gerstein HC, Wang Y, Yusuf S (1999) The relationship between glucose and incident cardiovascular events. A metaregression analysis of published data from 20 studies of 95,783 individuals followed for 12.4 years. Diabetes Care 22:233-40
Davidson MB and Peters AL (1997) An overview of metformin in the treatment of type 2 diabetes mellitus. Am J Med 102:99-110
DeFronzo RA (1999) Pathogenesis of type 2 diabetes: implications for metformin. Drugs 58 Suppl 1:29-30
DeFronzo RA and Goodman AM (1995) Efficacy of metformin in patients with non-insulin-dependent diabetes mellitus. The Multicenter Metformin Study Group. N Engl J Med 333:541-9
Dorella M, Giusto M, Da Tos V, Campagnolo M, Palatini P, Rossi G, Ceolotto G, Felice M, Semplicini A, Del Prato S (1996) Improvement of insulin sensitivity by metformin treatment does not lower blood pressure of nonobese insulin-resistant hypertensive patients with normal glucose tolerance. J Clin Endocrinol Metab 81:1568-74
Fagan TC, Deedwania PC (1998) The cardiovascular dysmetabolic syndrome. Am J Med 105: 77S-82S
Fanghanel G, Sanchez-Reyes L, Trujillo C, Sotres D, Espinosa-Campos J (1996) Metformin's effects on glucose and lipid metabolism in patients with secondary failure to sulfonylureas. Diabetes Care 19:1185-9
Fontbonne A, Charles MA, Juhan-Vague I, Bard JM, Andre P, Isnard F, Cohen JM, Grandmottet P, Vague P, Safar ME, Eschwege E (1996) The effect of metformin on the metabolic abnormalities associated with upper-body fat distribution. BIGPRO Study Group. Diabetes Care 19: 920-6
Fulgencio JP, Kohl C, Girard J, Pegorier JP (2001) Effect of metformin on fatty acid and glucose metabolism in freshly isolated hepatocytes and on specific gene expression in cultured hepatocytes. Biochem Pharmacol. 62:439-46
Gerich JE (1996) Pathogenesis and treatment of type 2 (noninsulin-dependent) diabetes mellitus (NIDDM). Horm Metab Res. 28:404-12
Giugliano D, De Rosa N, Di Maro G, Marfella R, Acampora R, Buoninconti R, D'Onofrio F (1993) Metformin improves glucose, lipid metabolism, and reduces blood pressure in hypertensive, obese women. Diabetes Care 16:1387-90
Henry RR (1998) Type 2 diabetes care: the role of insulin-sensitizing agents and practical implications for cardiovascular disease prevention. Am J Med. 105:20S-26S
Howlett HC and Bailey CJ (1999) A risk-benefit assessment of metformin in type 2 diabetes mellitus. Drug Saf 20:489-503
Klein R (1995) Hyperglycemia and microvascular and macrovascular disease in diabetes. Diabetes Care18:258-68
UK Prospective Diabetes Study (UKPDS) Group (1998) Intensive blood-glucose control with sulphonylureas or insulin compared with conventional treatment and risk of complications in patients with type 2 diabetes (UKPDS 33). Lancet 352:837-53
Lebovitz HE (1999) Effects of oral antihyperglycemic agents in modifying macrovascular risk factors in type 2 diabetes. Diabetes Care 22 Suppl 3:C41-4
Lee A (1998) Metformin decreases food consumption and induces weight loss in subjects with obesity with type II non-insulin-dependent diabetes. Obes Res 6:47-53
Makimattila S, Nikkila K, Yki-Jarvinen H (1999) Causes of weight gain during insulin therapy with and without metformin in patients with Type II diabetes mellitus. Diabetologia. 42: 406-12

Mather KJ, Verma S, Anderson TJ (2001) Improved endothelial function with metformin in type 2 diabetes mellitus. J Am Coll Cardiol 37:1344–50

Perriello G (1995) Mechanisms of metformin action in non-insulin-dependent diabetes mellitus. Diabetes Metab Rev 11 Suppl 1:S51–6

Perriello G, Misericordia P, Volpi E, Santucci A, Santucci C, Ferrannini E, Ventura MM, Santeusanio F, Brunetti P, Bolli GB (1994) Acute antihyperglycemic mechanisms of metformin in NIDDM. Evidence for suppression of lipid oxidation and hepatic glucose production. Diabetes 43: 920–8

Reaven GM, Laws A: Insulin resistance, compensatory hyperinsulinemia, and coronary heart disease. Diabetologia 37:948–952, 1994

Schneider J (1990) Effects of metformin on dyslipoproteinemia in non-insulin-dependent diabetes mellitus. Diabete Metab 17:185–90

Snorgaard O, Kober L, Carlsen J (1997) The effect of metformin on blood pressure and metabolism in nondiabetic hypertensive patients. J Intern Med 242:407–12

Stumvoll M, Nurjhan N, Perriello G, Dailey G, Gerich JE (1995) Metabolic effects of metformin in non-insulin-dependent diabetes mellitus. N Engl J Med 333:550–4

Pyorala K, Laakso M, Uusitupa M (1987) Diabetes and atheroslerosis: an epidemiologic view. Diabetes Metab Rev 3:463–524

Tooke JE and Hannemann MM (2000) Adverse endothelial function and the insulin resistance syndrome. J Intern Med 247:425–31

Turner RC, Millns H, Neil HA, Stratton IM, Manley SE, Matthews DR, Holman RR (1998) Risk factors for coronary artery disease in non-insulin dependent diabetes mellitus: United Kingdom Prospective Diabetes Study (UKPDS: 23) BMJ 316:823–8

Wiernsperger NF, Bailey CJ (1999) The antihyperglycaemic effect of metformin: therapeutic and cellular mechanisms. Drugs 58 Suppl 1:31–9

Zimmet P, Collier G (1999) Clinical efficacy of metformin against insulin resistance parameters: sinking the iceberg. Drugs 58 Suppl 1:21–8

CHAPTER 7

Dyslipidemia and Cardiovascular Risk in Diabetes

R. Carmena, J.F. Ascaso

Diabetes mellitus, due to its rising incidence world wide, and its increased risk for the development of cardiovascular complications, represents a significant public health problem [1]. In this chapter, we will focus on the impact on cardiovascular risk of lipid abnormalities, a frequent finding in type 2 diabetic patients.

It is well known that, antedating the increased risk for microvascular complications, diabetics have an elevated risk for developing macrovascular complications. In fact, at the time of diagnosis of type 2 diabetes, between 20-40% of subjects show some type of cardiovascular complications [2, 2a]. This finding has led to the hypothesis that the clock for atherosclerosis and macrovascular complications starts ticking long before the diagnosis of type 2 diabetes can be established [3], underlying the importance of the pre-diabetic or abnormal glucose tolerance state. Abnormalities like insulin resistance, lipid disorders, and hypertension, which are frequently present in such state and precede in time the onset of chronic hyperglycemia, have definite importance as risk factors for cardiovascular complications.

Main Metabolic Abnormalities in Type 2 Diabetes Mellitus

Although the primary defect underlying type 2 diabetes remains to be elucidated, the main metabolic characteristics of the disease are well known and include hyperglycemia, insulin resistance, increased hepatic glucose production and impaired secretion of insulin by the pancreatic beta cells. Lipid abnormalities are common in type 2 diabetes, hypertriglyceridaemia is found in 20-60% of cases and is frequently associated with low HDL-cholesterol and small, dense LDL particles [4]. This cluster of lipid abnormalities, also known as diabetic dyslipidemia, is thought to play a causal role in the macrovascular complications. In addition, lipid abnormalities (mainly hypertriglyceridaemia) may precede by years the onset of hyperglycemia in type 2 diabetics.

Lipid metabolism in diabetes is modulated by a series of factors among which, the degree of glycemic control and the presence of insulin resistance are the two most prominent players. Insulin resistance is at the basis of the pathophysiologic mechanisms of diabetic dyslipidemia, being closely linked to hypertriglyceridaemia and forming a vicious cycle with atherogenic potential [5].

Insulin Resistance and Lipid Metabolism in Type 2 Diabetes Mellitus

Insulin resistance can be defined as a diminution of the biological response to a given concentration of insulin. Although the term insulin resistance was originally used to indicate impaired insulin action on glucose metabolism in diabetic patients [6], it also has been observed in nondiabetic persons and is characterised by hyperinsulinaemia in the presence of normal or elevated plasma glucose levels [7]. Insulin resistance can be genetic and/or acquired, and has a broad clinical spectrum that includes rare genetic syndromes, abdominal obesity, polycystic ovary syndrome, glucocorticoid or growth hormone excess, uraemia, and glucose intolerance, among others [8, 9]. The most important acquired factors that contribute to insulin resistance are abdominal obesity, physical inactivity and smoking [10]. In the last decade, the insulin resistance syndrome has been recognised as an important factor predisposing to several chronic diseases, including hypertension, hyperuricaemia, hyperglycaemia, dyslipidaemia, and atherosclerosis [11, 12].

If the capacity of the pancreas to compensate is normal, resistance to the glucoregulatory actions of insulin leads to compensatory hyperinsulinaemia and, as a consequence, insulin resistant individuals with normal glucose tolerance are hyperinsulinaemic. Plasma insulin concentrations are related to the severity of insulin resistance [13]. Accordingly, hyperinsulinaemia in the presence of normal or elevated levels of blood glucose can be considered a marker of tissue insulin resistance [14]. Thus, the plasma insulin concentration has been used in epidemiological studies in non-diabetic populations as a surrogate for insulin resistance.

The different methods used to measure insulin action in vivo have been extensively reviewed [15]. Strictly speaking, insulin sensitivity is measured as the inverse of insulin resistance. All methods have their problems and their main difficulties have been recently highlighted [5]. The insulin suppression test, the first method used, and the euglycaemic hyperinsulinaemic clamp technique and its variations, considered by some authors as the reference method for measurement of insulin resistance, are rather laborious and complex and have been used in small experimental studies [16, 17]. The minimal model approach, introduced by Bergman [18], avoids the procedural difficulties of the clamp technique by utilising a computer program, and measures the dynamic insulin response to a glucose injection. It is now widely used in clinical research and, in well-defined groups of patients, is considered a valuable alternative to the glucose clamp technique for the assessment of insulin sensitivity [7, 12 – 13].

One major difficulty in the study of insulin resistance is that there is not yet available a quantitative definition of insulin resistance. Numerous studies have shown that in an apparently healthy population, the range of insulin sensitivity is remarkably large, 3 to 7-fold variations having been reported. As much as 25 % of the normal population is as insulin resistant as are subjects with impaired glucose tolerance or type 2 diabetes mellitus [7, 19]. An ethnic difference in the role of the insulin resistance/hyperinsulinemia syndrome in determining blood pressure levels has been established and could possibly be associated to other manifestations of the syndrome, such as lipid abnormalities [20, 21]. More studies are needed to further evaluate this issue.

Several well-characterized alterations of lipid metabolism are commonly associated with insulin resistance (Table 7.1), although there are difficulties in interpreting

Table 7.1. Alteration of lipid metabolism in type 2 diabetes mellitus

Hypertriglyceridaemia (increased VLDL-TG and VLDL-apoB concentrations)
Decreased HDL-cholesterol
Decreased HDL2 and HDL2/HDL3 ratio
Elevation of free fatty acids in fasting and postprandial situation
LDL phenotype B (small and dense LDL particles)
Decreased lipoprotein-lipase activity
Increased hepatic triglyceride-lipase activity
Prolonged postprandial lipemia
Increased Lp(a) in the presence of diabetic nephropathy

these associations in terms of cause and effect. One important consequence of insulin resistance is the loss of the suppressive effect of insulin on fat mobilization from adipose tissue. As a result, there is an increase in free fatty acids (FFA) flux owing to reduced suppression of lipolysis (Fig. 7.2). The failure to suppress FFA in the postprandial period, due to the decreased activity of lipoprotein lipase (LPL), and the elevated plasma FFA due to increased adipocyte lipolysis, a well known phenomenon among type 2 diabetics, may explain the increased hepatic VLDL-TG secretion [22]. It has been shown that insulin acutely inhibits hepatic secretion of VLDL-TG and apoB-100, and in insulin resistance states like type 2 diabetes, an increase in VLDL-TG and VLDL-apoB secretion is usually observed [23].

Insulin exerts an important effect on LPL activity [24], consequently, in insulin resistance states there is impaired postprandial TG clearance and decreased transfer of cholesterol into HDL due to deficient LPL action combined with increased hepatic lipase activity. This complex of lipoprotein disturbances tends to increase the plasma concentrations of the small, dense LDL particles, the so-called "type B phenotype", which is considered atherogenic [25]. These alterations explain the lipid abnormalities in type 2 diabetes, that include elevated plasma VLDL-TG and VLDL-apoB concentrations, decreased HDL-cholesterol, elevation of plasma FFA (both fasting and postprandial), and presence of small, dense LDL particles. These changes have been described as the "atherogenic lipoprotein phenotype" (ALP) [26].

Although the association between hypertriglyceridaemia and both glucose intolerance and hyperinsulinaemia was described some decades ago [27, 28] the elucidation of cause and effect remains a major challenge; i.e. are lipid changes secondary to insulin resistance or viceversa?

Several mechanisms must be considered in order to explain the association between insulin resistance and both glucose and lipoprotein abnormalities. As stated above, one implicit assumption has been that insulin resistance is the underlying factor and that the changes in lipid metabolism are secondary [9]. This assumption is based on evidence suggesting that hypertriglyceridaemia is a consequence of insulin resistance, irrespective of the glucose tolerance status [29], and on the recent demonstration, in two prospective studies [30, 31], that fasting hyperinsulinaemia precedes hypertriglyceridaemia and low plasma HDL-cholesterol concentrations. Other authors found that fasting FFA concentration explain 83% of variation in plasma triglyceride concentration, indicating that subjects with endogenous hypertriglyceridaemia are resistant to both the antilipolytic and glucoregulatory actions of insulin and the increased flux of FFA as a result of insulin resistance [32].

It has been hypothesized that the primary event could be insulin resistance initially localized in adipose tissue. This situation would increase FFA efflux and amplify insulin resistance in muscle and liver. In fact, in visceral obesity, the elevated flux of FFA to the liver is associated with insulin resistance [33].

On the other hand, abnormal lipid and lipoprotein concentrations could impair the insulin action at muscle level in the diabetic [34]. There is evidence that hypertriglyceridaemic type 2 diabetic subjects, with plasma triglycerides levels between 3–18 mmol/L are more insulin resistant than matched type 2 diabetic subjects without hypertriglyceridaemia [35]. Since Randle's report [36], it is known that high plasma concentrations of FFA result in a decreased systemic glucose uptake in the muscle and liver and impaired insulin sensitivity. The hypertriglyceridaemia can lead to insulin resistance even without concomitant obesity or type 2 diabetes mellitus, and those high plasma VLDL concentration down-regulate insulin receptors [5]. Moreover, overexpression of plasma apolipoprotein CIII causes severe hypertriglyceridaemia in transgenic mice and in some patients. This variant was defective in its response to insulin and contributes to the development of hypertriglyceridaemia and insulin resistance [37, 38].

Apolipoprotein E polymorphisms may influence the well-established relations of hypertriglyceridaemia to hyperinsulinaemia in insulin resistant/hyperinsulinaemic conditions. It has been shown that, in contrast to apoE2 and apoE3 carriers, who showed higher plasma triglyceride concentrations with fasting hyperinsulinaemia, healthy premenopausal women with the apoE4 isoform had similar plasma triglyceride concentrations at high and low fasting insulin levels [39]. In another study, conducted in nondiabetic subjects from a biethnic population, the apoE 3/2 phenotype was associated with lower plasma levels of fasting and 2 h post-prandial insulin [40]. Therefore it seems that apoE polymorphism could explain some of the lipid variations observed in the insulin resistance syndrome in different populations.

The association between insulin action and lipid metabolism could also be influenced by factors affecting both glucose and lipid metabolism, like obesity, abdominal distribution of fat, physical activity, diet, smoking habits, age, gender, etc. The amount of visceral fat is an important factor modulating the degree of insulin sensitivity and the lipid profile and may explain the major metabolic differences between men and women [41]. Obesity is very frequently found in type 2 diabetics and the impact of obesity on insulin resistance and diabetic dyslipidemia is well established. Studies conducted by our group have shown that with elevated plasma FFA the peripheral insulin sensitivity, expressed as the Si index, is significantly reduced both in lean and obese subjects. The reduction is more accentuated in the group with BMI > 27. Thus, obesity is a risk factor for type 2 diabetes and has become an important therapeutic target in its prevention.

To summarize, the effects of insulin resistance on lipid metabolism in type 2 diabetics include: (1) Lack of activity of lipoprotein lipase, which explains the increased postprandial lipaemia characteristic of these patients; this is associated with decreased exogenous and endogenous triglyceride clearance and low plasma levels of HDL-cholesterol. (2) Increased hepatic lipase activity, which favors the production of small, dense LDL particles. (3) Increased lipolysis, with an elevated flux of FFA to the liver and increased triglyceride and apo B secretion. The increase in FFA (Fig. 7.1) has important consequences, i.e. hypertriglyceridaemia, hyperglycemia (due to less

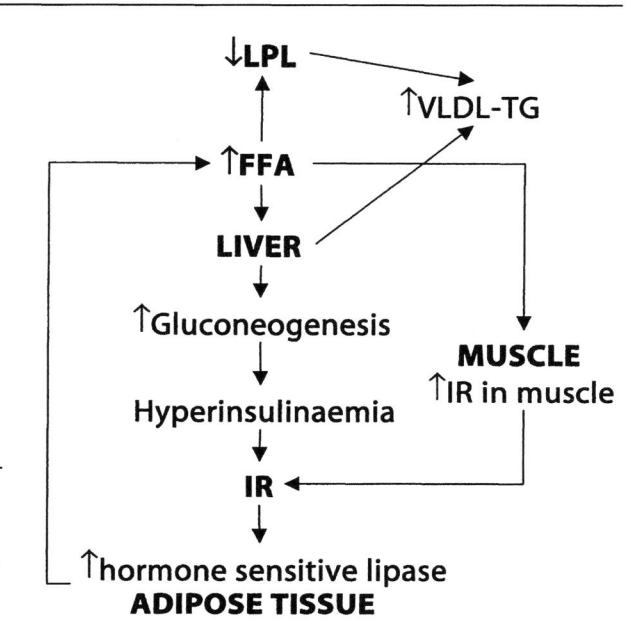

Fig. 7.1. Free fatty acid metabolism and insulin resistance. *LPL*, lipoprotein lipase; *VLDL-TG*, very low-density lipoprotein tryglicerides; *FFA*, free fatty acids; *IR*, insulin resistance

peripheral utilization and increased hepatic production), and hyperinsulinaemia and insulin resistance.

Dyslipidemia and Cardiovascular Risk in Type 2 Diabetes Mellitus

The incidence of cardiovascular diseases among type 2 diabetics has been shown to be elevated in different epidemiological studies. In the Framingham Study [42], the incidence of cardiovascular diseases and deaths due to cardiovascular complications was almost double in diabetic men and triple in diabetic women when compared to sex and age-matched controls (Table 7.2). In the Münster Heart Program (PROCAM) [43, 44], diabetes is one of the independent risk factors identified and the prevalence of cardiovascular complications among diabetics is significantly higher than in non diabetics.

Table 7.2. Incidence (×1,000) of cardiovascular diseases (CVD) and cardiovascular mortality in type 2 diabetes; Framingham Study (adapted from Kannel and McGee 1979)

	Diabetic men	Control men	Diabetic women	Control women
Any type of CVD	39.1	19.1	27.2	10.2
Death due to CVD	17.4	8.5	17.0	3.6
Intermitent claudication	12.6	3.3	8.4	1.2
Thrombotic stroke	4.7	1.9	6.2	1.7
CHD	24.8	14.9	17.8	6.9

CVD, cardiovascular disease; CHD, coronary heart disease.

Moreover, as Stamler et al. [45] have reported, at the same level of major cardiovascular risk factors (hypercholesterolemia, smoking, and diastolic hypertension), diabetic subjects have triple cardiovascular mortality than non diabetics, stressing the importance of factors which are characteristic of the diabetic state, like chronic hyperglycemia and insulin resistance. Thus, the "classic" risk factors do not seem to account for the excess risk of atherosclerosis in type 2 diabetes and new approaches to explain the connection of diabetes and accelerated atherosclerosis are needed. As some have proposed [46], a more profound understanding of the atherogenic effect of diabetic dyslipidemia may provide the means for prevention of premature vascular disease in diabetic patients.

The dominant features of diabetic dyslipidemia are hypertriglyceridemia and low HDL cholesterol concentrations. Increased production of VLDL by the liver, high TG concentrations after a fatty meal, and low LPL activity lead (Fig. 7.2) to raised concentrations of TG-rich lipoproteins (TRL) in plasma [44]. These changes, together with an increase in hepatic lipase activity, lead to qualitative changes in HDL and LDL, with preponderance of small and dense particles, easier to oxidize and more atherogenic. In addition the impaired catabolism of TRL permits its enrichment in cholesterol and their conversion into more atherogenic particles.

The elevation of remnant particles (TRL) in plasma, both fasting and postprandially, is a well known characteristic of diabetic dyslipidemia [47]. Postprandial lipid metabolism could play an important role in the development of atherosclerosis, as pointed out by Zilversmit [48] years ago. The rise in the plasma concentration of TRL particles after a fat-containing meal is greater in type 2 diabetics than in non-diabetic subjects [49]. Most studies have shown that hypertriglyceridemia in the fasting state is a major predictor of the magnitude of postprandial lipemia. However, postprandial

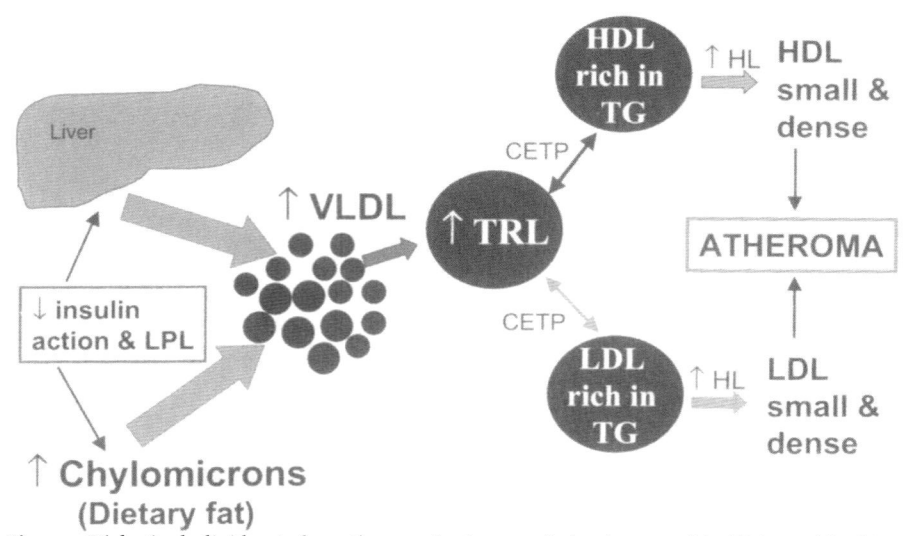

Fig. 7.2. Diabetic dyslipidemia has atherogenic characteristics: increased in TRL, enriched in cholesterol and predominance of small, dense HDL and LDL particles. *LPL*, lipoprotein lipase; *HL*, hepatic lipase; *TRL*, triglyceride-rich lipoproteins; *CETP*, cholesterol ester transfer protein

hypertriglyceridemia and insulin resistance have been observed in normoglycemic first-degree relatives of patients with type 2 diabetes with normal fasting triglycerides [50]. These findings indicate the important role of insulin resistance in affecting lipid metabolism in subjects with genetic predisposition to diabetes.

As previously stated subjects with impaired glucose tolerance or prediabetic state show hyperinsulinemia and dyslipidemia before the onset of clinical diabetes, at a time when glucose concentrations are relatively normal. Cardiovascular risk factors are increased, especially increased blood pressure and triglyceride and decreased HDL cholesterol, before the onset of type 2 diabetes [51], suggesting that not only is hyperglycemia responsible for the dyslipidemia in the diabetic state but also other factors such as insulin resistance [3].

In the U.S., over the past decade, there have been declines of 36 and 27% in CVD mortality among men and women without diabetes. Diabetic subjects, however, have shown a decrease of only 13% among men and an increase of 23% among women [52]. The treatment and prevention of cardiovascular disease in individuals with type 2 diabetes remains an enormous clinical challenge. Cardiovascular disease accounts for approximately 70% of deaths in these patients. Thus, bigger efforts should be made to treat and lower CVD risk factors earlier and more aggressively in diabetics. Epidemiological studies support the evidence that for CVD the clock starts ticking before the diagnosis of diabetes [53]. Thus, there is a consensus of opinion in favor of early intervention with diet, exercise and drugs in the prediabetic state.

Lipid-Lowering Trials in Diabetes

Besides treatment for hyperglycaemia, blood pressure control, obesity, etc., active intervention to reduce the risk for macrovascular disease should also include treating diabetic dyslipidemia with diet and drugs. According to the American Diabetes Association, current priorities of drug choices include the HMG-Co reductase inhibitors (statins) and fibrates [54]. Although LDL cholesterol levels are usually not significantly different in type 2 diabetic and normoglycemic subjects, LDL composition is markedly smaller and denser and more atherogenic in type 2 diabetic subjects. For reasons given below, lowering of LDL cholesterol becomes a priority and, according to ADA and NCEP guidelines, the recommended LDL cholesterol levels in diabetics, especially in those with cardiovascular disease, should be ≤100 mg/dL.

Several large, prospective studies (4S, CARE, LIPID) using statins (pravastatin and simvastatin) have shown a significant decreased in LDL cholesterol and in coronary artery disease events in diabetic subgroups [55]. In addition, aggressive lipid-lowering with atorvastatin in patients with angina pectoris (of whom 15% had diabetes), significantly reduced the incidence of ischemic events [56]. There are several ongoing statin trials including a large number of diabetic patients, like the Heart Protection Study (simvastatin) and the Collaborative Atorvastatin Diabetes Study, and the Atorvastatin as Prevention of Coronary Heart Disease in Patients with Type 2 Diabetes [57]. Interestingly, a post hoc analysis of the WOSCOPS data has shown evidence for a protective treatment effect of pravastatin in the development of diabetes mellitus [58]. Assignment to pravastatin therapy resulted in a 30% reduction in the hazard of becoming diabetic.

Concerning fibrates, one recent prospective study in men with coronary heart disease treated with placebo or gemfibrozil has shown a significant benefit in the subgroup of 627 diabetics treated with gemfibrozil [59]. A significant reduction in the combined endpoint of CHD death, non-fatal MI and confirmed stroke, with a relative risk reduction of 24 % was observed. The small group of diabetic men included in the Helsinki Heart Study also showed a beneficial effect of gemfibrozil, non-significant given the small numbers involved [60]. The Diabetes Atherosclerosis Intervention Study, the first trial performed specifically in a diabetic population, is an angiographic study of 418 type 2 diabetics (in the press), has shown the benefits of treating with fenofibrate this mixed (primary and secondary prevention) group of patients.

In conclusion, with the evidence available at the time of writing, diabetic dyslipidemia should be treated vigorously with diet and hypolipidemic drugs. In most patients, the first therapeutic option are the statin drugs, while fibrates could be of benefit as monotherapy in patients with a profile similar to the VA-HIT participants.

References

1. Zimmet PZ, Alberti KGMM: The changing face of macrovascular disease in non-insulin-dependent diabetes mellitus: an epidemic in progress. Lancet 1997; 350 (suppl I): 1-4
2. Perry RC, Baron AD: Impaired glucose tolerance: why is it not a disease?. Diabetes Care 1999; 22: 883-885
2a. Stratton IM, Adler AI, Neil HA, Matthews DR, Cull CA, Hadden D, Turner RC, Holman RR: Association of glycaemia with macrovascular and microvascular complications of type 2 diabetes (UKPDS 35): prospective observational study. BMJ 2000; 321: 405-412
3. Haffner SM, Stern MP, Hazuda HP, Mitchell BD, Patterson J: Cardiovascular risk factors in confirmed prediabetic individuals: does the clock for coronary heart disease start ticking before the onset of clinical diabetes?. JAMA 1990; 263: 2893-2898
4. Position Statement, American Diabetes Association: Management of dyslipidemia in adults with diabetes. Diabetes Care 2002; 25 (Suppl 1): S74-S77
5. Steiner G, Vranic M: Hyperinsulinaemia and hypertriglyceridemia, a vicious cycle with atherogenic potential. Int J Obesity 1982; 6 (suppl 1): 117-124
6. Kahn CR: Insulin resistance: a common feature of diabetes mellitus. N Engl J Med 1986; 315:252-254
7. Reaven GM: Pathophysiology of insulin resistance in human disease. Physiol Rev 1995; 75: 473-486
8. Moller DE, Flier JS: Insulin resistance. Mechanisms, syndromes, and implications. N Engl J Med 1991; 325:938-948
9. Taskinen MR. Insulin resistance and lipoprotein metabolism. Curr Opin Lipidol 1995; 6: 153-160
10. Ruderman N, Chisholm D, Pi-Sunyer X, Schneider S. The metabolically obese, normal-weight individual revisited. Diabetes 1998; 47: 699-713
11. Reaven GM: The role of insulin resistance and hyperinsulinaemia in coronary heart disease. Metabolism 1992; 41 (suppl 1): 16-19
12. Chaour M, Théroux P, Gilfix BM, Campeau L, Lespérance J, Ghitescu M, Gélinas F, Solymoss BC. True fasting serum insulin level, insulin resistance syndrome and coronary artery disease. Coron Artery Dis 1997; 8: 683-688
13. Godsland IF, Stevenson JC: Insulin resistance: syndrome or tendency ? Lancet 1995; 346: 100-03
14. Stern MP: The insulin resistance syndrome: the controversy is dead, long live the controversy!. Diabetologia 1994; 37: 956-9
15. Scheen AJ, Paquot N, Castillo MJ, Lefèbvre PJ: How to measure insulin action in vivo. Diabet Metabol Rev 1994; 10: 151-88

16. Fulcher GR, Walker M, Alberti KGMM: The assessment of insulin action *in vivo*. In: International Textbook of Diabetes Mellitus, Alberti KGMM, DeFronzo RA, Keen H, and Zimmet P, Eds. John Wiley, Chichester, 1992, 513-529
17. Swan JW, Walton C, Godsland IF: Assessment of insulin sensitivity in man: a comparison of minimal model-and euglycemic clamp-derived measures in health and heart failure. Clin Sci 1994; 86: 317-322
18. Bergman RN, Finegoog DT, Ader M: Assessment of insulin sensitivity in vivo. Endrocr Rev 1985; 6: 45-86
19. Williams B: Insulin resistance: the shape of things to come. Lancet 1994; 344: 521-524
20. Ferrannini E, Haffner SM, Mitchell BD, Stern MP: Hyperinsulinemia: the key feature of a cardiovascular and metabolic syndrome. Diabetologia 1991; 34: 416-422
21. Zimmet PZ, Collins VR, Dowse GK, Alberti KGMM, Tuomilehto J, Knight LT, Gareeboo H, Chitson P, Fareed D, for the Mauritius Noncommunicable Disease Study: Is hyperinsulinemia a central characteristic of a chronic cardiovascular risk factor clustering syndrome ?. Mixed findings in asian, indian, creole and chinese mauritians. Diabetic Med 1994; 11: 388-396
22. Coppack SW, Evans RD, Fisher RM, Frayn KN, Gibbons GF, Humphreys SM, Kirk MJ, Potts JL, Hockaday TDR: Adipose tissue metabolism in obesity: lipase action in vivo before and after a mixed meal. Metabolism 1992; 41: 264-72
23. Lewis GF, Uffelman KD, Szeto LW, Weller B, Steiner G: Interaction between free fatty acids and insulin in the acute control of very low density lipoprotein production in humans. J Clin Invest 1995; 95: 158-166
24. Eckel RH: Lipoprotein lipase. A multifunctional enzyme relevant to common metabolic diseases. N Engl J Med 1989; 320: 1060-68
25. Austin MA, Horowitz H, Wijsman E, Krauss RM, Brunzell J: Bimodality of plasma apolipoprotein B levels in familial combined hyperlipidemia. Atherosclerosis 1992; 92: 67-77
26. Austin MA, King MC, Vranizan KM, Krauss RM: Atherogenic lipoprotein phenotype. A proposed genetic marker for coronary heart disease. Circulation 1990; 82: 495-506
27. Farquhar JW, Frank JW, Gross RC, Reaven GM: Glucose, insulin and triglyceride responses to high and low carbohydrate diets in man. J Clin Invest 1966; 45: 1648-1656
28. Avogaro P, Crepaldi G, Enzi G: Association of hyperlipidemia, diabetes mellitus and mild obesity. Acta Diabetol Lat 1967; 4: 572-590
29. Laakso M, Sarlund H, Mykkanen L: Insulin resistance is associated with lipid and lipoprotein abnormalities in subjects with varying degrees of glucose tolerance. Arteriosclerosis1990; 10: 223-31
30. Haffner SM, Valdez RA, Hazuda HP, Mitchell BD, Morales PA, Stern MP: Prospective analysis of the insulin-resistance syndrome (Syndrome X). Diabetes 1992; 41: 715-2
31. Mykkanen L, Kuusito J, Haffner SM, Pyorälä K, Laakso M: Hyperinsulinemia predicts multiple atherogenic changes in lipoproteins in elderly subjects. Arterioscler Thromb 1994; 14: 518-526
32. Yki-Järvinen H, Taskinen MR: Interrelationships among insulin's antilipolytic and glucoregulatory effects and plasma triglycerides in nondiabetic patients with endogenous hypertriglyceridemia. Diabetes 1988; 37: 1271-1278
33. Bjorntorp P: Fatty acids, hyperinsulinemia, and insulin resistance: which comes first ?. Current Opin Lipidol 1994; 5: 166-174
34. Zuñiga-Guarjardo S, Steiner G, Shumak S, Zinman B. Insulin resistance and action in hypertriglyceridemia. Diabetes Res Clin Pract 1991; 14: 55-61
35. Widen E, Ekstrand A, Salorante C, Franssila-Kallunki A, Eriksson J, Schalin-Jantti C, Groop L: Insulin resistance in type 2 (non-insulin-dependent) diabetic patients with hypertriglyceridemia. Diabetologia 1992; 35: 1140-1145
36. Randle PJ, Garland PB, Hales CN, Newsholme EA: The glucose fatty-acid cycle. Its role in insulin sensitivity and the metabolic disturbances of diabetes mellitus. Lancet 1963; i: 785-789
37. Li WW, Dammerman MM, Smith JD, Metzger S, Breslow JL, Leff T. Common genetic variation in the promoter of the human apo CIII gene abolishes regulation by insulin and may contribute to hypertriglyceridemia. J Clin Invest 1995; 96: 2601-2605
38. Hölzl B, Paulweber B, Sandhofer F, Patsch JR. Hypertriglyceridemia and insulin resistance. J Intern Med 1998; 243: 79-82
39. Despres JP, Verdon MF, Moorjani S, Pouliot MC, Nadeau A, Bouchard C, Tremblay A, Lupien

PJ: Apolipoprotein E polymorphism modifies relation of hyperinsulinemia to hypertriglyceridemia. Diabetes 1993; 42: 1474-1481
40. Valdez R, Stern MP, Howard BV, Haffner SM: Apolipoprotein E polymorphism and insulin levels in a biethnic population. Diabetes Care 1995; 18: 992-1000
41. Després JO: Dyslipidemia and obesity. Baillières Clin Endocrinol Metab 1994; 8: 629-660
42. Wilson PWF: Diabetes mellitus and coronary heart disease. Am J Kidney Dis 1998; 32 (Suppl 3): S89-S100
43. von Eckardstein A, Schulte H, Assmann G: Risk for diabetes mellitus in middle-aged Xcaucasian male participants and implications for the definition of impaired fasting glucose by the American Diabetes Association. Prospective Cardiovascular Münster. J Clin Endocrinol Metab 2000; 85: 3101-3108
44. Assmann G, Carmena R, Cullen P, Fruchart JC, Jossa F, Lewis B, Mancini M, Paoletti R: Coronary heart disease: reducing the risk: a worldwide view. International Task Force for the Prevention of Coronary Heart Disease. Circulation. 1999;100:1930-1938
45. Stamler J, Vaccaro O, Neaton JD, Wentworth D: Diabetes, other risk factors, and 12-year cardiovascular mortality for men screened in the Multiple Risk Factor Intervention Trial. Diabetes Care 1993; 16: 434-444
46. Syvänne M, Taskinen MR: Lipids and lipoproteins as coronary risk factors in non-insulin-dependent diabetes mellitus. Lancet 1997; 350 (suppl I) 20-23
47. Howard BV: Lipoprotein metabolism in diabetes mellitus. J Lipid Res 1987; 28: 613-628
48. Zilversmit DB: Atherogenesis: a postprandial phenomenon. Circulation 1979; 60: 473-485
49. Chen YD, Swami S, Skowronski R, Coulston A, Reaven GM: Differences in postprandial lipemia between patients with normal glucose tolerance and noninsulin-dependent diabetes mellitus. J Clin Endocrinol Metab 1993; 76: 172-177
50. Axelsen M, Smith U, Eriksson JW, Taskinen MR, Jansson PA: Postprandial hypertriglyceridemia and insulin resistance in normoglycemic first degree relatives of patients with type 2 diabetes. Ann Intern Med 1999; 131: 27-31
51. Mykkänen L, Kuusisto J, Pyörälä K, Laakso M: Cardiovascular disease risk factors as predictors of type 2 (non-insulin-dependent) diabetes mellitus in elderly subjects. Diabetologia 1993; 36: 553-559
52. Gu K, Cowie CC, Harris MI: Diabetes and decline in heart disease mortality in US adults. JAMA 1999; 281: 1291-1297
53. Zimmet PZ: Diabetes epidemiology as a tool to trigger diabetes research and care. Diabetologia 1999; 42: 499-518
54. American Diabetes Association. Management of dyslipidemia in adults with diabetes (supplement). Diabetes Care 1999; 22: S56-S59
55. Betteridge DJ, Colhoun H, Armitage J: Status report of lipid-lowering trials in diabetes. Current Opinion Lipidol 2000; 11: 621-626
56. Pitt B, Waters D, Brown WV, et al: Aggressive lipid-lowering therapy compared with angioplasty in stable coronary artery disease. N Engl J Med 1999; 341: 70-78
57. Betteridge DJ, Colhoun H, Armitage J: Status report of lipid-lowering trials in diabetes. Current Opinion Lipidol 2000; 11: 621-626
58. Freeman DJ, Norrie J, Sattar N, Neely DG, Cobbe SM, Ford I, et al. Pravastatin and the development of diabetes mellitus. Evidence for a protective treatment effect in the West of Scotland Coronary Prevention Study. Circulation 2001; 103: 357-362
59. Rubins HB, Robins SJ, Collins D et al: Gemfibrozil for the secondary prevention of coronary heart disease in men with low levels of high density lipoprotein cholesterol. N Engl J Med 1999; 341: 410-418
60. Koskinen P, Mänttäri M, Manninen V et al: Coronary heart disease incidence in NIDDM patients in the Helsinki Heart Study. Diabetes Care 1992; 15: 820-825

CHAPTER 8

Hypertension in Type 2 Diabetes Mellitus

M. Serrano Rios, M.T. Martinez Larrad

Introduction: Type 2 Diabetes Mellitus and Insulin Resistance

Type 2 Diabetes Mellitus (DM) is a heterogeneous collection of hyperglycaemic syndromes due to a variable combination of two basic physiopathological disturbances: A defective beta cell function and a decreased insulin sensitivity (insulin resistance) at specific target tissues: skeletal muscle, adipocytes. Type 2 DM, the most common form of Diabetes (over 90% of all cases) has become, as it has been Type 1 DM, a global problem with the characteristics of a worldwide epidemic due to the worrying increase in prevalence in the last 10 years. It has been estimated (Amos et al. 1997) that for year 2010 there will be over 221 million people affected with Type 2 DM as compared to the existing 124 millions in 1997. India, Pakistan, Africa, Asia and Latin America will be the hardest hit countries by this epidemic. The causes of Type 2 DM, and hence of the current increase in prevalence are many, including a complex interplay between a poligenic background, – likewise variable among different ethnic groups –, and a vast array of environmental factors related to inappropriate western-like ("cocacolonization") lifestyle: excessive caloric intake, lack of physical activity, diet rich in refined foods and poor in fibre; and often an excessive alcohol intake. A major outcome of these factors is also the parallel emergence of a "bad" companion of Type 2 DM: obesity. Of major relevance is the central or visceral type of obesity, a condition typically promoting insulin resistance (IR) and the clustering of many metabolic and non-metabolic disturbances that integrate the so-called insulin resistance syndrome X or metabolic syndrome X, originally described by G. M. Reaven (Reaven 1988, Reaven 1999) and others. This metabolic syndrome is a high-risk situation for the development of macrovascular (atherosclerosis) disease and its consequences. Traditionally, IR and its surrogate, compensatory hyperinsulinemia have been postulated as the link between the different components of the insulin resistance syndrome (IRS) and its relationship to cardiovascular (CV) disease. This issue is debatable and has deserved a recent meta-analysis (Ruige et al. 1998) However, the strength of that link does not necessarily have to be identical for every individual component: type 2 DM, dyslipidemia, arterial hypertension, pro-coagulation state, hypofibrinolysis and atherosclerosis. In fact, recent application of the factor analysis approach (Sakkinen et al. 2000), an statistical strategy that allows to reduce variables to a few cluster of pathophysiological significance, indicate that in non-diabetics as well as in diabetics (Type 2) individualized factors (e.g. visceral obesity, increased glucose/insulin levels, (↓ HDL, ↑ TG, ↑ PAI-1) cluster with IR and CV risk more strongly than other components (↑ systolic and ↑ diastolic) blood pressure (BP) (Lehto et al). Using the factor analysis approach in a large (902) population of non-insulin treated Type 2 DM in

Finland followed up for 7 years to examine the predictive value for CHD mortality of a so called "hyperinsulinemia cluster" (↑ BMI ,↑ TG, ↑ fasting insulin, ↓ HDL cholesterol) concluded that this situation significantly increased the risk of death due to CHD (Lehto et al. 2000).

Type 2 DM and CV Disease – Mortality and Morbidity

Type 2 DM "per se" (for review see: Jolk and Colwell 1997, Nathan et al. 1997) and likewise as a component of the IRS is a major cause of death all over the world (Kannel and McGee 1979, Kannel 2000, Head and Fuller 1990, Laakso and Lehto 1997, Laakso 1999). Thus, the overall life expectancy in persons with this Type of diabetes is about 25 % relatively less to the general population. The high prevalence of cardiovascular disease of Type 2 DM is to be blamed since age-adjusted mortality rate for coronary heart disease is 2–4 times higher in Type 2 diabetics than in the general population and it is responsible for about 60 % of all causes of death. Moreover, the risk of death in a 5 years period has been also shown to be similar in diabetics without a previous myocardial infarction (MI) to that in non-diabetics who have already suffered one episode of MI (Haffner et al. 1998). Furthermore, both, the immediate and long term risk of death following MI is greater in diabetics than in non-diabetics, and equal in both sexes. Cerebrovascular disease (Laakso and Lehto 1997) mostly of the atherothrombotic Type, also contribute to no less than 15 % of deaths in Type 2 DM. Increased morbidity in Type 2 DM is also contributed to by other macrovascular complications due to PVD (foot ulceration, gangrene). So that Type 2 DM is the first cause of non-traumatic amputation of lower limbs. Type 2 DM also cause great morbidity due to its microvascular complications. It is, in fact, the most common cause of blindness, with increasing prevalence of diabetic renal disease and endstage renal failure (ESRD). For all these reasons, Type 2 DM imposed an enormous burden on public and individual health and economic cost (direct and indirect) everywhere. The natural history of Type 2 DM is a very dynamic one and before overt hyperglycemia is identified, a long preceding stage of impaired glucose tolerance has passed undetected. However, that period (prediabetes) is clinically silent but not innocuous in terms of macro/micro vascular and nerve damage due to the eroding effect of glucose toxicity and to the accumulation of CV risk factors clustering in the IRS.

Hypertension and Type 2 DM: Prevalence

Hypertension is one of the most common morbid associations in Type 2 DM, with an average estimated prevalence of 40 %. Hypertension is an independent CV risk factor associated with Type 2 DM. (Cowie and Harris 1995, Elliot et al. 1995). It has been estimated, that the prevalence of hypertension in diabetics is about 2–5 times higher than in non-diabetic population, though varying in Type 1 and in Type 2 DM (Laakso and Lehto 1997, Stern and Tuck 2000). In Type 1 DM the prevalence of hypertension is mostly related to renal disease and is increasing after microalbuminuria is detected. In Type 2 microalbuminuric patients the prevalence of high blood pressure (HBP) is ≈ 70 % and might be even higher if current criteria for the definition of high blood pressure are applied. In Type 2 DM the prevalence of hypertension show wide interethnic variations being higher in Afro-Americans and Mexican-American but not in Pima Indians. Most important is that hypertension often precedes Type 2 DM, and may be present at a very early degree of glucose intolerance ($\approx$ 20 – 40 % in IGT) any age group. In fact, a high prevalence of BP have been detected in newly diagnosed Type 2 diabetics or very shortly after the clinical diagnosis was made. Thus in the United Kingdom Prospective Study (UKPDS 23) 32 % of men and 45 % of women with recently diagnosed Type 2 diabetes were already hypertensive. Also (Cowie and Harris 1995) in US adults entering the NHANES II (1976 – 1980) National Health and Nutrition Examination Survey with undiagnosed diabetes, 67 % had hypertension and half of them were uncontrolled. Interesting enough several epidemiological studies (see Ferrannini for review 1999) show that the increased prevalence of hypertension in diabetic subjects decreases from 70 years of age onwards. Conversely, the prevalence of impaired glucose tolerance (IGT) may be as high as 30 % in people with essential hypertension with a conversion rate after 10 years or more from normoglycemia (NG) to impaired glucose tolerance (IGT) occurring independently of other variables (age, race, sex, obesity). The coexistence of arterial hypertension and Type 2 DM in an individual patient conveys a three fold increased risk of CV mortality as compared to non-diabetic persons across all blood pressure levels as reported in the MRFIT Study (Stamler et al. 1993). Furthermore the UKPDS 23 (Turner et al. 1998) reported a hazard ratio of 1.72 for coronary heart disease in Type 2 diabetics with arterial hypertension particularly in those with systolic blood pressure over 142 mm Hg.

The WHO multinational Study demonstrated that in 4740 diabetics (over 80 %, of the Type 2) the appearance of hypertension and proteinuria increased the CV risk 5 in men and 8 folds in women when compared with normotensive normoalbuminuric diabetics. Moreover, recently available evidence point out that the hypertensive Type 2 diabetics with high systolic blood pressure (SBP) have an increased risk for cardiovascular heart disease (CHD) and that even single high BP values may be at long term of predictive value (cited in Ferrannini 1999). Arterial hypertension in Type 2 DM adds a very strong risk for stroke when compared to normotensive diabetics and non-diabetics, this added risk being independent of others such as obesity or dyslipidemia (Laakso and Lehto 1997, Laakso 1999). As shown by a recent case -control study in Finland including 10.068 diabetic patients, most of them with Type 2 DM followed up for 13.2 yrs, established that HBP was also a strong predictor of non-traumatic limb amputations. This interesting finding still requires confirmation and was not found in the WHO Multinational Study. Several studies have also shown that both diabetes and hypertension are strong risk factors for renal disease in either type of diabetes as well as for retinopathy. In fact, in Type 2 patients on haemodialysis the survival expectancies are dramatically shortened if hypertension supervenes, an scenario which is not rare since in US about 65 % of patients with advanced nephropathy are Type 2 diabetics. The UKPDS 38 (UKPDS 38, 1998) demonstrated that the tight control of HBP is as important as the meticulous glycemic control in reducing total mortality, any death related to diabetes and other diabetes related events. Abundant available clinical and epidemiological evidence (Stern and Tuck 2000) indicated that the coexistence of hypertension and diabetes significantly increased the risk of nephropathy and retinopathy in those patients. Even more important, reducing BP to < 150/85 mm Hg after 10 yrs of treatment also reduced the progression of microalbuminuria and retinopathy as well as the prevalence of stroke and MI.

Pathogenesis of Hypertension in Type 2 DM

The aetiology/pathogenesis (for review see DeFronzo 1995; Bakris 1995; Ferrannini 2000, Deewania 2000; Stern and Tuck 2000; Diabetic Nephropathy 2001 ADA recommendations) of hypertension in Diabetes is multifactorial but somehow different in Type 1 and in Type 2 DM. Most cases of hypertension in Type 2 DM are of the so called "essential" Type and secondary hypertension is not as common.

Renal Disease

Nephropatic hypertension is, however, a most important cause. The incidence of diabetic nephropathy (DeFronzo 1995) in Type 2 DM has been reported to be slightly less or equal (20 – 30 %) than in Type 1 DM (30 – 40 %) when variables such as age and BMI are controlled. Also the incidence of renal failure in large samples of Type 2 DM patients with remarkable interracial differences have been found to be about 30 %, by some authors, being much higher in Afro-Americans than in Caucasians in the US. The natural history of diabetic renal disease is less well characterised in Type 2 DM

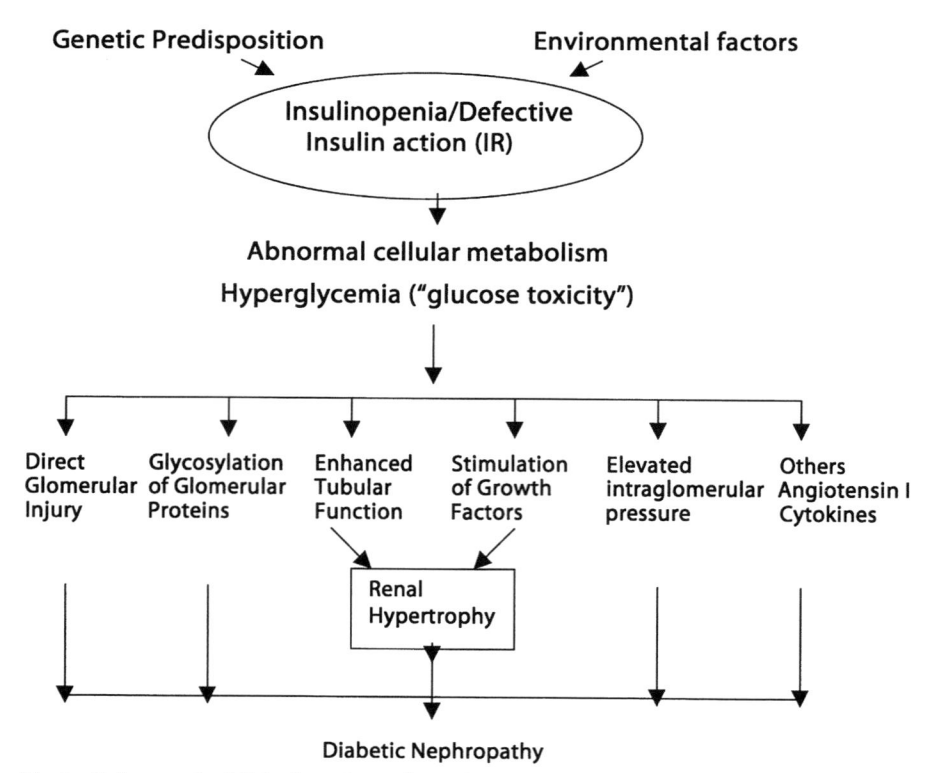

Fig. 8.1. Pathogenesis of diabetic nephropathy. In this scheme, one basic disturbance, insulin lack or insulin resistance, leads to a variety of alterations in cellular metabolism. This, in turn, leads to glomerular injury through multiple, diverse mechanisms. (Modified from DeFronzo 1995]

than in Type 1 DM. However, it has been reported that renal hypertrophy and hyperfiltration, typical of the earliest stages of renal disease in Type 1 DM, may also be found in newly diagnosed Type 2 DM and that it can be equally reversible by appropriate glycemic control. Available data show that it can microalbuminuria has a strong predictive value in Type 2 DM for progression to overt diabetic nephropathy in Caucasians, Japanese, Native Americans as well as in Pima Indians and Naurús these latter two groups, showing a high incidence of Type 2 DM and of diabetic renal disease. In the light of current clinical and Epidemiological evidence it must be stressed that the role of the diabetic nephropathy should not be underestimated as it is a most important aetiology of arterial hypertension in Type 2 DM (Fig. 8.1).

Insulin Resistance and Hypertension in Type 2 (Bakris 1995; Ferrannini 1999)

The most interesting but still highly debated hypothesis postulates that in the absence of renal disease, IR and hyperinsulinemia might be the common link for both conditions. The landmark works of Ferranini et al. (Ferrannini et al. 1987, 1997) are of paramount importance since these authors were the first to demonstrate by the precise measurement of insulin sensitivity using the euglycemic hyperinsulinemic clamp that normoglycemic non-obese with essential hypertension, often have a remarkably impaired insulin mediated glucose uptake or IR. An updated critical review of this issue has been recently published by E. Ferrannini (Ferrannini 1999). According to recent data, it has been calculated that in normal individuals of either sex a weight gain as low as 1 kg. would results in 0.1 – 0.3 mm Hg rise in blood pressure. Recent data from the EGIR (European Group for the Study of Insulin Resistance) using an extensive data base including 422 "clamp" studies collected in several European Countries, demonstrated that systolic, diastolic and mean blood pressure are higher in insulin-resistant than in insulin-sensitive subjects independently of age, sex or Body Mass Index (BMI). Contrariwise, other data do not favour a cause-effect relationship between insulin resistance-hyperinsulinemia and both Type 2 DM and arterial hypertension: classical but rare examples are the low prevalence of high blood pressure in the hyperinsulinemic state of insulinoma neither in the genetic syndromes with extreme insulin resistance nor in the polycistic ovary syndrome in women. Furthermore available epidemiological evidence in several ethnic groups discover a striking discrepancy between the prevalence of insulin resistance in Type 2 DM and its associations with arterial hypertension as it happens in non-insulin resistant people in Mauritius, Alaskan; or in Pima Indians. Still it cannot be denied that hypertension, insulin resistance and Type 2 DM may share a common "soil" or genetic predisposition that may only surface under the impact of environmental factors associated to sedentary lifestyle habits (over nutrition, poor physical activity...) In favour of this hypothesis are some data as noted by Ferrannini (Ferrannini 1999): 1) IR has been reported in offspring of normoglycemic with essential hypertension. 2) Specific alleles (A1, A2) of the enzyme glycogen synthase (chromosome 19), a strong candidate gene for IR have been found in Type 2 diabetics with hyperinsulinemia and high BP (Groop et al. 1993). 3) Transgenic Knockout heterozygous mice for either Glut 4 (Stenbit et al. 1997) or IRS2 genes (Whithers et al. 1998) develop insulin resistance, impaired glucose tolerance and hypertension. The recent discovery that a point mutation in one of the exons of the PPARγ gene is associated with IR, hypertension and Type 2 DM (Barroso et al. 1999) is exciting but require further investigation. Even more exciting is the recent discovery of the new hormone resistin that appears to be a link between obesity and Type 2 DM (Steppan et al. 2001) but whose potential role in the pathogenesis of the insulin resistance syndrome is still far from being elucidated. From a mechanistic point of view the understanding of the reciprocal relationships between insulin resistance, hypertension and Type 2 DM (or diabetes in general) is fundamental to evaluate the impact of hyperinsulinemia as well as of IR on the physiological (central/peripheral) haemodinamic factors that normally control the blood pressure. Those actions of insulin that are of potential pathogenic significance include: 1) Vascular effects: Abundant experimental and clinical data indicate that insulin intervenes in the regulation of vascular tone(artery/ vein) by direct interaction with the endothelium and the smooth muscle of the arterial wall in which interaction NO(nitric oxide) and $Na^+K^+ATPase$ are the effectors leading to vasodilatation. Baron (Baron 1993) first advanced the hypothesis that these vasodilator action of insulin will be impaired in the presence of IR states (obesity and Type 2 DM) postulating that in these situations the insulin induced recruitment of capillaries in critical tissues (skeletal muscle) will be altered and consequently glucose uptake sharply reduced. However, many discrepancies of the haemodinamic changes induced by insulin in healthy and in diabetic subjects have been reported including not only vasodilatation but also the opposite effect: vasoconstriction.

It has been indicated that these effects are pharmacological rather than physiological. On the other hand, insulin mediated endothelium vasodilatation and endothelial dysfunction are neither systematically correlated with the metabolic alteration nor with the degree of insulin sensitivity in normotensive or hypertensive subjects. Other effects of insulin on the CV system include vasoconstriction of post venous capillary vessels, an increase (10 – 15 %) in cardiac output and stroke volume, release of catecholamines as well as changes in the peripheral vascular resistance, mediated by peripheral and central neural mechanisms. In this context a stimulating effect of insulin on the sympathetic nervous system may induce some times an increase in blood pressure. However, many unexplained facts still exist such as the findings in some animals (dogs) and in normoglycemic individuals that an increase in sympathetic nervous activity may be associated with a paradoxical decrease in BP and peripheral vascular resistance; or that hyperglycemic/hypertensive individuals sometimes respond to insulin with a decrease in BP induced by sympathetic stimulation (Bakris 1995). Other actions of insulin of potential relevance to the IR include an increased tubular reabsorption of sodium; Mitogenic effects, regulation of sodium and calcium homeostasis and of the angiotensin renin aldosterone system.

Definition of Hypertension in Diabetes

The threshold values for the definition of hypertension in the general population has been modified in the last few years. The VI J.C. (The Sixth Report of the Joint National Committee on Prevention, Detection, Evaluation and Treatment of High Blood Pressure, 1997) states that "Hypertension is defined by SBP of 140 mm Hg or greater, diastolic BP (DBP) of 90 mm Hg or greater or taking antihypertensive medication". Con-

Table 8.1. Risk stratification and treatment[a] (from The Sixth Report of the Joint National Committee on Prevention, Detection, Evaluation, and Treatment of High Blood Pressure, 1997)

Blood pressure stages (mm Hg)	Risk group A (No risk factors; no TOD/CCD[b])	Risk group B (At least 1 risk factor not including diabetes; no TOD/CCD)	Risk group C (TOD/CCD and/or diabetes with or without other risk factors)
High-normal (130–139/85–89)	Lifestyle modification	Lifestyle modification	Drug therapy[d]
Stage 1 (140–159/90–99)	Lifestyle modification (up to 12 months)	Lifestyle modification[c] (up to 6 months)	Drug therapy
Stages 2 and 3 (≥160/≥100)	Drug therapy	Drug therapy	Drug therapy

[a] For example, a patient with diabetes and a blood pressure of 142/94 mm Hg plus left ventricular hypertrophy should be classified as having stage 1 hypertension with target organ disease (left ventricular hypertrophy) and with another major risk factor (diabetes). This patient would be categorized as "Stage 1, risk group C", and recommended for immediate initiation of pharmacologic treatment. Lifestyle modification should be adjunctive therapy for all patients recommended for pharmacologic therapy.
[b] TOD/CCD indicates target organ disease/clinical cardiovascular disease.
[c] For patients with multiple risk factors, clinicians should consider drugs as initial therapy plus lifestyle modifications.
[d] For those with heart failure, renal insufficiency or diabetes.

sidering the imperative need of identifying and treating HBP in order to reduce its serious impact on CV morbidity and mortality, the same Committee proposes a stratification of BP in adults over the age of 18 who are not receiving antihypertensive medication nor suffering any type of acute illness. In diabetic patients both the ADA (American Diabetes Association) Clinical Recommendations 2000 and the IDF (International Diabetes Federation) (Guidelines for Diabetes Care 1999) accepted the values of 140/90 mm Hg to define hypertension what would correspond to the stage 1 hypertension of the VI Joint Committee. However in the light of recent trials (Hypertension Optimal Treatment [HOT, UKPDS]) it seems advisable in terms of potential CV risk to accept the figure of 130/80 mm Hg not only as an ideal therapeutic target but also as desirable "normal" limit of BP for non-nephropatic diabetics. Additionally it is appropriate to include DM in the evaluation of BP, according to the concept of risk stratification proposed by the VI JC (Table 8.1) and the task force for Prevention of Cardiovascular Diseases in Europe. This concept takes into account not only the actual figures of BP (blood pressure) but even most important the number of concomitant CV risk factors (central obesity, HDL, sedentary lifestyle, alcohol consumption) and the presence or not of identifiable organ damage (E.g.: left ventricular hypertrophy and dysfunctions). This global evaluation of BP is, indeed, essential to asses the risk for every individual patient and to establish the bases for every therapeutic strategy. As for normal people it should be stressed that blood pressure in diabetics is also a continuum and hence any cut-off limit is somewhat arbitrarily chosen and subject to modifications imposed by evidence-based criteria (ADA – American Diabetes Association).

CV Risk Assessment: Definition of Hypertension in Type 2 DM

The evaluation of CV risk in every newly (and established) patient with Type 2 DM demands an exhaustive medical history and clinical examination at baseline and at every follow-up visit. A Type 2 diabetic patient whether hypertensive or not is more than just a hyperglycemic individual. Detailed protocols for clinical practice are available from the European Consensus for the Management of Type 2 DM and the ADA Clinical Recommendation 2001. Emphasis is made on the measurement of BP both in supine, sitting and standing positions since in a number (25%) of Type 2 DM patients, some degree of misleading autonomic dysfunction may be present after 10 or more years from diagnosis. It is not uncommon the combination of systolic hypertension in the supine position with orthostatic hypotension. The appropriate condition for accurate clinical measurement of BP should be the one recommended by the Sixth report of the Joint Committee (1997). It is important to remember that BP readings usually change over time and that of course, "white coat" arterial hypertension may be present, requiring reconfirmation of the readings obtained at the office under well controlled conditions in the ambulatory setting. Continuous 24 hours (Holter) BP monitoring may be often required before or during treatment. Not uncommonly BP recordings during the night in diabetic patients show abnormal patterns with no evidence of a nocturnal BP fall (non-dippers). This latter phenomenon is often found in hypertensive diabetics and more so in those with microalbuminuria and established renal disease. This finding is important since the mean 24hr BP increase by a factor of 4 or more in microalbuminuric diabetic patients compared to normoalbuminuric and may be interpreted as a marker of progression to clinical diabetic renal disease.

Control of Hypertension in Type 2 DM

Goals. How Much Lowering Is Desirable?

The goals for control of Diabetes have been set in the past few years at <140/90 mm Hg, <140/85 mm Hg and currently to ≤130/80 mm Hg if nephropathy is not present. Still, in diabetic patients at any stage of renal disease strong efforts should be made to follow the concept that "The lower we can achieve the better". In children BP values should be reduced to the correspondent age -adjusted 90th percentile. (HOT, UKPDS) The ADA "Recommendations Clinical Practice" 2001 state that in patients with isolated systolic hypertension over 180 mm Hg, BP should be reduced to about or less than, 169 mm Hg, and that a further decrease of 20 mm Hg is recommended if systolic BP values lie between 160–179 mm Hg. Whenever possible (tolerance, maintenance) further decrease of elevated systolic BP values to 140 mm Hg or even less is recommended.

Non-pharmacological Measures

These measures are the cornerstone of any therapeutic strategy. The essentials of non-phamacological measures are those recommended by the VI Joint Committee and adapted by the Guidelines of the IDF (International Diabetes Federation). EASD

8 Hypertension in Type 2 Diabetes Mellitus

(European Association for the Study of Diabetes) (European Region): 1) Weight loss (at least 10% of the baseline) if overweight is present (BMI >27 in males, >26 in females). Restriction in saturated fat to less than 10% of the total fat content of the diet. A weight loss of 4-5 kg significantly decreases blood pressure at long term (1 year or more) in most individuals. Protein restriction should be appropriately adjusted in the presence of renal failure. 2) Restriction of sodium intake. A reduction of 75-100 mmol/day in sodium intake, lowers BP for weeks to years according to several well-controlled clinical trials. In hypertensive diabetics with nephropathy further reduction to 2-4 gr is desirable. Sodium reduction provides many benefits, other than a decrease in BP, namely: regression of left ventricular hypertrophy, reduction of urinary excretion of potassium and calcium. The intake of these two cations should be the one recommended by the Minimal Dietary Allowances. 3) Reduction of alcohol intake: It is most important since excessive alcohol ingestion is a significant risk factor for hypertension and stroke. Excessive alcohol consumption in Type 2 DM treated with oral hypoglycaemic drugs or insulin may enhance the risk of hypoglicemia due to its potent inhibition of neoglucogenesis. Furthermore alcohol provide extra calories (7 kcal/g) to the total daily caloric intake and may impair weight loss and worsen the (often) present hypertriglyceridemia. Reasonable limitations are no more than 300 ml of wine, 60 ml of whisky and no more than 720 ml of beer. For those treated with insulin or oral agents (in Type 2 DM) one must be more cautious and no more than one or two drinks of the less alcohol containing beverages (e.g. light beer or wine) should be allowed. 4) Caffeine may increase BP but there is no proven evidence of its influence on HBP. 5) Smoking: Is a bad habit that must be eradicated by appropriate educational programmes in any person with DM or without. 6) Physical activity: Regular aerobic individualized programmed physical activity, is essential in implementing successful lifestyle modification in the general population, in non-diabetic hypertensive and in Type 2 hypertensive patients. The multiple health benefits derived from long-term sustained daily exercise are beyond doubt and have been recently reviewed (American Diabetes Association: Clinical Recommendations 2000, American Diabetes Association: Clinical Practice. Recommendations 2001). According to this recent position statement of the ADA there is an urgent need for introducing exercise immediately after diagnosis of DM to stop or attenuate the progression of IR and the potential deterioration of IGT. A thorough medical evaluation is, of course, mandatory before recommending and planning exercise in Type 2 diabetics; and a thoughtful consideration of the risk benefit ratios is mandatory in the presence of high risk situations such as severe hypertension, and dyslipidemia and/ or retino-renal complications. The judicious use of well acknowledged guidelines is to be encouraged (ADA, IDF-EASD).

Pharmacological Treatment

A vast armamentarium of drugs is currently available for the pharmacological treatment of hypertension in non-diabetic as well as in diabetic patients. (See for review: Elliot et al. 1995/ The Sixth Report of the Joint National Committee on Prevention, Detection, Evaluation and Treatment of High Blood Pressure 1997/ MacLeod and Mclsy 1998/ Deewania P, 2000/ Yki-Järvinen 2000; de la Sierra and Ruilope 2000).

Table 8.2. Specific antihypertensive drugs: the main effect of most commonly used antihypertensive drugs in type 2 diabetics with hypertension (modified from MacLeod and McJoy 1998)

Drug	Glucose metabolism	Lipid metabolism TC/TG/HDL	IR	K+	PBF*	Micro-albuminuria	LVH	Sexual dysfunction
Diuretics	Controversial (high doses/ thiazides)	−/−/−	−	−	(−)	0, +	0, +	−
B-blockers								
Non-selective	−	(−)/−/−	−	0	−	0, +	+	(−)
Selective	(−)	0/(−)/0	(−)	0	(+)	0, +	+	+, +[d]
Calcium antagonists	0, (+)[a]	0/0/0	0	0	(+)	0[b], +	+	0
ACE inhibitors	0, (+)	0/0/0	(+)	0	0	++,+++	+	0
Angiotensin II antagonists	0	0/0/0	−	0	0	(+)[c], +	+	(−)
α-blockers	(+)	+/+/+	+	0	0	0	+	?
α2 receptor agonists	0	?/?/?	?	?	?	?	?	?

−, Adverse effect; +, positive, benefial effect; 0, no effect; (+)/(−), possible, not uniformly confirmed effect.
[a] May be with verapamil.
[b] Nifedipine.
[c] Results to be published (see text).
[d] More in non-hydropiridines.
K+ = potasium
PBF = peripheral blood flow
LVH = left ventricular hypertrophy
TG = trigicerides
TC = total cholesterol
HDL = high density lipoproteins

Specific Blood Pressure Lowering Drugs

Diuretics

Diuretics were the typical first choice drugs in the therapy of hypertension for many years in non-diabetic and in diabetic patients (Table 8.2). The benefit of diuretics, mostly low doses of thiazides, have been repeatedly proven in many controlled long-term clinical trials to favourably modify the risk of stroke, myocardial infarction and any type of cardiovascular events in the general population as well as in Type 2 diabetics. Thus in the SEPH (Systolic Hypertension in the Elderly Program Treatment, Curb et al. 1996), the effect of chlorthalidone was compared to placebo in an extensive subgroup of recently diagnosed Type 2 diabetics (12.5 – 25mgs) with isolated systolic hypertension chlortalidone induced a significant reduction in stroke (22%), cardiovascular events (34%) and (26%) in total mortality with no clinically meaningful adverse effects. However, some class of diuretics at high doses (thiazides) have been reported to deteriorate the long-term glycemic control in diabetics, likely due to hypokalemia.

On the other hand, potassium-sparing diuretics (triamterene) have been rarely used because of the potential risk of hyperkalemia. In contrast, loop-acting diuretics (e.g. furosemide) are now tested and widely used in combination with other antihypertensive drugs with good results. Still added to their benefits, thiazides at low but effective doses are cheaper and have negligible side-effects on metabolic parameters (glycemic/lipid profile) and may help in reducing the progression of renal disease in diabetics (MacLeod and McJoy 1998).

Alfa-receptor Antagonists

Several drugs compose this class of blood pressure lowering drugs (prazosin, terizosin, doxazosin and others) that also have a weak favourable impact on insulin sensitivity, lipid profile and glycemic control in diabetic patients. Their efficacy in the control of hypertension in both Types of DM have been proven in several studies but a positive effect on microalbuminuria or renoprotection has not been conclusively established and we have not enough comparative trials with other antihypertensives in DM. Lastly one must mention central receptor agonists: Monoxidine/Methyldopa. Inconsistent and scarce data are available concerning their long term efficacy in the control of hypertension, CV outcomes (morbidity/mortality) and diabetic renal disease.

Beta Adrenoreceptor Blockers

This family of antihypertensive agents that include more than 14 individual members is another classic group of drugs used to treat hypertension in non-diabetic patients but caution has been advised regarding its use in diabetes, on the basis of its adverse action on glucose and lipid metabolism, on peripheral blood flow and /or its potential to suppress alarm reactions, impairing patients' awareness of hypoglycaemia or worsening erectile dysfunction. Non-Selective Beta blockers (eg: propranolol, timolol, nadolol, labetalol) may impair insulin sensitivity apart from inhibiting insulin secretion, in non-diabetic and diabetic hypertensive people but these negative effects are probably less serious with low doses of cardioselective beta blockers (metoprolol, atenolol, bisoprolol, acebutolol). In fact, in the UKPDS 38, 39 (UK Prospective Study Group, 1998- UKPDS 38, 1998.) 1148 patients with Type 2 DM and hypertension using either Atenolol or an angiotensin converting enzyme (ACE) inhibitor (Captopril) showed a remarkable reduction in diabetes related end points by 24%, stroke by 44% and retinopathy by 37%. Atenolol and Captopril similarly reduced (at nine years from baseline) urinary albumin concentration to less than 50 mg and also the clinical proteinuria. Most interesting, the compliance was similar in Atenolol and Captopril treated patients in the first four years of treatment but in the follow up period more patients in the beta blocker group discontinued this medication due to impaired peripheral circulation or bronchospasm (6% vs. 0 in the Captopril group). Nonetheless the incidence of hypoglycemia was low and similar in both treatment groups. The UKPDS concluded that "no specific benefits nor adverse effects were detected with either drug and that both were considered equally effective and safe in lowering BP as well as in reducing the risk of fatal/non-fatal macro/microvascular complications in hypertensive Type 2 diabetic individuals". Interestingly enough in the UKPDS, albuminuria, when present, was of a comparable degree in patients treated with Atenolol or Captopril and there were no absolute differences concerning the risk for renal failure.

Angiotensin I Converting Enzyme Inhibitors

A wealth of observational and prospective placebo controlled clinical trials have firmly established Angiotensin I converting enzyme ACE inhibitors as first choice drugs in the treatment of hypertension in the general population and in hypertensive patients with either Type 1 or Type 2 DM (also for review: UKPDS 39, 1998., Zuanetti et al. 1997, Toto 2001). Apart of its efficacy in lowering blood pressure long term, ACE inhibitors have very potent renoprotective actions significantly reducing microalbuminuria and the progression of diabetic renal disease. ACE inhibitors are also active even if (as it often happens in Type 2 DM) the renin angiotensin system is suppressed. These drugs have no adverse effect on glucose and lipid metabolism although it is debatable whether they improve insulin sensitivity in Type 2 diabetics. The long-term and short-term renoprotective effects of the ACE inhibitors were first demonstrated with Captopril in Type 2 diabetics and later confirmed with other ACE compounds. Later all these compounds have been shown to reduce impressively the degree of proteinuria as compared with other blood pressure lowering drugs. The risk of precipitating acute renal failure with the ACE inhibitors therapy due to the inadverted presence of renal artery stenosis is much feared but not common. In the UKPDS 39, 400 Type 2 hypertensive patients were followed up for nine years and alocated to Captopril administered in stepwise increasing doses (25 mg/day to 50 mg/day) complemented with a sequence of BP lowering drugs (slow release Nifedipine, Methyldopa, Prazosin); the aims, in this study were to reach predefined values in SBP of < 150 / and DBP < 85 mm Hg. Captopril (as effectively as Atenolol) reduced the mean blood pressure to 144/83 mmHg and a remarkable compliance to Captopril was observed (78% of patients) 9 years after randomisation. Most common reason for non-compliance (88 out of 400 patients or 22%) were Captopril induced cough (4%) and "feeling dizzy or unwell" (4%). Despite the fact that 5 patients were withdrawn from Captopril treatment by an increase in plasma creatinine levels, renal artery stenosis was considered likely but unconfirmed and this fact a recent French study found a routine screening to search that probability unjustified. Moreover a remarkable reduction in diabetes related death and stroke (44%) was observed in other fatal/non-fatal combined macrovascular events (37%) as well as in microvascular complications (retinopathy, renal failure) in comparison with the less well controlled group. The HOPE Heart Outcomes Prevention Evaluation Study was not intended as an anti-hypertensive trial. The study reported the effects of the ACE inhibitor Ramipril versus placebo in 9297 subjects with high CV risk, aged 55 years old or more with evidence of vascular disease, diabetes and one other CV risk but no evidence of heart failure (HF) or ventricular low ejection fraction. Overall, the trial clearly demonstrated a significant reduction in the pre-established primary outcomes: myocardial infarction and stroke. In the MICROHOPE a subset of the HOPE including 3577 persons with Diabetes (98% Type 2 Diabetes) aged 66 yrs with mean SBP/DBP 141,7/80 mm Hg were included. Microalbuminuria was present in 31% and 56% of the diabetic patients who revealed a history of hypertension. A variable proportion of these patients were taking other antihypertensive drug: diuretics 19%, beta-blockers (29%), calcium channel blockers (45%). The reduction in the relative risk (RR) for the primary outcomes with Ramipril was impressive as compared to placebo: Combined macrovascular events (25%), MI (22%), stroke (33%) and CV death (37%). Reduction in total mortality (24% risk of revascularization (17%) and of overt nephropathy (24%) were less impressive but significant with Ramipril. Even more important was that these favourable effects of this ACE inhibitor were already detected 1 year after randomisation, increasing significantly (20%) in the second year; and maintained yet in the subsequent follow up. The trial was stopped earlier (4,5 yrs) than foreseen by an independent (Safety/Monitoring) board in view of the unequivocally beneficial effects of the drug. Few side effects were observed with Ramipril, they caused stopping the medication in only 7% (133 out of 808) of the patients.

Angiotensin II Receptor Blockers

As stated above BP control is a most significant goal when aiming to delay the onset or stop the progression of renal disease in DM. This specific issue is of paramount importance since DM is the first cause of end stage renal disease (ESRD) in the US, and in other countries. Arterial hypertension is indeed present in a vast majority of diabetic patients to account for about 25% of new cases of ESRD. On the other hand, microalbuminuria, a reliable indicator of progression for renal disease in Type 1 DM is also a marker for increased risk for CV death and hypertension in both Types of diabetes. Also, baseline proteinuria, an independent risk factor for progressive renal damage in non-diabetics correlates with the progression of diabetic nephropathy in Type 1 and also in Type 2 DM; and its reduction may be an indirect measure of effective blood pressure control (at least in non-diabetic individuals). Thus the coexistence of proteinuria and hypertension demands more strict end points for BP control: (e.g. 125/75 mm Hg).

The importance of the renin-angiotensin system (RAS) and the role of ACE inhibitors have already been discussed and its antihypertensive, antiproteinuric, cardio and renoprotective effects on both diabetic and non-diabetic patients are already well established. Also the effects of the vasoactive angiotensin II generated after activation of RAS may be suppressed by specific blocking of its AT1 receptor sub Type. In fact, Angiotension II in man has two sub Types of receptors named AT1 and AT2, the former being known to be mediating all the known physiologic action of Angiotensin II on cardiovascular structure and function such as: vasoconstriction, salt and water retention, and increased sympathetic activity at short term. At long-term, AT1 receptor stimulation may contribute to vascular wall and left ventricular hypertrophy, glomerular mesangial expansion (inflammation, fibrosis) thus leading to progressive renal damage. Selective blockade of this receptor sub Type AT1 allows the active peptide Angiotensin II to stimulate the AT2 receptors causing: vasodilatation, decreased intraglomerular pressure and inhibiting proliferation/fibrosis hence protecting the renal tissue from further damage. Currently a relatively wide range of angiotensin II receptor blocker (ARBs), the "Artans" are available : Losartan, Candesartan, Valsartan, Irbesartan, Eprosartan mesylate, Temisartan, being the most extensively used. The efficacy, tolerance and safety of these agents have been firmly established in animal models as well as in numerous clinical trials in humans, both non-diabetics and diabetics (see Burnier and Brunner 2000) both short-term and long-term. Currently available evidence confirm that ARBs are safe, well tolerated antihypertensive agents of similar efficacy to ACE inhibitors in decreasing high blood pressure in non-diabetic subjects and in diabetic patients. Some experimental and short-term clinical studies had also indicated that ARBs may have a comparable renoprotective (e.g.: reduction of proteinuria) effect but evidence of the long-term renal protection offered by ARBs has became available only very recently (Brenner et al. 2001; Parving et al. 2001).

The Prime Program (Program for Irbesartan Mortality and Morbidity Evaluation) included two Trials: IRMA 2 (Irbesartan Microalbuminuria Type 2 Diabetes Mellitus in hypertensive patients) and the IDNT (Irbesartan Diabetes Nephropathy Trial). The IRMA (Irbesartan in patients with type 2 DM with microalbuminuria) 2 is a multinational, multicenter, double blind, placebo controlled randomized (Parving et al. 2001) trial designed to evaluate the effectiveness of Irbesartan (either 150 mg or 300 mg/daily) to delay or prevent diabetic nephropathy in Type 2 hypertensive diabetics with persistent moderate microalbuminuria. A total of 590 overweighted Type 2 diabetic patients, hypertensive, aged 30–70 years old were randomized in three groups (placebo: n = 201; Irbesartan 150 mg/daily: n = 195; Irbesartan 300 mg/daily: n = 194) and followed up to two years. Target BP measures 3 months after randomization, were: 135/85 mmHg for all the three groups; other antihypertensive drugs were used as required but for ACE inhibitors.

The primary outcome, or primary efficacy measure, was the time to onset of diabetic nephropathy (e.g.: urinary albumin excretion: more than 200 µmg/min; and 30 % higher than the baseline rate confirmed in two consecutive visits). Secondary outcomes included changes in the degree of albuminuria, creatinine clearance and restoration (< 20 mg/min) of albumin excretion in the first visit. The result of this Trial conclusively proved that Irbesartan significantly reduced the progression from microalbuminuria to overt diabetic nephropathy in a great majority of patients and is dose-dependent in comparison with the control group (placebo and other antihypertensive agents). The restoration of normoalbuminuria by the last visit was observed more frequently in patients treated with the higher (300 mg/daily) dose of Irbesartan (34 % vs 21 % in the placebo group p < 0,006) but no significant differences

8 Hypertension in Type 2 Diabetes Mellitus

between the groups were detected in the decline (initial or sustained) of creatinine clearance. The average BP along the study period was similar in the placebo and the 150 mg Irbesartan groups but a significantly lower SBP than in placebo treated patients was obtained when combining the results of both Irbesartan arms of the trial. No significant differences between groups were observed other outcomes (e.g. non-fatal cardiovascular events) and a similarly modest increase in glycosylated hemoglobin was observed in all treatment groups. As a most important conclusion: "The IRMA study clearly demonstrates that Irbesartan could significantly benefit the hypertensive diabetic with microalbuminuria" as it was summarized by Dr. H. H. Parving, principal investigator of the study; and "the renoprotection by Irbesartan shown in this study was clearly independent of its antihypertensive effects".

The second trial of the PRIME Program, the IDNT Trial (Lewis et.al. 2001) was developed to determine whether the use of Irbesartan or the calcium antagonist amlodipine slowed the progression of nephropathy in Type 2 diabetic patients independently of its antihypertensive effects (Table 8.3). The trial was designed as prospective, randomized, double blind, conducted in 210 centres including 1715 Type 2 diabetic patients aged 30–70 years old, with established arterial hypertension (SBP>135 mmHg, DBP>85 mmHg while sitting (or documented antihypertensive treatment) and proven proteinuria (>900 mg urinary protein excretion in 24 hours). Patients were randomly assigned to 75–300 mg of Irbesartan, 2.5 to 10 mg/daily of amlodipine (n=579, n=567 patients) or placebo. Antihypertensive agents other than ACE inhibitors, ARBs or calcium blockers were used as required by patients in the three groups to reach the target BP values of: SBP of ≤135 mmHg (or 10 mmHg lower than that at baseline) and DBP of ≤85 mmHg. Primary end points were: a composite of a doubling of the baseline serum creatinine levels, the onset of ESRD (dialysis, renal transplanta-

Table 8.3. Clinical trials demonstrating that blood pressure lowering preserves renal function (modified from Toto 2001)

Source	Patient Population	BP control level (mmHg)	Renal outcome	ACEI Comparison	ACEI Superior
Petersen et al.	Non-diabetic	120/80	Slowed decline in GFR	No	...
Zucchelli et al.	Non-diabetic renal disease	140/80	Slowed decline in GFR	Yes	No
Hannedouche et al.	Non-diabetic renal disease	120/80	Slowed decline in GFR	Yes	No
Ihle et al.	Non-diabetic renal disease	130/80	Slowed decline in GFR	Yes	Yes
Lewis et al.	Type 2[a]	135/80	Decreasing progression nephropathy	No	...
Brenner et al.	Type 2[b]	140/90	35% Decline in proteinuria	No	...
Parving et al.	Type 2[c]	144/83	Renoprotection	No	...

BP, blood pressure; ACEI, angiotensin-converting enzyme inhibitor; GFR, glomerular filtration rate; Ccr, creatinine clearance.
[a] ARBs.
[b] Drug Losartan.
[c] Drug Irbesartan (see text).

tion, or death of any cause). Secondary end points include: a composite of death from CV events, non-fatal myocardial infarction, heart failure, lower limb amputations or neurological sequelae of stroke. Mean follow up period was 2.6 years.

The study demonstrated that Irbesartan treatment significantly decreased the risk of the composite primary end point when compared to both placebo and Amlodipine therapy groups whereas similar BP values were achieved. Furthermore, the death rates from cardiovascular events or other causes did not differ between Irbesartan, placebo or Amlodipine. Overall, the main relevant conclusion in IDNT is that "the ARB Irbesartan is more effective than Amlodipine in protecting from progression of established diabetic nephropathy in Type 2 hypertensive patients and that this favourable effect is obtained independently of the blood pressure lowering action of this drug". The results of a major third trial with the ARB Losartan (Brenner et.al. 2001) was the Renaal Study (Reduction of Endpoints in Non-insulin dependent diabetes mellitus with Angiotensin II Antagonist Losartan) were published simultaneously with the previous two trials. The Renaal trial was aimed "to determine whether Losartan used alone or in combination with currently available antihypertensive agents would "increase the time to doubling of the serum creatinine concentration, the onset of ESRD, of death". Other secondary end points assessed included: a comparison of the effects of Losartan and placebo on a composite of morbidity/mortality of CV cause, proteinuria and relative risk of progression of the nephropathy". The design was of a prospective, multinational, multicentre, randomized, double blind placebo trial including 1513 Type 2 diabetic patients with established renal disease. Although only the existence of nephropathy was the "sine qua non" criterion for inclusion in the study, almost all patients enrolled in the trial were hypertensive.

Initially the planned follow up period was 3.5 years but the study was discontinued earlier (3.4 years, mean: 2.3 – 4.6) by unanimous decision of the Steering Committee based on the incoming evidence suggesting that ACE inhibitors might reduce CV events in Type 2 DM with renal dysfunction. Patients were stratified according to their degree of proteinuria and randomized to be treated with either Losartan (50 mg/daily) or assigned to placebo (once daily) with subsequent dose adjustments (100 mg Losartan/day or its equivalent in placebo) in both groups according to the BP levels. After eight weeks antihypertensive drugs (but neither ACE inhibitors nor ARBs) were added at the adjusted dose required to achieve the target BP values. At the end of the trial it was shown that Losartan compared with placebo has significantly reduced the incidence of primary composite end points by 16 % with a risk reduction of ERSD by 28 %, ($p < 0.006$); and of the incidence of doubling the serum creatinine level by 25 % ($p < 0.002$).

Losartan also has a positive impact on the level of proteinuria with a 35 % higher decline ($p < 0.001$) than that seen with placebo. Some secondary outcomes (morbidity/mortality from cardiovascular events) were similarly affected by Losartan or placebo. Therefore, Losartan resulted in significantly renal protection in Type 2 diabetes with established nephropathy apart from its BP lowering effects. These benefits were also obtained by combining Losartan with conventional antihypertensive drugs (calcium channel antagonists, diuretics, α/β blockers, centrally acting agents). Overall, these three trials clearly establish that ARBs have strong renoprotective effects and delay the progression of diabetic nephropaty in Type 2 diabetics but particularly so in those with hypertension and/or renal disease.

Still many questions have yet to be answered. An important one is to asses the relative value of ACE inhibitors and ARBs by a direct comparison of their renoprotective and BP lowering effects at long-term in large populations of Type 2 diabetics from different ethnic groups with more endpoints related to cardiovascular events mortality to be evaluated. So far such studies are not yet available but an interesting ongoing trial is comparing the relative renoprotective effects in Type II diabetics of the ARB Temisartan with the ACE inhibitor Enalapril. The results of this Trial are expected to be available in 2004. Lastly, ACE inhibitors and ARBs have similar contraindications (e.g. hyperkalemia, pregnancy, renal artery stenosis) the latter having lesser adverse effects. Currently, an individual choice of any of these drugs must be done on this basis (Barnett 2001).

Calcium Channels Blockers (CCB; Cabezas-Cerrato et al. 1997)

The dihydropiridines (Nifedipine, Nicardipine, Isradipine, Felodipine, Amlodipine) among the best known, are of proven efficacy as antihypertensive drugs and also effective in reducing left ventricular hypertrophy. Nonetheless their renoprotective effects are less clearly established at long-term. Interclass differences exist regarding their efficacy on both renal functioning and in the control of HBP in the general population. Adverse effects are few but may be troublesome, such as peripheral oedema. The non-hydropiridines, Verapamil and Diltiazem are the most widely used agents of that subclass. Both have established efficacy as BP lowering drugs without neither significant adverse general cardiovascular effects nor a high incidence of orthostatic hypotension or of sexual dysfunction. However, its vasodilator effect may be deleterious in patients with postural hypotension (autonomic neuropathies, and also their negative inotropic action contraindicate contraindicates its use in those patients with advanced (classes II-IV NYHA) heart failure. Unlike dihydropiridine compounds, these calcium antagonists may be renoprotective at long term. Many observational and prospective controlled clinical trials have assessed the effects of both classes of CCB in Type 1 and in Type 2 diabetics: vs. placebo or in comparison with ACE inhibitors, diuretics, and other antihypertensive agents. The FACET (Fosinopril vs. Amlodipine cardiovascular event trial) a single centre trial, included 380 Type 2 diabetics who were randomly allocated to either Fosinopril (ACE arm) or Amlodipine (CCB). In this trial both agents showed comparable reduction in blood pressure groups without major impairment in glycemic control, nor in lipid profiles or in renal function. A major concern, however, was raised in this trial since patients treated with the calcium antagonist amlodipine had an unexpected higher incidence of fatal/non-fatal MI, hospitalization for angina pectoris and stroke. These adverse outcomes in the Amlodipine group were already apparent at 1.5 months of treatment. The issue of a harmful CV risk in this trial prompted the re-examination of previous trials with CCB and recent meta-analyses. Some authors (Pahor et al. 2000) confirmed the higher mortality in Nifedipine (7016) treated elderly hypertensive and case-control studies reported a greater risk for CV events with CCB treatment in Type 2 diabetics when compared to other treatment groups (ACE ihibitors, diuretics). Of more concern was the great number of coronary events in Nisoldipine treated (470) Type 2 diabetics with hypertension in the ABCD Trial (The Appropriate Blood pressure Control in

Diabetes Project: Nisoldipine vs. Enalapril) leading to stop the trial before the foreseen deadline for the follow-up period (5 years). On the basis of these and other studies on non-diabetic hypertensive MIDAS (Miocardial Infarction Data Acquisition System) and in diabetics (Type 2) with hypertension Syst Eur (Systolic Hypertension in Europe Trial) or with only impaired glucose tolerance (a small fraction of patients in MIDAS) Furberg (Furberg 1999) concluded that "long to intermediate action CCBs are inferior to ACE inhibitors and diuretics in reducing major CV events in this population"; and that one ought "be prudent to avoid all formulations of CCBs until large ongoing trials as the ALLHAT are available". These pessimistic views appear to be supported by one recent meta-analysis by Pahor et al. (Pahor et al. 2000) that recommended not to use calcium blockers as first choice drug or in combination with other anti-hypertensive therapies but for those instances of intolerance to ACEs, diuretics, or beta-blockers. On the contrary, the Blood Pressure Lowering Treating Hypertension Collaboration of Prospective Randomised Trialists Collaboration revised in the same issue of the Lancet a very large number of patients selected on the basis of HBP, DM and vascular (coronary heart, cerebrovascular and peripheral vascular disease) or renal disease. The Group, interpreted the results of the ACE inhibitors 4 trials and 2 CCBs trials: (Syst Eur; Prevent) as showing strong benefits in blood pressure lowering and even a significant reduction(30 – 40 %) of CCBs concerning the risk of stroke, CV death and major CV events. These discrepancies, between both simultaneous reports are difficult to interpret and make it difficult to adopt a definite position, regarding the use of CCBs in Type 2 DM but do not authorize to underestimate the value of CCBs as drugs useful in the hypertensive diabetic. Still we must wait until the results of large prospective trials on diabetic patients are available before deciding which is the "ideal drug of choice" that must provide simultaneously optimal control of hypertension in Type 2 DM, be renoprotective and significantly reduce the risk of macrovascular disease related events with negligible adverse effect. According to DeFronzo the ideal (if it would ever exist) antihypertensive drug must fulfill a strict series of criteria (Table 8.4).

Table 8.4. The ideal antihypertensive drug in diabetes (from DeFronzo 1995)

Is metabolically neutral and does not inhibit:
  Insulin secretion
  Insulin action
  Hepatic glucose production
  Counterregulation hormones

Does not:
  Cause or mask symptoms of hypoglycemia
  Aggravate hyperlipidemia
  Promote orthostatic hypotension
  Cause impotence
  Aggravate coronary/peripheral vascular disease

Specifically:
  Preserves renal function

Drug Choice and Therapeutic Strategies – Concluding Remarks

As already indicated it is currently accepted that all efforts should be made to set BP in hypertensive diabetics at less or equal to 130/80 mm Hg and in the presence of renal disease even at a lower: 120/80 mm Hg. Also current evidence indicates that low dose Thiazide, and ACE inhibitors may be recommended as first choice drugs. Cardioselective B_1 blockers are first line agents but they have a potentially negative influence on metabolic control and our hypoglycemia awareness, or in patients with erectile dysfunction should be taken into account in individual patients. B_1 cardioselective blockers are, indeed, better indicated for Type 2 diabetics who have coronary heart disease. It must be stressed on the basis of recent studies (HOT, UKPDS) that a small reduction of as little as 5 mm Hg in DBP (HOT) or of 8 mm Hg (UKPDS) or lower does make a significant difference in reducing CV risk. Any antihypertensive treatment in diabetes must be as aggressive as possible for hypertension as well as for other risk factors dyslipidemia, obesity, antiplatelet aggregation and must concomitandly include lifestyle changes.

In fact, drug treatment of hypertension in Type 2 DM is based on these principles:

1. It is "a must" to consider the simultaneous treatment of all the metabolic and nonmetabolic coexistent abnormalities: obesity, dyslipidemia, insulin resistance.
2. Any combination of antihypertensive drugs is aimed to control elevated blood pressure without having significant adverse side effect on glycemic control or any potential in deteriorating renal or cardiovascular functioning.
3. Major endpoints of antihypertensive treatment, apart from decreasing blood pressure in the diabetic patient, are the long-term prevention (and reduction) of all cause-mortality and morbidity due to cardiovascular complications and of course a major goal should be achieved as early and as efficiently as possible in order to stop the progression of renal disease.
4. The long-term control of hypertension in Type 2 hypertensive diabetics will surely require not only a single antihypertensive drug but a combination of two, three or even more drugs in order to obtain a lasting, satisfactory reduction of high BP in these patients. ACE inhibitors or ARB agents are recommended as first choice drugs alone or in combination with low dose Thiazides.

References

Agarval R.: Treatment of hypertension in patients with diabetes: lessons from recent trials. Cardiol-Rev. 9 (1): 36 – 44. 2001
American Diabetes Association: Clinical Practice. Recommendations 2001. Standards of Medical Care for patients with Diabetes Mellitus. Diabetes Care 24, Suppl 1,533-543. 2001
American Diabetes Association: Clinical Recommendations 2000.Diabetes Care 23(Supl. 11) S27-31.2000
Amos S.F., McCarthy D.J., Zimmet P. Diabet Med 14P: S1 – S85, 1997
Bakris G.L.:Pathogenesis of Hypertension in diabetes. Diabetes Reviews 3(3) 460-476. 1995
Barnett AH: The Role of Angiotensin II Receptor Antagonists in the Management of Diabetes. Blood Pressure 10 (Suppl I): 21-26. 2001
Baron A.D.: Cardiovascular Action of Insulin in humans. Implications for Insulinsensitivity and Vascular tone. In Ballieres Clinical Endocrinology and Metabolism. Insulin Resistance and Disease. Editor: E. Ferrannini. pp 961-988.Ballieri Tindall. Pha London.1993

Barroso I., Gurnell M.,Crowley V.E. Agostini M, Schwabel J.W., Soos MA et al. Dominant negative mutations in human PPARγ is associated with severe insulin resistance, diabetes mellitus and hypertension. Nature 402: 880-883. 1999

Baszilay J.J, Jones J.J., Davi B.R al for Allhat Collaborative Research Group: Baseline characteristics of the diabetic participants in the antihypertension and lipid lowering treatment to prevent Heart Attack. Trial (Allhat). Diabetes Care 24:654-658.2001

Blood Pressure Lowering Treatment Trialist's Collaboration: Effects of ACE inhibitors, calcium antagonist and other blood pressure lowering drugs: Results of prospectively designed overview of randomised trials. Lancet 355:1995-64.2000

Borhani N.O., Mercuri M., Borhani P.A et al. Final outcome results of the multicenter Isradipine Diuretic Atherosclerosis Study (MIDAS): A randomised controlled study. JAMA.276:785-91.1996

Brenner B.M., Cooper M.E., Zeeuw D., Keane W.F., Mitch W.E., Parving H.H., Remuzzi G., Snapinn S.M., Zhang Z., and Shahinfar S., for the RENAAL Study Investigators: Effects of Losartan on renal and cardiovascular outcomes in patients with Type 2 diabetes nephropathy. N Engl J Med 342 (12): 861-869. 2001

Burnier M., Brunner H.R.: Angiotensin receptor antagonists. Lancet 335: 637-645. 2000

Cabezas Cerrato J.,García Estévez D.A. Araujo D.: Insulin sensitivity and beta cell function in essential hypertensive and normotensive first degree relatives of hypertensive subjects. Diabetes and Metabolism.23:402-408.1997

Cabezas Cerrato J.,García Estévez D.A. Araujo D:Lack of Association both in insulin resistance and in insulin levels with blood pressure values in essential hypertension. Horm Metab Res.29:561-565.1997

Cabezas-Cerrato J., García-Estévez D.A., Araujo D., Iglesias M: Insulin sensitivity, glucose effectiveness, and beta-cell function in obese with essential hypertension: investigation of the effects of treatment with a calcium channel blocker (diltiazem) or an angiotensin-converting enzyme inhibitor (quinapril). Metabolism 46:173-178.1997

Cowie C.G., Harris M: Physical and Metabolic characteristics of persons with Diabetes. Diabetes in America.2nd Edition Chapter 7 pp117-164. National Institute of Health. NIH Publications n95.1468.1995

Curb J.D., Pressel S.L., Cutler J.A., Savage P.J., Applegate W.B., Black H., Camel G., Davis B.R., Frost P.H., Gonzalez N., Guthrie G., Oberman A., Rutan G.H., Stamler J.: Effect of diuretic-based antihypertensive treatment on cardiovascular disease risk in older diabetic patients with isolated systolic hypertension. Systolic Hypertension in the Elderly Program Cooperative Research Group. JAMA 276(23):1886-1892.1996

Davis B.R., Cutler J.A., Gordon D.J., et al: Rationales and Design for the Antihypertensive and Lipid lowering treatment to prevent Heart Attack Trial (ALLHAT) Am J Hypertens 9:342-60.1996

Davis B.R., Furberg C.D., Wright J.I. et al: Major cardiovascular events in hypertensive patients to Doxazosin vs. Chlortalidone.The Antihypertensive and Lipid lowering treatment to prevent Heart Attack Trial (ALLHAT) JAMA 283:1967-1975.2000

De La Sierra A., Ruilope L.M.: Treatment of hypertension in diabetes mellitus. Hypertension Reports 2:335-342. 2000

Deewania P: Hypertension and Diabetes. Arch. Intern Med. 160:1585-1594.2000

DeFronzo R.A.: Diabetic nephropathy: etiologic and therapeutic considerations. Diabetes Reviews 3: 510-564. 1995

Diabetes Control and Complications Trial Research Group: The effect of intensive treatment of Diabetes on the development and progression of long-term complications in Insulin dependent Diabetes Mellitus. N. Engl. J. Med.329:977-86.1993

Diabetic Nehropathy. ADA Recommendations 2001: S73-S76. 2001

Elliot J.W., Stein P.P, Black H.R.: Drug treatment of hypertension in patients with Diabetes. Diabetes Reviews 3(3) 477-509,1995

Ferrannini E, Natali A,Copaldo B et al. Insulin resistance hyperinsulinemia and blood pressure. Role of age and Obesity. Hypertension 30:1144-1149.1997

Ferrannini E., Buzzigoli G., Bonadonna R. et al. Insulin resistance in essential hypertensión. N. Engl. J. of Med.317:350-357.1987

Ferrannini E.: Insulin Resistance and Blood Pressure in Insulin Resistance. The Metabolic Syndrome X. Editors: G.M. Reaven, A.Laws. Part III Chapt 15, pp:281-308. Humana Press. Totowa. N.J. 1999

Furberg C.D.: Hypertension and Diabetes: Current Issues. Am. Heart J.138:400-405.1999

Groop L.C., Kankuri M., Shalin-Jantti C., Ekstrand A, Nikula-Ijas P., Widen E, Kuismanen E., Eriksson J., Franssila-Kallunki A, Saloranta C., et all: Association between polymorphism of the glycogen shyntase gene and non insulin-dependent diabetes mellitus. N. Eng. J. Med. 328:10-14.1993

Guidelines for Diabetes Care. A Desktop Guide to Type 2 Diabetes Mellitus. IDF (European Region). Brussels 1999

Haffner S.M., Lehto S., Ronnemaa T et al.: Mortality from coronary heart disease in subject with Type 2 diabetes and in nondiabetic subjects with and without prior myocardial infarction. N Engl J Med 339: 229-234.1998

Hannedouche T., Landais P., Goldfarb B., et al. Randomised controlled trial of enapril and beta blockers in non-diabetic chronic renal failure. BMJ. 309: 833-837. 1994

Hansson L., Zanchetti.A., Carruthers S.G. et al.: Effects of intensive blood- pressure lowering and low-dose aspirin in patients with hypertension: principal results of the Hypertension Optimal Treatment (HOT) randomised trial. HOT Study Group. Lancet 351:1755-1762.1998

Hansson L.,Zanchetti.A., Carruthers S.G. et al: Effects of intensive blood- pressure lowering and low-dose aspirin in patients with hypertension: principal results of the Hypertension Optimal Treatment (HOT) randomised trial. HOT Study Group. Lancet 351:1755-1762.1998

Hansson. L., Lindholm L .H., Ekbom T., Dahlof B., Lanke J., Schersten B., Wester P.O., Hedner T., de Faire U.: Randomised trials of old and new antihypertensive drugs in elderly patients: cardiovascular mortality and morbidity in the Swedish trial in old patients with hypertension 2 study. Lancet 1354:1751-1756.1999

Head J., Fuller J.H.: International variation in mortality among diabetic patients: The WHO multinational Study of Vascular Disease in Diabetics. Diabetología 3:477-481.1990

Heart outcomes prevention evaluation (HOPE) study investigators. Effect of angiotensin converting enzyme inhibitor Ramipril on cardiovascular events in high-risk patients. New Eng.J.Med.342: 145-153.2000

Heart outcomes Prevention Evaluation (HOPE) Study Investigators: Effects of Ramipril on cardiovascular and microvascular outcomes in people with Diabetes Mellitus: Results of the HOPE and the MICROHOPE substudy. Lancet 355:253-59.2000

Ihle B.U., Whitworth J.A., Shahinfar S., Cnaan A., Kincaid-Smith P.S., Becker G.J. Angiotensinconverting enzyme inhibition in nondiabetic progressive renal insufficiency: a controlled double-blind trial. Am J Kidney 27: 489-495. 1996

Jolk J, Colwell J.A. Arterial Thrombosis and Atherosclerosis in Diabetes. Diabetes Reviews 5(4) 316-352.1997

Kannel W.B., McGee D.L: Diabetes and Cardiovascular Disease. The Framingham Study. JAMA 241:2035-38.1979

Kannel W.B: Fifty years of Framingham Studies: Contribution to understand Hypertension .J. Human Hypert.14: 183-90.2000

Laakso M., Lehto S.: Epidemiology of macrovascular disease in Diabetes. Diabetes Reviews 5(4) 294-315,1997

Laakso M.: Hyperglicemia and cardiovascular disease in Type 2 Diabetes. Diabetes 48:937-42.1999

Letho S, Rönmena A, Pyöräläk K, Laakso M: Cardiovascular risk factors clustering with endogenous hyperinsulinemia predict death from coronary heart disease in patients with Type 2 Diabetes. Diabetología 43:148-55.2000

Lewis E.J., Hunsicker L.G., Clarke W.R., Berl T., Pohl M.A., Lewis J.B., Ritz E., Atkins R.C., Rohde R., and Raz I., for the Collaborative Study Group. Renoprotective Effect of the AngiotensinReceptor Antagonist Irbesartan in Patients with Nephropathy due to Type 2 Diabetes. N Engl J Med 345 (12): 851-860. 2001

MacLeod M., McJoy J.: Drug treatment of hypertension complicating Diabetes Mellitus. Drugs: 56(2) 189-199.1998

Nathan D.M., Meighs J., Singer D.E.: The epidemiology of Cardiovascular Disease in Type 2 Diabetes Mellitus. How sweet it is...or is it?. Lancet 350 (Suppl): 4-9,1997

Pahor M., Psaty B.M., Alderman M.H., Applegate W.B., Williamson J.D., Cavazzini C., Furberg

C.D.: Health outcomes associated with calcium antagonist compared with other first-line antihypertensive therapies: a meta-analyses of randomised controlled trials. Lancet 356:1949-54.2000
Parving H.H., Lehnert H., Bröchner-Mortersen J., Gomis R., Andersen S., and Arner P., for the Irbesartan in Patients with Type 2 Diabetes and Microalbuminuria Study Group: The effect of Irbesartan on the Development of Diabetic Nephropathy in Patients with Type 2 Diabetes. N Engl J Med 345 (12): 870-876. 2001
Peterson J.C., Adler S., Burkart J.M., et al.. Blood Pressure control, proteinuria, and the progression of renal disease: the modification of diet in renal disease study. Ann Intern Med. 123:754-762. 1995
Reaven G.M. Role of Insulin Resistance in Human Disease. Diabetes 37:1495-1607.1988
Reaven G.M. The pathophysiological consequences of adipose tissue insulin resistance. Insulin Resistance. The Metabolic Syndrome X. Editor: G.M. Reaven, A .Laws. Part II. Chapter 12. pp 233–246.Humane Press.Inc. Totowa N.J.1999
Ruige J.B., Assendelft W.J., Dekker J.M., Kostense P.J., Heine R.J., Bouter L.M.: Insulin and risk of cardiovascular Disease. A meta-analysis. Circulation 97(10):996 – 1001, 1998
Sakkinen P.A.,Wahl P., Cushman M. et al: Clustering of procoagulation, inflammation and fibrinolysis variables with metabolic factors in the insulin resistance syndrome.Am.J.Epidem.10,897-907.2000
Stamler J.Vaccaro O., Neaton J.D. et all for the multiple risk factor intervention trial research group. Diabetes, other risk factors and 12yr cardiovascular mortality for men screened in the multiple risk factor intervention trial. Diabetes Care 16:434–44.1993
Stenbit E.A, Tsauts L.J., Barcelin R. et all: Glut 4 heterogeneous knockout mice develop muscle insulin resistance and Diabetes. Nature Med 10:1096-1101.1997
Steppan C.M., Baile S.T., Bhat S., Brown E.J., et al.: The hormone resistin links obesity to diabetes. Nature 409: 307-312. 2001
Stern N., Tuck M.:Pathogenesis of Hypertension in Diabetes Mellitus. A fundamental and Clinical Text.2nd Edition.Part IX Chap 94.pp943-953.Editors D.L. Le Roith, S.I. Taylor and S.M Olesky. Lippincot Williams and Wilkins P. Baltimore 2000
The Sixth Report of the Joint National Committee on Prevention, Detection, Evaluation and Treatment of High Blood Pressure. Arch. Intern. Med. 157:2413-2445.1997
Toto R.: Angiotensin II subType 1 receptor blockers and renal function. Arch Intern Med 161 (12): 1492-9. 2001
Turner R.C., Mills H., Neil H.A.W.; Stratton I.M., Manlegse Mathews D.R., Holman R.R. for the United Kingdom prospective Study Group :Risk Factors for coronary artery disease in non insulin dependent diabetes mellitus: United Kingdom prospective diabetes study (UKPDS 23)BMJ 316:823-8.1998
UK Prospective Study Group: Efficacy of the atenolol and captopril in reducing risk of macrovascular and microvascular complications in Type 2 Diabetes. UKPDS 39. BMJ 317.713-20.1998
UKPDS 38: Tight blood pressure control and risk of macrovascular and microvascular complications in Type 2 Diabetes. UK Prospective Diabetes Study Group. BMJ 317:703-713.1998
Whithers O.J., Gutierrez J.S., Teolwery H. et al. Disruption of IRS-2 causes Type 2 Diabetes in mice.Nature.391:900-904.1998
Yki-Järvinen H. Management of Type 2 Diabetes Mellitus and Cardiovascular Risk. Lessons from the Intervention Trials. Drugs 60(5): 975-983.2000
Zuanetti G., Latini R., Maggoni A.P. et al for the GI SS 3 investigators. Effect of the ACE inhibitor lisinopril on mortality in diabetic with acute myocardial infarction. Data from the GISS 3 study. Circulation 96:4239-45.1997
Zucchelli P., Zuccala A., Borghi M. et al. Longterm comparison between captopril and nifedipine in the progression of renal insufficiency. Kidney Int. 42: 452-458. 1992

CHAPTER 9

Microalbuminuria and Cardiovascular Disease in Type 2 Diabetes

M. Massi Benedetti, M. Orsini Federici

Introduction

People with type 2 diabetes show an excess morbidity, mortality and disability compared with non-diabetic people; the excess mortality in western countries is mainly due to a higher incidence of macrovascular accidents. In the London cohort of the WHO Multinational Study of Vascular Disease in Diabetics (CVD), myocardial infarction, other ischemic heart diseases and other cardiac diseases accounted for 45.6%, 8.8% and 4.3% of deaths respectively and all cardiovascular diseases represented the 58% of causes of death [1]. The Multifactorial Primary Prevention Trial has confirmed that, mortality for all cardiovascular disease was significantly higher in people with diabetes than in non diabetic individuals (30.4 versus 8.3 deaths per 1000 observation-years respectively, in middle-aged Swedish men) [2].

The higher prevalence of CVD in type 2 diabetes can be secondary to the disease itself; in fact. hyperglycaemia, hyperinsulinemia and insulin resistance may contribute to the onset and development of atherosclerotic lesions thus rendering diabetes an independent risk factor for CVD [3]. Moreover, other risk factors for CVD, dyslipidemia, hypertension and visceral obesity are commonly concurrent with type 2 diabetes. In the late 1980s all these abnormalities, correlated with an elevated risk of CVD, were associated to the so-called X syndrome [4]. More recently, new applicants for the X syndrome were proposed: high levels of plasminogen activator inhibitor-1, hyperuricemia and microalbuminuria [5].

Definition of Microalbuminuria

About one third of diabetic patients develop diabetic nephropathy during their life. The presence of a level of proteinuria above 0.3 g/24 h (>300 mg/24 h) indicates the diagnosis of diabetic nephropathy [6]. Even though, in the initial stage, renal function is usually normal, the natural history of diabetic nephropathy foresees a progressive decline of functionality toward end-stage renal disease. Clinical diabetic nephropathy is usually preceded in years, by a condition of a slight increase in urinary excretion of albumin below the threshold for overt proteinuria, called "microalbuminuria" [7].

Macroalbuminuria is defined as a urinary albumin excretion rate (UAER) in the range of 20–200 µg/min (30–300 mg/24 h) [8].

The appearance of microalbuminuria is consequent to an increased leakage of albumin through the basement membrane of the glomeruli. Two mechanisms can lead to this increased leakage. The first one is an increased intraglomerular capillary pressure that is a typical condition in diabetes mellitus and that is also present in hypertension [9]. Furthermore, a hyperglycaemic condition can produce a loss of negative charges on the basement membrane of the glomeruli with the consequence of an increased capillary permeability to negatively charged proteins such as albumin [10].

Originally microalbuminuria was only considered as an early predictor of risk for development of diabetic nephropathy; in fact up to 80% of diabetic patients with microalbuminuria, if not adequately treated, show a progression towards macroalbuminuria [11].

More recently several studies have indicated that microalbuminuria is an independent risk factor for cardiovascular morbidity and mortality in diabetes.

Epidemiology of Microalbuminuria and Cardiovascular Disease

In the past two decades, different investigations have demonstrated the correlation between microalbuminuria and excess mortality in type 2 diabetes, mainly for cardiovascular disease.

Jarrett and colleagues demonstrated, in a retrospective analysis of 44 type 2 diabetic patients with AER measured from a single overnight urine collection, that subjects with AER greater than 30 µg/min had an increased risk of early death (all causes but chiefly cardiovascular); moreover Albumin excretion Rate (AER) resulted independent of age, sex, diabetes duration and blood pressure values, as risk factors for mortality. A similar correlation was also found when they considered the threshold of 10 µg/min [12].

A larger retrospective study of 232 type 2 diabetics, from Mogensen et al., confirmed the importance of microalbuminuria as a predictive factor for premature mortality. In this study the mortality risk was found to be correlated with the increasing level of urinary albumin concentration (UAC) determined on early morning urine samples: an UAC of 15 µg/ml corresponded to an increased risk of 37% with respect to the normal controls and an UAC comprised between 30–140 µg/ml to a risk of 148%. At the lower level of UAC, the mortality risk was independent of age, sex, plasma glucose and blood pressure, while in the range 30–140 µg/ml UAC also predicted the development of overt proteinuria [13].

Schmitz and Vaeth retrospectively investigated the role of microalbuminuria and other risk factors (age, sex, age at diagnosis, diabetes duration, blood pressure, fasting plasma glucose, weight, serum creatinine, retinopathy, treatment) in the prediction of increased mortality in a Danish population of 503 subjects with diabetes mellitus, of whom 265 died during the 10 years of observation. They showed that UAC above the limit of 40 µg/ml was an independent risk factor as far as age, serum creatinine and duration of diabetes. The hazard ratio for UAC between 40–200, after correction for the other independent risk factors, was 2.28 ($p < 000002$) relative to the normal group. In the 58% of the subjects who have died during the study period, cardiovascular disease was the cause of death, while only 3% died from uraemia [14].

On the basis of these three retrospective studies that showed a clear correlation between AER and an increased risk for cardiovascular disease, it was concluded that microalbuminuria was an independent risk factor for CVD mortality. Otherwise retrospective studies could be affected by several bias, especially source errors, so that they cannot be use to exactly define the causal relationship. Several prospective studies have been subsequently performed to assess the real predictive power of microalbuminuria for cardiovascular mortality.

Mattock et al. followed 141 type 2 diabetic subjects without overt proteinuria during the years 1985–1987 analysing the predictive power of several risk factors; at the end of the follow up the mortality rate was significantly higher ($p<0.001$) in the group of patients with microalbuminuria (28%, 8.2% per year) than in the one without microalbuminuria (4%). Increased mortality was also correlated to hypercholesterolemia, hypertriglyceridemia and pre-existing coronary heart disease, but the predictive capability of microalbuminuria was still maintained even when adjusted for the effects of these other major risk factors [15].

The high mortality rate per year evidenced by the previous study was not confirmed in another similar experience from Gall et al. In fact they found a mortality rate of 3.8% per year in the microalbuminuric cohort. While the age and the presence of other risk factors were comparable, the only difference was in the ethnic composition of the two populations studied. 100% of subjects in the Gall study were Caucasians with respect to the 39% of Afro-Caribbean and Indian Asians and 61% of Caucasians in the study from Mattock, thus indicating a possible role of race in the excess mortality in microalbuminuric subjects [16].

Neil and colleagues studied 236 type 2 diabetic patients for a period of 6-years assessing AER with a random daytime urine specimen. During the considered period 93 subjects died, mostly due to CVD disease. The relative risk of death for the patients with UAC of 40–200 µg/l was 2.2 with respect to subjects with UAC below 40 µg/l. Different studies have shown strict correlation of AUC from early morning samples and of the albumin/creatinine ratio with the overnight AER, while random daytime specimens presented a lower correlation due to the possible influence of different confounding factors such as exercise or on standing. An important finding from the study of Neil et al. was the evidence that microalbuminuria correlated with an increased risk of mortality regardless of the collection procedure used for the measurement of UAC [17].

Another prospective study was performed by McLeod et al. on a population of 153 type 2 diabetic people with different levels of abnormal urinary albumin excretion and of 153 controls with normal albumin excretion (AER <10.5 µg/min). This study confirmed the predictive value of microalbuminuria for increased mortality rate (Odds Ratio 1.47, $p<0.001$ vs. controls) and mostly highlighted that the difference in mortality rates raise with increasing levels of AER, from just outside the normal range to the upper levels for microalbuminuria criteria. Risk Ratios for all causes of death, at a multivariate analysis, were equal to 5.7, 6.8 and 8.8 for AER of 15, 20 and 30 µg/min respectively [18].

Pathogenetic Mechanisms for the Association of Microalbuminuria to Cardiovascular Disease

Even though the above reported and several other studies have clearly demonstrated that microalbuminuria is an important independent risk factor for cardiovascular morbidity and mortality, the causal link between the loss of albumin in urine and the development of cardiovascular disease is still not clear.

Endothelial Dysfunction and Haemostasis Disturbances

It is well known that endothelium has a central role in the vascular functionality being involved in the regulation of vessel tone and permeability, haemostatic and fibrinolytic processes, synthesis of matrix proteins and growth factors. Thus several disturbances of the endothelium structure and of its function are at the basis of the development of the atherosclerosis [19].

In this light one of the first hypothesis on the correlation of microalbuminuria to the origin of cardiovascular disease is that the increase of the AER could be associated to a generalised dysfunction of the endothelium.

Different plasma markers of endothelium function or of endothelium damage have been identified: von Willebrand factor (VWF), endothelin-1, angiotensin-converting enzyme, adhesion molecules such as ICAM-1 or VCAM-1 and e-selectin [20].

Stehouwer et al. have analysed the concentration and the change in concentration of the von Willebrand Factor, a glycoprotein that is released by damaged endothelial cells, in three groups of type 2 diabetic patients with different history of urinary albumin loss [21]. Patients of the first group had normal UAER at baseline and remained normal at the end of the follow up, while subjects of the second group that were normal at baseline, resulted microalbuminuric at the end of the study. The third group comprised patients that presented microalbuminuria at baseline. In the first group VWF levels did not change during the follow-up whereas both groups two and three showed a significant increase of VWF with respect to baseline (219 vs 116 % and 207 vs 157 % respectively). VWF baseline levels and changes during the study resulted strictly correlated with the development of albuminuria; the correlation between VWF concentrations and cardiovascular risk was seen only in the subgroup of patients with VWF levels above the median. The results indicated that in type 2 diabetic patients the pathogenesis of microalbuminuria, and cardiovascular disease are related to endothelial dysfunction and specifically that microalbuminuria was associated with increased risk of cardiovascular disease only in the presence of endothelium damage as showed by the more elevated levels of VWF in patients who developed CVD events.

Similar results were obtained by Collier et al. who found elevation of VWF and t-PA levels in type 2 diabetic patients with microalbuminuria with respect to the normoalbuminuric ones. Moreover, they also demonstrated in microalbuminuric patients an increase in the concentrations of malondialdehyde, which is a marker of lipid peroxidation. No differences were found between the two groups of diabetic patients for the markers (nonperoxide-conjugated diene isomer of linoleic acid PL-, 11LA') of the free radical activity even though in both groups they were higher with respect to the control group of healthy subjects [22].

Microalbuminuria and cardiovascular disease can thus be considered as two different aspects of endothelium damage. Endothelial cells of the glomerular capillary barrier are involved in glomerular function and particularly in the filtration of protein; the loss of albumin, typical of microalbuminuria, consequently may be due to glomerular endothelial damage. These results confirm the "Steno hypothesis" that in type 1 diabetic patients albuminuria reflects widespread vascular damage with the simultaneous involvement of the glomeruli, the retina and the intima of large vessels. The latter localisation of the vascular damage can explain the higher incidence of cardiovascular events in patients with associated elevation of albumin excretion rate [23].

More recently a 5-year follow up of the Horn Study has strongly confirmed the presence of a generalised atherosclerosis in type 2 diabetic patients at the basis of microalbuminuria and cardiovascular disease [24]. In fact the study showed a clear correlation of microalbuminuria and peripheral arterial disease, generally recognised as a marker of widespread atherosclerosis; moreover the presence of both microalbuminuria and peripheral arterial disease predicted cardiovascular and allcause mortality independently from other risk factors.

Endothelial cells, such as smooth muscle cells and tissue macrophage expresses different cellular adhesion molecules that play an important role in the formation and development of the atherosclerotic plaques, enhancing the binding of monocytes and leukocytes to the endothelium and the migration of the latter ones into the arterial intima [25]. Plasma levels of vascular cell adhesion molecule-1 (VCAM-1), representing the expression of membrane bound VCAM-1, have been found elevated in diabetic patients by several authors as .a result of endothelial damage. This finding was confirmed by Jager et al. who analysed a sample population of the Horn Study [26]. Patients in the middle and upper tertiles of VCAM-1 levels presented 2-3 fold increased cardiovascular risk respect to the population in the lower tertile. In this experience VCAM-1 levels were positively associated to the presence of microalbuminuria with a risk ratio for cardiovascular mortality in macroalbuminuric subjects of 3.38 (95% Confidential Interval: 1.71-6.68) with respect to normoalbuminuric individuals.

Fioretto et al. have described the existence of two different types of microalbuminuria in type 2 diabetic patients. The first one was associated with increased von Willebrand Factor levels, higher incidence of retinopathy and established renal injury, both diabetic glomerulopathy and tubulo-interstitial and arteriolar changes. In contrast the second type presented normal levels of von Willebrand Factor, lower incidence of retinopathy and conserved renal structure. They postulated that only the first type may express a status of generalised endothelial dysfunction with consequent association of higher risk for cardiovascular disease [27]. More recently similar results were also produced by Jager et al. that confirmed that in type 2 diabetic patients microalbuminuria occurs both in the presence or in the absence of a widespread endothelial damage and that the presence of endothelial dysfunction defines a much more malignant pattern for the future possible development of cardiovascular disease [28].

The presence of a pro-thrombotic status related to microalbuminuria was shown by Bruno et al., who studied an Italian population of 1967 type 2 diabetic patients with a follow-up period of 3-4 years, using the plasma fibrinogen levels as a marker of enhanced coagulation. Mean plasma fibrinogen levels in the studied population was higher (3.6 ± 0.9 g/l) than the control group of 200 normal persons (2.5 ± 0.5 g/l). In diabetic patients plasma fibrinogen was significantly correlated to both HbA1c level and albumin excretion rate; the association with AER was independent of other cardiovascular risk factors such as age, sex, hypertensive status, smoking habit, body mass index and total cholesterol level [29].

An enhanced activation of the clotting system was also demonstrated in type 2 diabetic patients by Gabazza et al. as a consequence of an altered anticoagulant activities [30]. Plasma levels of activated protein C–protein C inhibitor complex were elevated and the anticoagulant response to exogenous thrombomodulin was reduced in diabetic patients with respect to the control group of healthy individuals. Within diabetic patients the presence of microalbuminuria was associated with a low plasma level of activated protein C–protein C inhibitor complex and lower response to exogenous thrombomodulin than in the normoalbuminuric patients.

Lipid Abnormalities

Dyslipidemia is a common finding in type 2 diabetes with advanced nephropathy. Several studies also demonstrated the association of lipid abnormalities with microalbuminuria [31]. Moreover, a 5-year prospective studies of a population of newly diagnosed type 2 diabetic patients showed that microalbuminuria was prior to the development of lipid disturbances [32]. Dyslipidemia in microalbuminuric subjects is characterised by the presence of elevated VLDL, total and LDL cholesterol and apolipoprotein-B levels and reduced HDL cholesterol levels; this pattern of abnormalities is highly atherogenetic and exposes subjects to a higher risk of cardiovascular disease. Furthermore, microalbuminuria has been demonstrated to be a marker of a widespread vascular damage with increased vascular permeability; this condition permits a greater penetration of lipoprotein particles into the arterial wall. Thus the simultaneous presence of dislypidemia worsened the prognosis towards an accelerated atherogenesis.

More recently a study by Jerums et al. established a correlation between microalbuminuria and the highly atherogenic apoprotein(a) [33]. They demonstrated that apoprotein(a) levels increased linearly with increasing albuminuria in type 2 diabetic patients and that this increase is not correlated with metabolic control or hypertension. The presence of albuminuria increased the hepatic synthesis of different proteins including apoprotein(a) and the apopotrein(a) can worsen vasculopathy enhancing the albumin loss. The rise of apoprotein(a) was documented also at microalbuminuric state. They concluded that apoprotein(a) could be an important mediator between microalbuminuria and cardiovascular disease through its thrombogenic and atherogenic properties.

Blood Pressure Levels

Several authors described an important association between microalbuminuria and arterial blood pressure that is another well known cardiovascular risk factor. Pinkney et al. reported a close correlation between albumin excretion rate and blood pressure ($r=0.57$, $p<0.001$) in type 2 diabetic patients [34]. Patients with microalbuminuria presented 24-h, daytime systolic and diastolic blood pressure higher than the normoalbuminuric ones. No differences were noted in nocturnal dips between the two groups while microalbuminuria was associated with a blunted nocturnal decline of pulse rate. The correlation between albumin excretion rate and blood pressure was the same for the office blood pressure and the 24-h continuous monitoring. But this finding was in contrast with a previous experience from Schmitz et al. that showed in type 2 diabetic patients a superiority of the 24-h monitoring blood pressure with respect to the casual ambulatory readings in studying the correlation between microalbuminuria and blood pressure [35].

Impaired reduction of nocturnal blood pressure is associated with higher prevalence of complications by hypertension and predicts cardiovascular events. More than 50% of type 2 diabetic patients with nephropathy present an impaired nocturnal reduction thus presenting a superior risk for cardiovascular disease. A recent study by Nielsen et al. elucidated the correlation between diabetic nephropathy and nocturnal hypertension in type 2 diabetics [36]. Contrary to previous investigations that postulated a nocturnal overhydratation, due to the nephropathy, as the basis for the lack of reduction of blood pressure, they demonstrated that the mechanism behind this phenomenon was a sustained adrenergic activity during sleep mediated through a deficiency in peripheral vasodilatation. Another important study showed that in type 2 diabetic patients left ventricular hypertrophy was more frequent and severe in subjects who presented microalbuminuria [37]. This association is very important because left ventricular hypertrophy represents a worse prognostic value for cardiovascular events. Left ventricular hypertrophy was also associated with blunted reduction of nocturnal blood pressure.

Insulin Resistance and Hyperinsulinemia

Another hypothesis on the correlation between microalbuminuria and cardiovascular disease is that microalbuminuria reflects or is intimately related to the presence of insulin resistance and hyperinsulinemia. This correlation was highlighted by Niskanen and Laakso and by Nosadini et al. who showed that microalbuminuria, in a population of type 2 diabetic patients, identified the more insulin resistant individuals [38, 39]. Moreover, a higher insulin resistance was seen in first-degree relatives of type 2 diabetic patients with microalbuminuria with respect to the relatives of normoalbuminuric patients [40]. A strict correlation between microalbuminuria and hyperinsulinemia was also noted in non-diabetic subjects. Kuusisto et al. demonstrated, in a Finnish population of elderly non-diabetic individuals, a higher risk of coronary heart disease (CHD) mortality and events in those who were allocated in the upper quintiles of fasting insulin and urinary albumin/creatinine ratio [41]. Furthermore, the risk was noticeably increased in the group of subjects in which both hyperinsulinemia and AER were in the upper quintiles (CHD Mortality 12.5%; CHD events 18.8%, $p<0.001$) The association hyperinsulinemia/microalbuminuria remained highly predictive of CHD mortality and events even after the adjustment for other risk factors such as sex, current smoking, obesity, blood pressure and HDL cholesterol. Despite such findings this association identified a group of subjects with highly adverse pattern of CHD risk factors: elevated levels of triglycerides, low levels of HDL cholesterol and presence of hypertension. Similar results were also shown in the Insulin Resistance Atherosclerosis Study where insulin sensitivity was inversely related to the prevalence of microalbuminuria. An interesting finding was that within microalbuminuric individuals there was no difference in this association between hypertensive and normotensive subjects even though they both have higher BP values then normoalbuminuric subjects. These results indicated that hypertension did not account completely for the association of insulin resistance to microalbuminuria [42].

Different explanations could be hypothesized for the strengthening effect of the association between microalbuminuria and hyperinsulinemia on the cardiovascular risk both in type 2 diabetic patients and in non-diabetic subjects. Insulin and microalbuminuria have atherogenic effects. Insulin is a pleiotropic factor that can enhance smooth muscle cells proliferation, LDL binding to smooth muscle cells, fibroblast and monocytes and cholesterol synthesis in monocytes thus affecting the arterial wall in an atherogenetic way. Microalbuminuria has been found to be associated with accumulation of extracellular matrix in glomeruli and large vessel wall; the accumulation of matrix in large vessels wall was also discovered in atherosclerotic plaques. The alterations of the large vessels wall related to the presence of microalbuminuria could be worsened by the simultaneous effects of the hyperinsulinemia, accelerating the atherosclerosis. The second explanation is that the contemporary presence of microalbuminuria and hyperinsulinemia only identify a subgroup of people with a worse pattern of cardiovascular risk factors. Lastly, microalbuminuria has been proposed as a marker of the insulin resistance syndrome that usually presents an elevated risk of cardiovascular events and mortality.

Pickup et al. analysed the correlation between different features of the metabolic "syndrome X" and microalbuminuria with acute phase/stress reactants in order to elucidate the role of the innate immune system's response to environmental stress in the pathogenesis of the metabolic disturbances. They demonstrated that microalbuminuria was associated with the acute phase response and, more importantly, that microalbuminuria segregated with syndrome X [43].

This hypothesis, that microalbuminuria may be considered as an applicant of the syndrome X, was not confirmed by Jager et al. from the analysis of data from the Horn Study [44]. They found, in multiple logistic regression analysis, that microalbuminuria was independently associated with diabetes, hypertension and obesity (indicated by the waist to hip ratio) but not with impaired glucose tolerance, hyperinsulinemia or insulin resistance and dyslipidemia. It was concluded that microalbuminuria is a complication that is consequent to the presence both of diabetes and hypertension and not another feature of the insulin resistance syndrome.

Hyperomocysteinemia

A new potential link between microalbuminuria and cardiovascular disease has been identified in plasma homocysteine. Plasma homocysteine levels are commonly elevated in patients with renal failure secondary to the relevant role of the kidney in homocysteine catabolism. Moreover hyperomocysteinemia is recognised as an independent cardiovascular risk factor [45]. The importance of hyperomocysteinemia in type 2 diabetic patients has been investigated by Chico et al. [46]. They found higher plasma levels of homocysteine in type 2 diabetic patients with respect to the control group. Considering different features of the disease such as metabolic control, presence of complications, lipid profile and renal parameters, homocysteinemia presented the strongest association with the albumin excretion rate. Furthermore homocisteine plasma levels were higher in patients with nephropathy than in those without nephropathy and homocysteinemia increased linearly with the increase in severity of nephropathy. However the most important and new evidence was that in type 2 diabetic patients both incipient and overt proteinuria, in the absence of renal failure, were associated with elevations of plasma homocysteine levels. This suggests the possible role of hyperomocysteinemia in the correlation between microalbuminuria and cardiovascular disease.

Chronic Inflammation

Microalbuminuria has been associated with a status of chronic inflammation [47]. C-reactive protein and fibrinogen, two markers of chronic inflammation, were positively related to urinary albumin-to-creatinine ratio and both were higher in the presence of microalbuminuria. The two markers are also elevated in atherosclerosis. During chronic inflammation several cytokines are produced or released; these cytokines may affect the metabolism of glycosaminoglycans of the basal membrane of the glomeruli and of the vascular endothelium creating damage that can lead both to microalbuminuria and macrovascular disease. Thus chronic inflammation may be considered as a potential mediator between microalbuminuria and cardiovascular diseases.

Treatment of Microalbuminuria

Microalbuminuria is to some extent reversible secondary to an appropriate treatment for glycemic and blood pressure control. Moreover as illustrated before, microalbuminuria is a strong risk factor for cardiovascular disease. In this light cardiovascular risk factors must be intensively treated and a target pressure of 140/85 or lower should be reached, in microalbuminuric patients.

The treatment of hypertension and the achievement of the therapeutic goals are of particular importance as they allow a reduction in the risk of cardiovascular mortality and in the progression towards renal failure.

The Systolic Hypertension in the Elderly Study demonstrated improved cardiovascular outcomes in diabetic patients who received antihypertensive treatment [48]. A better prognosis with a reduction of all cardiovascular events and mortality was also shown in the Syst Eur Trial, in the UKPDS and in the Facet Study [49–51].

Strict blood pressure control is also essential to prevent the renal deterioration in hypertensive microalbuminuric type 2 diabetic patients. All classes of drugs that allow the achievement of blood pressure control should be used in theory. Nevertheless, the choice should be focused on the therapy that does not further impair renal function but, on the contrary, produces benefits. Several studies have shown the efficacy of the ACE-inhibitors in reducing blood pressure and simultaneously preventing deterioration of renal function [52, 53].

The possibility of delaying the progression of renal impairment with the utilisation of ACE-inhibitors has highlighted the necessity to start treatment in diabetic patients with microalbuminuria but no evidence of hypertension or even before in normoalbuminuric patients who presented risk factors for the development of nephropathy [54].

However a recent meta-analysis showed no difference in decreasing renal complications between ACE-inhibitors and calcium channel blockers [55].

Finally an interesting finding come from Tonolo et al. who founded a reduction in albumin excretion rate (25% less respect to the basal) in microalbuminuric hypercholesterolemic type 2 diabetic patients without hypertension, after long-term treatment with simvastatin [56]. This evidence corroborates the idea that microalbuminuria might be considered as a renal manifestation of a disseminate vascular damage related to the presence of lipid abnormalities.

Conclusions

Microalbuminuria in type 2 diabetes is a strong and independent predictor of cardiovascular events and mortality while its importance in predicting the development of diabetic nephropathy is lower, contrary to the finding in type 1 diabetes.

Despite this clear evidence, the mechanism of the link between microalbuminuria and cardiovascular disease has still not been completely identified. Microalbuminuria may express a widespread vascular and especially endothelial damage, a phenomenon which is also at the basis of the atherogenetic process. Moreover microalbuminuria is often associated with other important cardiovascular risk factors such as hypertension and lipid abnormalities. The inclusion of microalbuminuria in the insulin resistance syndrome is still controversial.

Due to the high preventive value of the presence of microalbuminuria for cardiovascular event, therapeutic interventions for glycaemic and blood pressure control are of crucial interest. All the different categories of antihypertensive drugs that can produce an effective reduction of blood pressure levels can be used even though several studies have demonstrated that ACE inhibitors should be the first choice. A new and important indication should also be the ACE-inhibition treatment in microalbuminuric patients regardless the presence of hypertension.

References

1. Morrish NJ, Stevens LK, Head J, Fuller JH, Jarrett RJ, Keen H. A prospective study of mortality among middle-aged diabetic patients (the London cohort of the WHO Multinational Study of Vascular Disease in Diabetics): causes and death rates. Diabetologia 1990;33:538–541.
2. Adlerbeth AM, Rosengreen A, Wilhelmsen L. Diabetes and long-term risk of mortality from coronary and other causes in middle-aged Swedish men. A general population study. Diabetes Care 1998;21:539–545.
3. Massi Benedetti M, Orsini Federici M. Cardiovascular risk factors in type 2 diabetes: the role of hyperglycaemia. Exp Clin Endocrinol Diabetes 1999; 107(suppl 4):S120-S123.
4. Reaven GM. Role of insulin resistance in human diseases. Diabetes 1988;37:1495–1607.
5. Reaven GM. A syndrome of resistance to insulin-stimulated glucose uptake (syndrome X): definition and implications. Cardiovasc Risk Fact 1993;3:2–11.
6. American Diabetes Association. Diabetic Nephropathy. Diabetes Care 1997;20:S24-S27.
7. Mogensen CE, Christensen CK, Vittinghus E. The stages in diabetic renal disease: with emphasis on the stage of incipient diabetic nephropathy. Diabetes 1983; 32(suppl 2): 64–78.
8. Mogensen CE, Keane FW, Bennett PH, Jerums G, Parving HH, Passa P, Steffes MW, Striker GE, Viberti GC. Prevention of diabetic renal disease with special reference to microalbuminuria. Lancet 1995; 346: 1080–1084.
9. Brenner BM, Hoestetter TH, Humes HD. Molecular basis of proteinuria of glomerular origin. N Engl J Med 1978; 298: 826–833.
10. Shimomura H, Spiro RG. Studies on macromolecular components of humen glomerular basement membrane and alterations in diabetes. Decreased levels of heparan sulfate proteoglycan and laminin. Diabetes 1987; 36: 374–381.

11. Viberti GC, Hill RD, Jarret RJ, Argyropoulos A, Mahmud U, Keen H. Microalbuminuria as a predictor of clinical nephropathy in insulin-dependent diabetes mellitus. Lancet 1982, I;1430-1432.
12. Jarrett RJ, Viberti GC, Argyropoulos A, Hill RD, Mahmud U, Murrells TJ. Microalbuminuria predicts mortality in non insulin dependent diabetes. Diabet Med 1984; 1: 17-19.
13. Mogensen CE. Microalbuminuria predicts clinical proteinuria and early mortality in maturity onset diabetes. N Engl J Med 1984; 310: 356-360
14. Schmitz A, Vaeth M. Microalbuminuria: a major risk factor in non-insulin-dependent diabetes. A 10-year follow-up study of 503 patients. Diabet Med 1988; 5: 126-134.
15. Mattock MB, Morrish NJ, Viberti GC, Keen H, Fitzgerald AP, Jackson G. Prospective study of microalbuminuria as predictor of mortality in NIDDM. Diabetes 1992; 41: 736-741.
16. Gall MA, Borch-Johnsen K, Hougaard P, Nielsen FS, Parving HH. Albuminuria and poor glycemic control predict mortality in NIDDM. Diabetes 1995; 44: 1303-1309
17. Neil A, Hawkins M, Potok M, Thorogood M, Cohen D, Mann J. A prospective population-based study of microalbuminuria as a predictor of mortality in NIDDM. Diabetes Care 1993; 16(7): 996-1003.
18. MacLeod JM, Lutale J, Marshall SM. Albumin excretion and vascular deaths in NIDDM. Diabetologia 1995; 38: 610-616.
19. Vane JR, Angaard EE, Botting RM. Mechanisms of disease: regulatory function of the vascular endothelium. N Engl J Med 1990; 323: 27-36.
20. Feldt-Rasmussen B. Microalbuminuria, endothelial dysfunction and cardiovascular risk. Diabetes Metab 2000; 26: 64-66.
21. Stehouwer CDA, Nauta JJP, Zeldentrust GC, Hackeng WHL, Donker AJM, den Ottolander GJH. Urinary albumin excretion, cardiovascular disease and endothelial dysfunction in non-insulin dependet diabetes mellitus. Lancet 1992; 340: 319-323.
22. Collier A, Rumley A, Rumley AG, Patterson JR, Leach JP, Lowe GDO, Small M. Free radical activity and hemostatic factors in NIDDM patients with and without microalbuminuria. Diabetes 1992; 41: 909-913
23. Deckert T, Feldt-Rasmussen B, Borch-Johnsen K, Jensen T, Kofoed-Enevoldsen A. Albuminuria reflects widespread vascular damage. The Steno hypotesis. Diabetologia 1989; 32: 219-226.
24. Jager A, Kostense PJ, Ruhè G, Heine RJ, Nijpels G, Dekker JM, Bouter LM, Stehouwer CDA Microalbuminuria and peripheral arterial disease are independent predictors of cardiovascular and all-cause mortality, expecially among hypertensive subjects. Five-year follow-up of the Horn Study. Arterioscler Thromb Vasc Biol 1999; 19: 617-624.
25. Davies MJ, Gordon JL, Gearing AJ, Pigott R, Woolf N, Katz D, Kyriakopoulos A. The expression of the adhesion molecules ICAM-1, VCAM-1, PECAM and E-selectin in human atherosclerosis. J pathol 1993; 171: 223-229]
26. Jager A, Van Hinsberg WM, Kostense PJ, Nijpels G, Dekker JM, Heine RJ, Bouter LM, Stehouwer CDA. Increased levels of soluble Vascular Cell Adhesion Molecule 1 are associated with risk of cardiovascular mortality in type 2 diabetes. Diabetes 2000; 49:185-191.
27. Fioretto P, Stehouwer CDA, Mauer M, Chiesura-Corona M, Brocco E, Carraro A, Bortoloso E, van Hinsberg VWM, Crepaldi G, Nosadini R. Heterogeneous nature of microalbuminuria in NIDDM: studies of endothelial function and renal structure. Diabetologia 1998; 41: 233-236.
28. Jager A, Van Hinsberg WM, Kostense PJ, Emeis JJ, Nijpels G, Dekker JM, Heine RJ, Bouter LM, Stehouwer CDA. Prognostic implications of retinopathy and high plasma von Willebrand factor concentration in type 2 diabetic subjects with microalbuminuria. Nephrol Dial Transplant 2001; 16: 529-536.
29. Bruno G, Cavallo-Perin P, Bargero G, Borra M, D'Enrico N, Pagano G. Association of fibrinogen with glycaemic control and albumin excretion rate in patients with non-insulin dependent diabetes mellitus. Ann Intern Med 1996; 125(8): 653-657.
30. Gabazza EC, Takeya H, Deguchi H, Sumida Y, Taguchi O, Murata K, Nakatani K, Yano Y., Mohri M, Satu M, Shimu T, Nishioka J, Suzuki K. Protein C activation in NIDDM patients. Diabetologia 1996; 39:1455-1461.
31. Seghieri G, Alviggi L, Caselli P, De Giorgio LA, Breschi C, Gironi A, Niccolai M. Sgruma lipids and lipoproteins in type 2 diabetic patients with persistent microalbuminuria. Diabetic Med 1990; 7: 810-814

32. Niskanen L, Uusitupa M, sarlund H, Siitonen O, Voutilainen E, Penttila I, Piolara K. Microalbuminuria predicts the development of serum lipoproteins abnormalities favouring atherogenesis in newly diagnosed type 2 (non insilun-dependent) diabetic patients. Diabetologia 1990; 33: 237–243.]
33. Jerums G, Allen TJ, Tsalamandris C, Akdeniz A, Sinha A, Gilbert R, Cooper ME. Relationship of progressively increasing albuminuria to apoprotein(a) and blood pressure in type 2 (non insulin-dependent) and type 1 (insulin-dependent) diabetic patients. Diabetologia 1993; 36: 1037–1044.
34. Pinkney JH, Foyle WJ, Denver AE, Mohamed-Ali V, McKinlay S, Yudkin JS. The relationship of urinary albumin excretion rate to ambulatory blood pressure and erythrocyte sodium-lithium countertransport in NIDDM. Diabetologia 1995; 38: 356–362.
35. Schmitz A, Pedersen MM, Hamsen KW. Blood pressure by 24-h ambulatory recordings in type 2 (non insulin-dependent) diabetics. Relationship to urinary albumin excretion. Diabete Metab 1991; 17: 301–307
36. Nielsen FS, Hansen HP, Jacobsen P, Rossing P, Smidt UM, Christensen NJ, Pevet P, Vivien-Roels B, Parving H. Increased sympathetic activity during sleep and nocturnal hypertension in type 2 diabetic patients with diabetic nephropathy. Diabetic Med 1999; 16: 555–562.
37. Rutter MK, McComb JM, Forstet J, Brady S, Marshall SM. Increased left ventricular mass index and nocturnal systolic blood pressure in patients with type 2 diabetes mellitus and microalbuminuria. Diabet Med 2000; 17: 321–325.
38. Niskanen L, Laakso M. Insulin resistance is related to albuminuria in patients with type II (non-insulin dependent) diabetes mellitus. Metaboliosm 1993; 42: 1541–1545.
39. Nosadini R, Solini A, Velussi M, Muollo B, frigato F, Sambataro M, Cipollina ME, De Riva F, Brocco E, Crepaldi G. Impaired insulin-induced glucose uptake by extrahepatic tissue is hallmark of NIDDM patients who have or will develop hypertension and microalbuminuria. Diabetes 1994; 43: 491–499.
40. Forsblom CM, Eriksonn JG, Ekstrand AV, Teppo AM, Taskinen MR, Groop LC. Insulin resistance and abnormal albumin excretion in non diabetic first degree relatives of patient with NIDDM. Diabetologia 1995; 38: 363–369.
41. Kuusisto J, Mykkanen L, Pyorala K, Laakso M. Molecular and cellular cardiology: hyperinsulinemic Microalbuminuria: a new risk indicator for coronary heart disease. Circulation 1995; 91(3): 831–837.
42. Mykkanen L, Zaccaro DJ, Wagenknecht LE, Robbins DC, Gabriel M, Haffner SM. Microalbuminuria is associate with insulin resistance in nondiabetic subjects. The Insulin Resistance Atherosclerosis Study. Diabetes 1998; 47: 793–800.
43. Pickup JC, Mattock MB, Chusney GD, Burt D. NIDDM as a disease of the innate immune system: association of acute-phase reactants and interleukin-6 with metabolic syndrome X. Diabetologia 1997; 40: 1286–1292.
44. Jager A, Kostense PJ, Nijpels G, Heine RJ, Bouter LM, Stehouwer CDA. Microalbuminuria is strongly associated with NIDDM and Hypertension but not with the insulin resistance syndrome: the Horn Study. Diabetologia 1998; 41: 694–700.
45. Arnesen E, Refsum H, Bonaa KH, Ueland PM, Forde OH, Nordrehaug JE. Serum total homocysteine and coronary heart disease. Int J Epidemiol 1995; 24: 704–709.
46. Chico A, Pereze A, Cordoba A, Arcelus R, Carreras G, de Leiva A, Gonzales-Sastre F, Blanco-Vaca F. Plasma homocysteine is related to albumin excretion rate in patients with diabetes mellitus: a new link between diabetic nephropathy and cardiovascular disease? Diabetologia 1998; 41: 684–693.
47. Festa A, D'Agostino R, Howard G, Mykkanen L, Russell P, Haffner T, Haffner SM. Inflammation and microalbuminuria in nondiabetic and type 2 diabetic subjects: the Insulin Resistance Atherosclerosis Study. Kidney Int 2000; 58: 1703–1710.
48. Curb JD, Pressel SL, Cutler JA, Savage P, Applegate WB, Black H et al. Effect of diuretic-based antihypertensive treatment on cardiovascular disease risk in older diabetic patients with isolated systolic hypertension. Systolic Hypertension in the Elderly programme Cooperative Research Group. JAMA 1996; 276: 1886–1892.
49. The Systolic Hypertension in Europe (Syst-Eur) Trial Investigators. Randomised double-blind comparison of placebo and active treatment for older patients with isolated systolic hypertension. Lancet 1997; 350: 757–764.

50. UK Prospective Diabetes Study Group. Tight blood pressure control and risk of macrovascular and microvascular complications in type 2 diabetes: UKPDS 38. BMJ 1998; 317: 703–713.
51. Tatti P, Pahor M, Byington RP. Outcome results of the Fosinopril versus Amlodipine Cardiovascular Events Trial (FACET) in patients with hypertension and NIDDM. Diabetes Care 1998; 21: 597–603.
52. HOPE Study Investigators. Effects of ramipril on cardiovascular and microvascular outcomes in people with diabetes mellitus: results of the HOPE study and MICRO-HOPE substudy. Lancet 2000; 355: 253–259.
53. UK Prospective Diabetes Study Group. Efficacy of atenolol and captopril in reducing risk of macrovascular and microvascular complications in type 2 diabetes. UKPDS 39. BMJ 1998; 21: 597–603.
54. Ravid M, Brosh D, Levi Z, Bar-Dayan J, Ravid D, Rachmani R. Use of enalapril to attenuate decline in renal function in normotensive normoalbuminuric patients with type 2 diabetes mellitus: a randomised controlled study. Ann Intern med 1998; 128(12): 982–988.
55. Nosadini R, Abaterusso C, Dalla Vestra M, Bortoloso E, Saller A, Bruseghin M, Sfriso A, Trevisan M. Efficacy of antihypertensive therapy in decreasing renal and cardiovascular complications in diabetes mellitus. Nephrol Dial Transplant 1998; 13 (suppl 8): 44–48.
56. Tonolo G, Ciccarese M, Brizzi P, Puddu L, Secchi G, Calvia P, Atzeni MM, Melis MG, Maioli M. Reduction of albumin excretion rate in normotensive microalbuminuric type 2 diabetic patients during long-term simvastatin treatment. Diabetes Care 1997; 20(12): 1891–1895.

CHAPTER 10

Cardiovascular Risk in Obese Type 2 Diabetes Mellitus Patients

G. Roman, X. Formiguera, N. Hâncu

Abstract. Abdominal obesity and Type 2 diabetes mellitus represent a frequent association, leading to an increased morbidity and mortality from atherogenic macrovascular disease. The key feature which links visceral obesity, Type 2 diabetes mellitus and cardiovascular risk is considered to be insulin resistance. It induces a cluster of metabolic, vascular, prothrombotic anomalies, known as metabolic syndrome. The cardiovascular risk related to metabolic syndrome consists of an amplified action of each component, leading to high and early probability of developing atherosclerotic pathology. As demonstrated by clinical trials, most of the newly-diagnosed obese Type 2 diabetic patients have a high cardiovascular risk due to the presence of cardiovascular risk factors. To reduce cardiovascular risk, an aggressive approach is required, in terms of risk factor identification, global risk evaluation, targeted and multifactorial interventions. Structured programme as: therapy, education, monitoring, evaluation should be applied. Weight loss is a major therapeutic goal. Lifestyle optimization, through hypocaloric diet and physical activity and specific medication for obesity, are methods to be considered.

Introductory Remarks

Obesity and Type 2 Diabetes mellitus frequently occur together. They are closely linked by commonality of aetiology and pathogenesis (genetics, insulin resistance and lifestyle), clinical and therapeutical features. Both of these chronic diseases are major causes of morbidity and mortality from atherogenic macrovascular disease and they are independent factors for coronary heart disease, resulting also in increased economic costs. Their complex connection support the term "diabesity", proposed by A. Satrap and N. Finer (2000).

Obesity is the strongest risk factor for the development of Type 2 Diabetes mellitus. Together with overweight with abdominal fat distribution, they play the major etiological role in about 80–90% of cases and represent a major obstacle to the successful long-term management of the disease. The risk for developing diabetes rises steadily once BMI exceeds 24 kg/m². Weight gain after the age of 21 significantly increases the risk of developing diabetes (Chan et al. 1994). Considering BMI at age 18, a 20-kg weight gain increases the risk for diabetes 15-fold. (Bray 1998). Women with a BMI 24–25 kg/m² have a 5-fold increased risk for developing type 2 diabetes and a BMI > 35 kg/m² increases the risk 93-fold (Han et al. 1997). On this basis, obesity could be considered the most important problem in Type 2 Diabetes care world-wide (Wilding and Williams 1998).

The risk of developing Type 2 Diabetes and cardiovascular disease is highly associated with abdominal (visceral) fat distribution. The clinical marker of visceral fat deposition is waist circumference. It has been found to be a strong predictor of diabetes (Chan et al. 1994). Obesity is involved in determining the cardiovascular risk both as an independent factor and as part of the metabolic X syndrome (Reaven 1988), where it is highly associated with hypertension, dyslipidaemia, increased prothrombotic status and endothelial dysfunction. The combination of insulin resistance and hyperinsulinemia is considered to be the main pathophysiological link of this association. The presence of Type 2 Diabetes mellitus completes the feature and multiplies the cardiovascular risk by adding a significant burden through specific metabolic and haemorrheological disturbances. For more data, see Chapter 21.

The first part of this chapter summarises the main aspects of cardiovascular risk related to Type 2 Diabetes and obesity, in terms of pathogenesis and epidemic. In addition, the impact of obesity in the clinical management of diabetes is discussed, together with recommendations and strategies suggested for weight management.

Cardiovascular Risk in Obese Type 2 Diabetes Patients

Pathogenetic Background

The key feature which links visceral obesity, Type 2 Diabetes mellitus and cardiovascular risk status is considered to be insulin resistance and hyperinsulinemia, developed in the first phase.

Insulin Resistance/Hyperinsulinaemia

Insulin resistance has a double determination: genetic and acquired. Both types of factors interact determining a post insulin receptor mechanism mainly at skeletal muscle level. The fat deposits at this level, have an important role in this mechanism. A genetic determination of body fatness and fat distribution is discussed. Genes anomalies refer to insulin receptors or intracelular signaling, glycogen sinthetasis, hexokinaza II, GLUT-4 glucose transporter, GLUT-2. Their expression is under acquired factors such as hypercaloric diets, rich in fat, poor in fibres and antioxidants and low physical activity.

Visceral adipocytes have a high secretory activity, acting like an endocrine organ: free fatty acids, leptin, lipoprotein lipase, angiotensinogen, TNF-α (tumor necrosis factor-alpha) and sR (soluble receptors), PAI-1(plasminogen activator inhibitor 1), IGF-1 (insulin-like growth factor-1), IL 6 (interleukin) and sR (soluble receptors), Apo E, prostaglandins, steroids, adipsin, adiponectin, adipophilin, tissue factor, resistin (Bray 1998, Frühbeck 2001). Visceral fat depots determine a high bazal and catecolamine-induced lypolitic activity. As a result, an increased flow of free fatty acids is directed towards periphery, acting: 1) directly on the liver to interfere with glucose handling, insulin clearance and increasing lipoprotein synthesis, and 2) on skeletal muscle, where are preferential oxidized, leading to the development of insulin resistance. Hyperinsulinaemia, developed as a compensation, maintains normoglycaemia in the first phase, but induces a cascade of metabolic, haemodynamic and haemorrheological disturbances.

Lipid Disorders and Oxidative Stress

Changes in plasma lipoproteins are influenced by insulin resistance, hyperinsulinaemia and altered sex steroid and glucocorticoid levels, seen in visceral obesity. Both qualitative and quantitative changes occur (Despres 2001).

- Quantitative alterations:
  - Hypertriglyceridaemia (VLDL and IDL increase)
  - Postprandial hyperlipidaemia
  - Decrease of HDL-2 (reduced lipoprotein lipase activity)
  - Increased total cholesterol/HDL-cholesterol ratio
  - Increased Apo-B concentration
- Qualitative alterations:
  - Increase of triglycerides-rich lipoproteins, more susceptible to hepatic lipase, leading to an increased number of LDL particles which are smaller and more dense, with a higher probability to be oxidized and thus to be more atherogenic
  - High percentage of small and dense HDL particles, with low cholesterol removal capacity

Haemodynamic Effect

Hyperinsulinaemia and visceral obesity are considered independent risk factors for hypertension. The mechanisms involved refer to: high sodium and water retension, enhanced sympathetic nervous system activity, increased sodium-pompe activity in skeletal muscle, arterial walls hypertrophy IGF-1 induced.

Haemorrheological Effects

Insulin resistance/hyperinsulinaemia are associated with the inhibition of fibrinolysis and hypercoagulability, with impact on cardiovascular and macrovascular disease (Juhan-Vague 1991, Carter 1997, Agewal 1999). These haemorrheological alterations consist of the elevation in: (1) Plasminogen activator inhibitor 1 (PAI-1), leading to fibrinolysis inhibition, (2) Plasminogen activator tissue antigen (tPA), (3) Fibrinogen, (4) von Willebrand factor, (5) Factor VII and 6) High blood viscosity and erythrocyte aggregability (Serrano-Rios 1998).

Atherogenic Effects

Endogenous hyperinsulinaemia is involved in atherogenesis by: (1) stimulating mitosis and DNA synthesis in endothelium and smooth muscular cells, (2) increasing plasminogen activator inhibitor 1 (PAI-1), (3) increasing intracellular cholesterol, (4) inducing foam cells, (5) increasing procoagulation factors (Sowers JR et colab. 1994). The insulin effects are mediated through IGF-1 receptors.

Endothelial Dysfunction

Endothelial dysfunction is one of the major factors involved both in the progression of atheroma plaque and in its instability, favouring the development of intravascular thrombosis (Serrano-Rios 1998, Ferrara LA et colab. 1993).

Metabolic X Syndrome

The concept of the Metabolic X Syndrome, introduced by Reaven (1998), recently called "dysmetabolic syndrome" (Valantine 2001, Groop 2001), includes the association of the following features:

- Insulin resistance/hyperinsulinaemia, recognised as the etiopathogenic element
- Glucose intolerance or Type 2 Diabetes mellitus
- Hypertriglyceridaemia
- Postprandial hyperlipidaemia
- Low HDL-cholesterol
- Hypertension
- Abdominal obesity (De Fronzo and Ferranini 1991)
- Hyperuricemia
- Sedentary lifestyle
- Low fibrinolysis activity through PAI-1 increased plasmatic level
- Prothrombotic tendency
- High level of small and dense LDL particles
- Endothelial dysfunction
- Microalbuminuria
- Hyperleptinaemia (Leyva et al. 1998)
- Low chronic inflammation state (raised interleukin 6 and C reactive protein (Despres 2001)
- Nonalcoholic fatty liver disease (Marchesini et al. 2001)

This cluster of the above mentioned anomalies substantially increases the risk of coronary heart disease in affected persons. The cardiovascular risk related to metabolic syndrome consists of the high and early probability of developing atherosclerotic pathology and is a result of the specific action of each component, amplified by their association (Hâncu and Roman 1999).

In accordance to the World Health Organization proposal, the diagnosis of the metabolic syndrome in persons with Type 2 Diabetes is confirmed if two of the following criteria are fulfilled (Alberti 1998):

- Hypertension (systolic blood pressure > 160 mm Hg, and diastolic blood pressure > 90 mm Hg) or antihypertensive treatment
- Dyslipidaemia, defined as triglycerides ≥ 1.7 mmol/l (150 mg/dl) and/or HDL cholesterol < 0.9 mmol/l (35 mg/dl) in men and 1.0 mmol/l (38 mg/dl) in women
- Obesity
- Microalbuminuria (urinary albumin excretion rate-AER ≥ 20 µg/min)

In persons without diabetes a positive diagnosis requires the presence of insulin resistance, defined as the highest quartile of the $HOMA_{IR}$ index (Alberti 1998).

According to The Third Report of the National Cholesterol Education Program (NCEP) Expert Panel on Detection, Evaluation, and Treatment of High Blood Cholesterol in Adults – Adult Treatment Panel III (ATP III), the metabolic syndrome is diagnosed if three of the following five criteria are fulfilled:

- Abdominal obesity, defined as waist circumference > 102 cm (> 40 in) in men and > 88 cm (> 35 in) in women
- Triglycerides ≥ 150 mg/dl (1.7 mmol/l)
- HDL-cholesterol < 40 mg/dl in men and < 50 mg/dl in women
- Blood pressure ≥ 130/≥ 85 mm Hg
- Fasting glucose ≥ 110 mg/dl

In men, waist circumferences of 94–102 cm (37–39 in) can be associated with increased metabolic risk.

Obesity makes a significant contribution to the morbidity and mortality associated with Type 2 diabetes. The risk of premature death is 10-fold greater in a diabetic person with BMI > 35 kg/m^2, compared with a non-obese diabetic person (Williams 1999). The mortality ratio for individuals whose body weight is 20–30% above ideal is 2.5–3.3 times higher than for those with normal weight, and for those with body weight more than 40% above ideal, the mortality ratio is 5.2–7.9 times higher (Maggio and Pi-Sunyer 1997). Obesity acts both as an (1) independent risk factor: increases peripheral resistance, leading to hypertension, left-ventricular hypertrophy and increases stroke volume, leading to cardiac output and left-ventricular hypertrophy, increases the renin-angiotensin activity and enhance the simpathetic nervous system, and (2) as a promoter in developing other cardiovascular risk factors. It exacerbates the insulin resistance and glucose intolerance, raises blood pressure, induces dyslipidaemia, induces prothrombotic status and it may predispose to micro- and macrovascular diabetic complications.

Dyslipidaemia is extremely atherogenic. The lipid profile is frequently characterized by (Grundy 1998):

- Moderate total hypercholesterolaemia (220–249 mg/dl)
- Hypertriglyceridaemia (> 150 mg/dl)
- Low HDL-cholesterol (< 40 mg/dl in men and < 50 mg/dl in women)
- Postprandial hyperlipidaemia
- High level of small and dense LDL particles

Hypertension in combination with obesity predisposes to heart failure, through eccentric ventricular dilatation, left-ventricular hypertrophy and diastolic dysfunction (Bray 1998). Hypertension is frequently associated with Type 2 diabetes (30–50%) and represents an independent predictive factor for ischemic heart disease, strokes, peripheral amputations. More than 75% of cardiovascular complications can be attributed to hypertension.

Hyperglicaemia represents a predictive factor for cardiovascular mortality, ischemic heart disease, strokes and peripheral amputations caused by obliterant arterial disease (EARPG 1997).

According to UKPDS, the quintet of major risk factors for ischemic heart disease are: LDL-cholesterol, HDL-cholesterol, HbA1c, systolic blood pressure and smoking.

Metabolically obese, normal weight (MONW) concept refers to the presence of insulin resistance/hyperinsulinaemia, subsequently metabolic disorders and high cardiovascular risk, in non-obese individuals (Ruderman et al. 1998). MONW individuals characteristics are: BMI = 20–27 kg/m², moderate weight gain (2–10 kg of adipose mass) in adult life, central fat distribution and enlarged fat cells, physical inactivity and a low level of fitness, high prevalence in general population and high risk of developing Type 2 Diabetes, dyslipidaemia, hypertension and cardiovascular disease. Other potential factors related to MONW individuals might be low birth weight and genetic predisposition. The therapeutic consequence is that optimizing the lifestyle, significantly reduces the entire cluster of metabolic and haemostatic abnormalities.

Epidemiological Data

The risk for developing Type 2 Diabetes is directly related to BMI: it is 80-fold greater for a BMI > 40 kg/m² compared to BMI < 22 kg/m². The life-time risk for acquiring Type 2 Diabetes is approximately 50% in persons with morbid obesity (Williams 1999). In Type 2 Diabetes, 75% of mortality is caused by coronary heart disease. Diabetic persons are twice as likely to die from a heart attack or a stroke than non-diabetic persons, and 17 times more likely to suffer an amputation due to peripheral vascular disease (Astrup and Finer 2000). Compared to the general population, in Type 2 Diabetes, ischemic heart disease is doubly more frequent in men and four times more frequent in women, heart failure is five times more frequent in men and eight times more frequent in women; cerebrovascular disease is three times more frequent in men and doubled in women and myocardial infarction is two-three times more frequent, leading to double the chance of mortality (Laakso and Leato 1997).

When Type 2 Diabetes is diagnosed, other insuline resistance syndrome components already exist. According to the Diabetes Intervention Study (DIS), 70% of newly-diagnosed Type 2 Diabetic patients presented components of metabolic syndrome, 80.5% of men and 85% of women were obese. Cardiac mortality among them was 25.9%.

The study conducted by Isomaa, on 4,483 individuals participating in the Botnia study, identified the metabolic syndrome in 42% women, respectively 64% men with impaired fasting glucose or impaired glucose tolerance and in 78% women and 84% men, with Type 2 Diabetes mellitus. The risk for coronary heart disease, stroke and cardiovascular mortality were markedly increased in subjects with the metabolic syndrome ($p < 0.001$) (Isomaa et al. 2001).

Suggestive data have been shown by "EPIDIAB" (Epidemic of diabetes), an ongoing Romanian study. The EPIDIAB Program, started in January 2000 and designed to last five years, has as objectives to analyze the newly-diagnosed cases of diabetes, in terms of epidemic, quality and costs of care and to develop strategic prediction. In 2000, 15,057 persons and in 2001, 16,394 persons, from a population of 7 millions, were diagnosed with diabetes, 90%, respectively 93% of them with Type 2 Diabetes. Analyzing the prevalence of cardiovascular risk factors among Type 2 Diabetes patients, the following data have been found (Hâncu et al. 2001):

a. *Prevalence of overweight and obesity in newly diagnosed type 2 diabetic patients* (Fig. 10.1). As we expected, a high prevalence of overweight, obesity and abdominal fat distribution was demonstrated.
b. *Prevalence of cardiovascular risk factors (CVRF) according to BMI*, was calculated for 870 Type 2 newly diagnosed diabetic patients. Obesity is correlated to a higher degree with dyslipidaemia, hypertension and family history of metabolic and cardiovascular disease (Fig. 10.2). Overall prevalence of cardiovascular risk factors in newly-diagnosed type 2 diabetic patients is presented in Fig. 10.3.
c. *Distribution in clinical risk classes* was made by adjusting BMI according to other cardiovascular risk factors (dyslipidaemia, hypertension, glycaemia, presence of cardiovascular disease) (Bray 1998). Due to the association of these factors, 67 % of the patients were included in the high risk clinical class (Fig. 10.4).

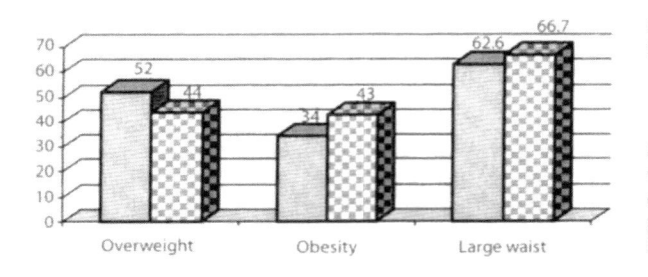

Fig. 10.1. Prevalence of overweight and obesity in newly diagnosed Type 2 diabetes patients. (EPIDIAB Study, N. Hâncu et al. 2001)

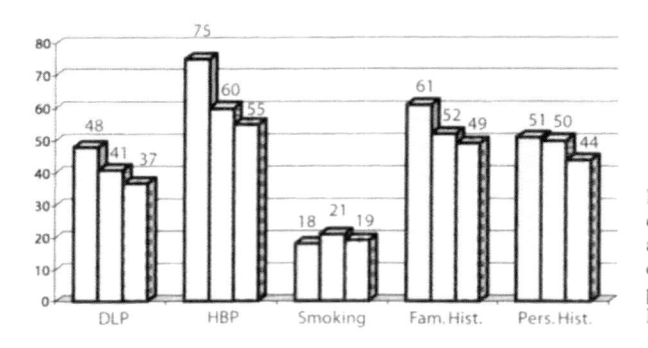

Fig. 10.2. Prevalence of cardiovascular risk factors according to BMI, in newly diagnosed Type 2 diabetic patients. (EPIDIAB Study, N. Hâncu et al. 2001)

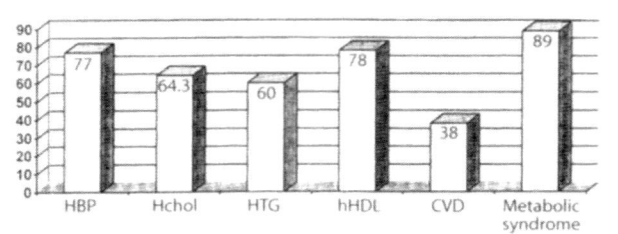

Fig. 10.3. Prevalence of cardiovascular risk factors in newly diagnosed Type 2 diabetic patients. *HBP*, high blood pressure; *Hchol*, hypercholesterolemia; *HTG*, hypertriglyceridaemia; *hHDL*, hypoHDL-cholesterolemia; *CVD*, cardiovascular disease. (EPIDIAB Study, N. Hâncu et al. 2001)

d. *Distribution of cardiovascular risk factors and cardiovascular risk according to BMI and waist circumference.* 333 patients were studied in order to evaluate the number of cardiovascular risk factors (Fig. 10.5) and the cardiovascular risk related to BMI and waist (Figs. 10.6, 10.7). To estimate the cardiovascular risk the Euro '98 Chart was used.

Due to the presence and association of cardiovascular risk factors, more than half of newly-diagnosed Type 2 diabetic patients have high cardiovascular risk (Fig. 10.8).

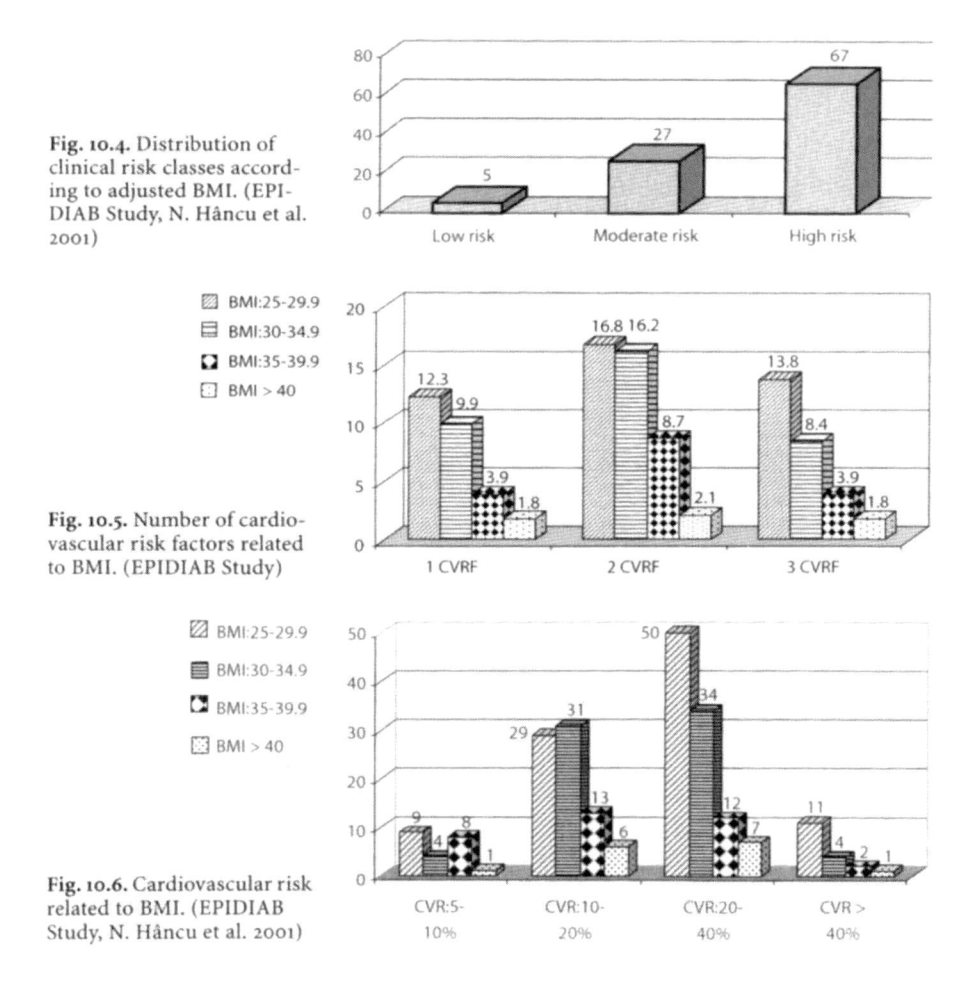

Fig. 10.4. Distribution of clinical risk classes according to adjusted BMI. (EPIDIAB Study, N. Hâncu et al. 2001)

Fig. 10.5. Number of cardiovascular risk factors related to BMI. (EPIDIAB Study)

Fig. 10.6. Cardiovascular risk related to BMI. (EPIDIAB Study, N. Hâncu et al. 2001)

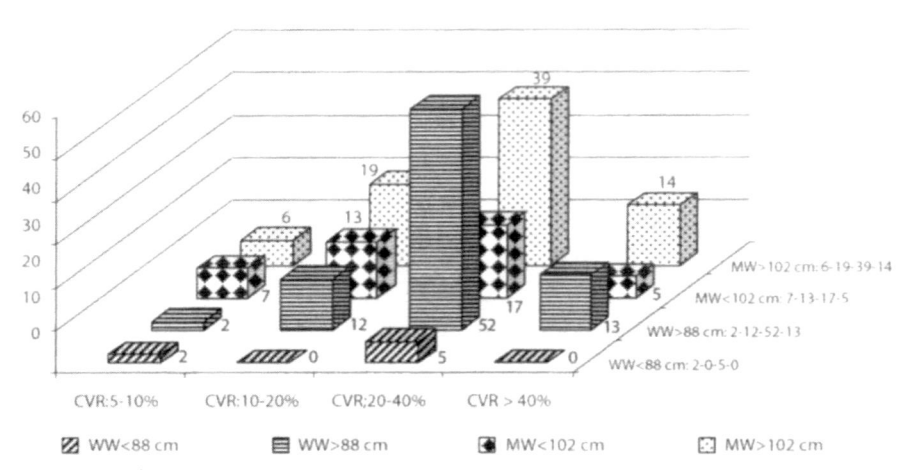

Fig. 10.7. Cardiovascular risk related to waist. *WW*, women waist; *MW*, men waist. (EPIDIAB Study, N. Hâncu et al. 2001)

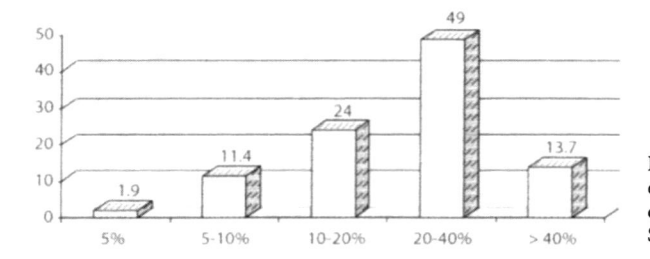

Fig. 10.8. Cardiovascular risk of newly diagnosed Type 2 diabetic patients. (EPIDIAB Study)

Clinical Significance

The clinical significance of the metabolic syndrome is related to its putative impact on cardiovascular morbidity and mortality.

To reduce the high rate of cardiovascular disease events and mortality in individuals with Type 2 Diabetes, an aggressive approach is required, in terms of risk factor identification, global risk evaluation and targeted interventions (see Chapter 21). Weight loss should be considered a major objective of the clinical management. The effect of intensional weight loss on mortality has been demonstrated by a study on the 12-year mortality of 4,970 overweight, Type 2 diabetic persons (Williamson et al. 2000). Intensional weight loss was reported by 34% of the patients, leading to a 25% reduction in total mortality and a 28% reduction in cardiovascular disease and diabetes mortality.

Suggested Recommendations for the Clinical Management of Obesity in Type 2 Diabetes Mellitus

General Considerations

As we have seen in the previous chapters, most individuals with Type 2 Diabetes are overweight or obese. Insulin resistance, associated with hyperglycemia, hyperlipidemia and hypertension, is directly related to body weight and adiposity. Therefor, weight loss may be one of the most important therapeutic objective for individuals with Type 2 Diabetes.

There is strong evidence (level A) supporting that in insulin resistant individuals, reduced energy intake and modest weight loss reduce insulin resistance, glycaemia, lipids, blood pressure in the short-term (Franz and Associates, 2002).

Goals for the Clinical Management of Overweight and Obesity

Weight control (weight loss and new weight maintenance) has a key role in the clinical management of Type 2 Diabetes. Moderate weight loss results in improvement of all major obesity related co-morbidities, including Type 2 Diabetes. The obese Type 2 diabetic persons face extra impediments to weight loss, including the effects of diabetic medication, poor glycaemic control and diabetes-related complications.

The goals can be stratified as:
- Short-term goals:
  - One cycle "weight loss – new weight maintenance", represented by a moderate weight loss, of 5–10%, in 3–6 months, followed by the new weight maintenance, for 6–9 months
  - Lifestyle optimization
  - Reduction of other cardiovascular risk factors
  - Reduction of obesity complications
- Long-term goals:
  - Successive cycles "weight loss-weight maintenance", untill a reasonable weight is achieved; the reasonable weight is associated with the lowest risk and an optimum quality of life
  - Long-term maintenance of reasonable weight
  - Weight regain prevention
  - Lifestyle changes maintenance
  - Quality of life maintenance
  - Control of cardiovascular risk factors and complications

Benefits of Weight Loss

A 5–10% weight reduction is associated with important medical benefits (Bray 1998, Donato 1998, Lean 1998, NIH, NHLBI 1998, Hâncu and Roman 1999, Kopelman 1999, Williamson 2000):

- Each kilo lost, mainly in the first year after diagnosis increases the life expectancy by 3–4 months

- The amount of weight loss in the first 12 months after diabetes diagnosis is related to life expectancy
- Weight loss in overweight diabetic persons is associated with 25% reduction in overall mortality over a follow-up period of 12 years
- A loss of 1-9 kg reduces the overall mortality by 30-40%
- Significant reduction of fasting plasma glucose (50%) and glycated hemoglobin (15%); the amount of improvement in glycaemic control is related to the magnitude of weight loss; to normalize glycaemia, a 20% decrease in body weight may be required (Wing 2001)
- Reduction in triglycerides (5-45%), LDL-cholesterol (15-25 mg/dl), total cholesterol (4-14%)
- Increase of HDL-cholesterol with 5-17%
- Decrease in blood pressure
- Decrease in insulin resistance
- Reduction of global cardiovascular risk
- Reduction of hypoglycaemic medication

Long-term data assessing the extent to which these improvements can be maintained are not available. The most successful long-term weight loss was reported by Diabetes Treatment Study, with a 9-kg weight loss maintained over 6 years (Franz and Associates 2002).

General Strategy of Clinical Management

The therapeutic approach of overweight or obese individuals with diabetes follows the same rules applied in non-diabetic obese persons, but it should be more sustained and more aggressive in terms of intention and methods. The clinical management must be goal directed and patient centered, taking into consideration lifestyle changes the individual can make and maintain. Involvement of patient in the decision-making process is strongly recommended.

The general strategy supposes two successive stages: (Fig. 10.9)
- Initial approach
  - Identification, global assessment and selection in the clinical risk classes
  - Short-term objectives setting
  - First cycle "weight loss – weight maintenance"
    Persons with newly diagnosed diabetes may be more likely to lose weight than those with a longer duration of diabetes, perhaps because the diagnosis serves as a "trigger" (Franz and Associates 2002).
- Long-term approach. Realistic methods should be adapted and applied according to medical criteria and patients possibilities. The following possibilities may be considered:
  - Maintenance of the new weight as long as possible
  - Further cycles "weight loss – maintenance" to achieve the desired weight
  - Long-term maintenance of the desired weight
  - Control of cardiovascular risk factors and complications

```
┌─────────────────────────────────────────────────────────┐
│         IDENTIFICATION, GLOBAL ASSESSMENT               │
│                                                         │
│  ┌──────────────────┐    ○  SHORT-TERM OBJECTIVES       │
│  │ INITIAL APPROACH │       - weight loss - 3- 6 months │
│  │ FIRST YEAR       │       - weight maintenance - 6 – 9 months │
│  └──────────────────┘  ○                                │
│                        ↓                                │
│  ┌──────────────────┐     LONG-TERM OBJECTIVES:         │
│  │ LONG-TERM        │  ○ - weight maintenance - one more year │
│  │ APPROACH         │    - new steps "weight loss-maintenance" │
│  └──────────────────┘                                   │
│      WEIGHT          ○         NEW STEPS                │
│      MAINTENANCE            „WEIGHT LOSS-MAINTENANCE"   │
│                                                         │
│        ○                  ○   ○   ○                     │
│            ┌─────────────────────┐                      │
│            │  REASONABLE WEIGHT  │                      │
│            └─────────────────────┘                      │
│              • LOW RISK                                 │
│              • GOOD QUALITY OF LIFE                     │
│              • LONG-TERM MAINTENANCE                    │
└─────────────────────────────────────────────────────────┘
```

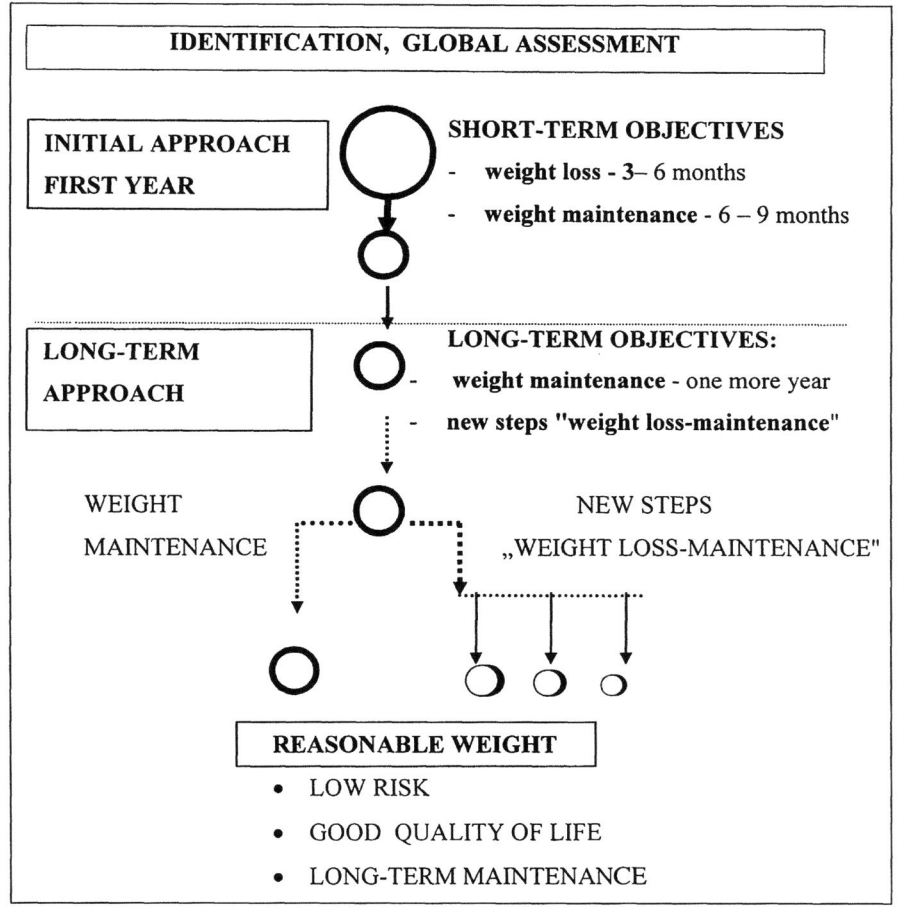

Fig. 10.9. Practical approach of persons with obesity and Type 2 diabetes. (Modified after Hâncu 2001)

Methods

The clinical management consists of a structured intervention based on the THEME Programmes (therapy, education, monitoring, evaluation) (Hâncu 2001) (Table 10.1).

Clinical Management

Therapy

Therapy refers to lifestyle optimization, medication and surgical intervention. Lifestyle optimization programmes involve diet, exercise and behavioural changes proved to produce about 7% decrease in body weight and significant changes in fasting blood glucose and other cardiovascular risk factors (Wing 2001). Strong evi-

Table 10.1. Clinical management of obesity: THEME programmes (Hâncu et al. 2000)

THEME Programmes	Comment
Therapy: Lifestyle and behavioural changes: – hypocaloric diet – standard – ULCD* – physical exercise – alcohol and smoking avoidance	→ Always recommended * Could be used for short period in patients at high risk, or BMI > 35 kg/m^2
Pharmacological therapy: – Sibutramine – Orlistat	→ To be considered
Gastric-reduction surgery	→ Limited at patients with very high risk
Therapeutic education and behavioural therapy	→ Compulsory to implement the therapy
Monitoring *Evaluation*	→ Recommended for continous communication with the patient and for quality of care assessment

dences (level A), sustain that structured programmes that emphasize lifestyle changes, including education, reduced fat (< 30 % of daily energy) and energy intake, regular physical activity and regular participant contact, can produce long-term weight loss of 5 – 7 % of starting weight (Franz and Associates 2002)

Diet

Weight Loss

To achieve this objective, a reduced caloric intake should be prescribed, dietary fat being the most important nutrient to be restricted. Reduced-fat diets, when maintained long term, contribute to modest weight loss and improvement of dyslipidaemia (evidence level B). When used alone, standard weight-reduction diets are unlikely to produce long-term weight loss; intensive lifestyle intervention is necessary (evidence level A) (Franz and Associates 2002).

Standard weight-reduction diets, 1,200 – 1,800 kcalories per day provide 500 – 1,000 fewer calories than are estimated to be necessary for weight maintenance. The result will be a weight loss of 1 – 2 kg per week or 10 % of initial body weight (Bray 1998, Donato 1998, Hâncu and Roman 1999). Use of foods made with nondigestible fat (olestra) may be considered in order to reduce the energy intake. Alcohol must be avoided.

Diet composition should be kept balanced. The following structure is now considered (Franz and Associates 2002):

- Carbohydrate and monounsaturated fat should together provide 60 – 70 % of energy intake (level E – expert consensus)
- Saturated fat should provide < 10 %, unless specific lipid target, when < 7 % is recomended (level A)

- Polyunsaturated fat should be approximately 10 % of energy intake (level C)
- Dietary cholesterol intake should be < 300 mg/day or less (level A)
- Protein intake should be 15 – 20 % of total daily energy (level E)
- Consumption of dietary fiber is to be encouraged (level B)

With very-low-calorie diets (VLCD), providing 800 kcalories or less per day, the caloric deficit and the rate of weight loss are approximately 2 to 3 times higher that of conventional diets. VLCD can produce substantial weight loss and rapid improvements in glycaemia (even before significant weight loss) and lipaemia. However, it has limited utility when considered as a long-term approach, due to the high percentage of recidivism and reduced patient compliance. A possibility is that VLCDs could be used intermittently and repetitively for short periods.

Vitamins and minerals supplementation might be considered.

Another option could be the structured meal replacements, that provide a defined amount of energy (200 – 300 calories), most of it derived from protein and carbohydrate. Use of meal replacements once or twice daily can result in significant weight loss (Franz and Associates 2002).

For a better adherence, the diet recommendations should be individualized and negotiated with the patient, in order to meet his/her preferences and possibilities. The nutrition prescription should consider treatment goals and lifestyle changes the person is willing and able to make. Therapeutic education should enssure and facilitate healthy choices.

When hypoglycaemic medication is associated (sulfonylureas or insulin), specific indications (amount of carbohydrates, meal timing) should be made to avoid hypoglycaemic episodes.

Weight Maintenance

Recomendations to be given during this phase reffer to the possibility of adding 200 – 300 more calories, while physical activity is increased and weight is carefully observed (Hâncu and Roman 1999).

Analysing individuals who successfully lost weight and maintained it long term, predictors of success have been identified: continuous consumption of low-energy and low-fat food (average energy consumption of 1,400 kcalories/day, with 24 % of energy derived from fat), average energy expenditure through added physical activity of 2,800 kcalories/week, meaning 1.5 hours of exercise daily (Shick 1998).

Physical Exercise

Weight Loss

Physical exercise improves insulin sesnsitivity, acutely lowers blood glucose and improves cardiovascular status. It is unanimously accepted that regular physical activity is a cornerstone in the treatment of patients with obesity and Type 2 Diabetes. It is adjunct to diet for weight reduction and maintenance and increased fat loss. Unfortunately long-term adherence to regular physical activity programmes is reduced. In a study of Mattfeldt-Beman et al. (1999) evaluation of a weight loss programme revealed that exercise is considered by the patients the least useful in the treatment programme. As the main effect of exercise is in maintaining of weight loss and cardiovascular fitness, physical activities must be chosen to be safe, sustainable and pleasant for long-term adherence.

The exercise prescription consists of four components: type, intensity, frequency and duration, which must be adjusted to the patient's medical condition, preferences and possibilities, after negotiating with the patient (Donato 1998).

- Type:
  - Aerobic exercise involving repetitive submaximal contractions of large muscle groups are preferred (brisk walking, cycling, swimming)
  - Recent studies report that mild but frequent exercise improves insulin sensitivity and can contribute to weight loss
  - Where appropriate, moderate resistance exercise should be considered in addition, with good effect on insulin sensitivity, hypertension, lipids, and glucose tolerance
- Intensity:
  - Should be progressively increased according to blood pressure increased rate (<200 mm Hg) and maximum pulse rate (220-age)
  - Starts at 40–50% of the patient's maximal aerobic capacity (maximal pulse rate) with gradual increments to 60–70% over 6–8 weeks
  - Special precautions should be taken for patients with complications or cardiovascular disease
  - Initiation of high exercise intensity must be avoided
- Duration and frequency:
  - 20–60 minutes daily, preferable during the morning, at least 5 days/week
  - Accumulation of smaller amounts of exercise, wherever feasible represents an equivalent alternative which increase adherence
- Programme: When a structured programme of exercise is prescribed, mainly when a high intensity exercise is included, following steps should be considered at each session:
  - Stretching 5–10 min
  - Warm up 5–10 min
  - Exercise 20–45 min
  - Warm down 10 min
- Special precautions:
  - Feet should be inspected daily and always after exercise
  - Exercise should be avoided in extreme hot or cold environments
  - Avoid postprandial exercise in patients with coronary artery disease and ortostatic hypotension
  - Special information should be provided in order to avoid hypos

Weight Maintenance

The greatest benefit of physical exercise seems to be in the maintenance of weight loss (Wing 2001) and cardiovascular fitness. An increase in duration and frequency of physical exercise in this period is recommended, in order to maintain weight and to allow a moderate increase of caloric intake.

Pharmacological Therapy

Use of specific medication enhances the weight loss. Weight-loss drugs are an important new approach in the treatment of obese patients. Available data suggest that weight loss medication, in conjunction with lifestyle strategies, may be useful in the treatment of patients with obesity and Type 2 Diabetes. However, the effect of this medication is modest.

Medication to be considered is:

Orlistat, a pancreatic lipase inhibitor blocks gastrointestinal absorbtion of about 30% of ingested fat.

In a 1-year randomized, double-blind, placebo-controlled study, the weight loss with orlistat was 6.2%, compare to placebo 4.3% ($p < 0.001$) (Hollander et al. 1998). Other effects were (Sjostrom et al. 1998, Heymsfield et al. 2000):

- Significant reduction of fasting glycaemia, glycated hemoglobin, total cholesterol, LDL-cholesterol, triglycerides and LDL/HDL-cholesterol ratio
- Reduction of fasting insulinaemia
- Reduction of sulphonylures doses

Sibutramine, a serotonin (5-HT) and noradrenaline reuptake inhibitor, has a dual mechanism of action: it reduces food intake by enhancing post-ingestive satiety and increase energy expenditure through enhancing thermogenesis. In addition, its metabolites reduce insulin resistance.

Randomized, double-blind, placebo-controlled studies, using sibutramine 15 mg/day, 12 and 24 weeks have obtained:

- A higher percentage of patients losing >5% of baseline body weight
- A significant decrease in body weight
- A significant improvement of glycemic control (decrease of 2-hour postprandial plasma glucose level and serum insulin level, decrease in HbA1c), compared to placebo use (Finer 2000).

Existing data suggest that these drugs maintain their efficacy only as long as they are taken. A meta-analysis of randomized clinical trials of medication for obesity, demonstrates that sibutramine has large effect sizes of weight loss even in drug-free follow-up period (Haddock et al. 2002). Even if there is no evidence of the efficacy and safety of a long-term medication in patients with Type 2 Diabetes, pharmacological therapy should be considered. Obesity medications can result in important reductions in overall medication use and net costs associated with obesity-related comorbidities (Haddock et al. 2002).

Gastric Reduction Surgery

At present gastric-reduction surgery seems to be the most effective weight-loss treatment, offering major sustained weight loss.

The Gothenburg-led Swedish Obese Subjects (SOS) study of primary prevention of severe obesity by bariatric surgery, demonstrated a sustained weight loss of more than 20 kg and a 2–32 fold reduction of 2-year incidence of diabetes, hypertension, hypertriglyceridaemia and hypo-HDL. The 10-year incidence of Type 2 diabetes was five-fold reduced. Thus bariatric surgery is an effective way to improve most cardiovascular risk factors (Sjöström 2000).

However it is recommended that such surgery should be considered only in Type 2 diabetic patients with BMI > 35 kg/m² (NIH 1991, Campbell and Rössner 2001).

Vertical banded gastroplasty is the preferable surgical procedure. Long-term data comparing the benefits and risks of gastric reduction surgery to those of medical therapy are not available.

Therapeutic Education and Behavioural Therapy

Both are methods that should be integrated in the clinical management in order to provide knowledge and to induce motivation and skills. To be efficient, both education and behavioural therapy must be individualized and adapted to the patient and systematically and continuously applied. A combination of individual and group therapy, associated with written material seems to be the most efficient approach.

Important behavioural approaches are self-control, self-observation, stimulus control to promote cues for healthy lifestyle and family and social support.

Monitoring

It assures the quality and the continuity of clinical management. Parameters to be followed are:

- Weight, waist circumference, BMI
- Lifestyle: adherence to diet, physical activity
- Glycemic control, lipids profile, blood pressure
- Cardiovascular status
- Adverse events
- Quality of life

Increasing the length of treatment contact appears to improve long-term outcome and markedly reduces weight regain. The frequency of these contacts may be more important than their content: biweekly visits seem to be more effective than monthly contact (Wing 2001).

An important parameter to be monitored and controled is the weight gain related to hypoglicemic medication, which could be considered the price paied for the glycemic control. Use of sulphonylurea drugs and insulin treatment are associated with weight gain. Due to its mechanism of action, metformin is free in weight gain effect. The glitazone class of drugs, act on glycemic control by increasing insulin sensitivity, but subsequently promote weight gain by stimulating adipogenesis. It seems that in this case the body fat gained is in the subcutaneous layer, not in the visceral and therefore should have less deleterious metabolic impact (Campbell and Rössner 2001).

Evaluation

A periodically global assessment is necessary in order to adjust and coordinate the clinical management.

Concluding Remarks

Obesity and Type 2 Diabetes mellitus are frequently associated. There incidence is accelerating throughout the world.

Along with hypertension, dyslipidaemia, characterized by a low HDL-cholesterol level, small, dense low-density lipoprotein cholesterol and high triglyceride levels, increased prothrombotic and antifibrinolytic factors, visceral obesity and Type 2 Diabetes are components of a risk factor constellation, termed "insulin resistance syndrome", "syndrome X", "metabolic" or "dysmetabolic" syndrome. Insulin resistance and hyperinsulinaemia associated with the syndrome, appear to play a central role and are considered the etiopathogenic elements. Genetic and environmental factors are disscussed to be involved in developing insulin resistance, which is recognized as the common soil for the development of both diabetes and coronary heart disease.

The clinical importance of the metabolic syndrome is related to its putative impact on cardiovascular morbidity and mortality. Newly-diagnosed Type 2 diabetic patients associate at least one cardiovascular risk. Screening for associated comorbid conditions and aggressiv control of all cardiovascular risk factors should be major objectives of the clinical management.

All efforts should be made to achieve weight loss and weight control, as proved to be beneffic. Structured THEME programmes (therapy, education, monitoring and evaluation) should be applied. Lifestyle optimization, through low-fat hypocaloric diet, physical activity and behaviour changes, associated with weight-loss inducing medication are methods to be considered.

References

1. Agewal S (1999) Insulin sensitivity and haemostatic factors in men at high and low cardiovascular risk. The Risk Factor Intervention Study Group. J. Intern. Med. 246(5): 489–495
2. Alberti KGMM, Zimmet PZ (1998) Definition, diagnosis and classification of diabetes mellitus and its complications. Part 1: Diagnosis and classification of diabetes mellitus, provisional report of a WHO consultation. Diabet Med 15: 539–553
3. Astrup A, Finer N (2000) Redefining Type 2 diabetes: "Diabesity" or "Obesity Dependent Diabetes Mellitus" ?. Obesity Reviews 1:57–59
4. Bantle J. B. (1999) Weight – loss Treatments for Overweight Individuals with Diabetes. American Diabetes Association Guide to Medical Nutrition Therapy for Diabetes. In Marion J. Franz, Bantle J. B (eds), Clinical Education Series, pp 69–85
5. Bray GA (1998) Contemporary Diagnosis and Management of Obesity. Handbooks in Health Care Co.,N Newton, Pennsylvania
6. Campbell L, Rössner S (2001) Management of obesity in patients with Type 2 diabetes. Diabet Med 18: 345–354
7. Carter AM, Grant PJ (1997) Vascular homeostasis adhesion molecules and macrovascular disease in non-insulin-dependent diabetes mellitus. Diabetic Med 14:423–432
8. Chan JM, Stampfer MJ, Ribb EB, Willet WC, Colditz GA (1994) Obesity, fat distribution and fat gain as risk factors for clinical diabetes in man. Diabetes Care 17:961–969
9. Consensus Development Conference Panel: Gastrointestinal surgery for severe obesity (1991). Ann Intern Med 115: 956–961
10. Donato K.A. (coordinator) (1998) Executive summary of the clinical guidelines on the identification, evaluation and treatment of the overweight and obesity in adults. Arch. Int. Med.158 (Sept.): 1855–1867
11. De Fronzo R.A., Ferranini E (1991) Insulin resistance: a multifocal syndrome responsible for

NIDDM, obesity, hypertension, dyslipidemia and atherosclerotic cardiovascular disease. Diabetes Care 14:173–194
12. Despres J-P, Isabelle Lemieux, Denis Prud'homme (2001) Treatment of obesity: need to focus on high risk abdominally obese patients. BMJ 322:716–720
13. European Arterial Risk Policy Group (1997) A strategy for arterial risk assessment and management in type 2 diabetes mellitus. Diabetic Med 14: 611–621
14. Expert Panel on Detection, Evaluation, and Treatment of High Blood Cholesterol in Adults: Executive Summary of the Third Report of the National Cholesterol Education Program (NCEP) Expert Panel on Detection, Evaluation, and Treatment of High Blood Cholesterol in Adults (Adult Treatment Panel III). JAMA 285: 2486–2497
15. Ferrara LA, Mancini M, Celentano A, Galderisi M, Iannuzi R, Marotta T, Gaeta I (1993) Early changes of the arterial carotid wall in hyperinsulinemia, hypertriglyceridemia versus hypercholesterolemia. Arterioscler Thromb 13:367–370
16. Finer N, Bloom SR, Frost GS, Banks LM, Griffiths J (2000) Sibutramine is effective for weight loss and diabetic control in obesity with type 2 diabetes: a randomised, double-blind, placebo-controlled study. Diabetes, Obesity Metab, 2: 105–112
17. Frühbeck G (2001) Adipose tissue as an endocrine organ. Obesity Matters 1: 16–20
18. Groop L, Orho-Melander M (2001) The dysmetabolic syndrome. J Intern Med 250 (2): 105–120
19. Grundy SM (1998) Hypertriglyceridemia, atherogenic dyslipidemia and the metabolic syndrome. Am J Cardiol 81 (4 A): 18B-25B
20. Haddock CK, Poston WSC, Dill PL, Foreyt JP, Ericsson M (2002). Pharmacotherapy for obesity: a quantitative analysis of four decades of published randomized clinical trials. Int J Obesity 26: 262–273
21. Han TS, Richmond P, Avenell A, Lean MEJ (1997) Waist circumference reduction and cardiovascular benefits during weight loss in women. Int J Obesity 21:127–134
22. Hauptman J (1998) Role of orlistat in the treatment of obese patients with type 2 diabetes: a 1-tear randomized double-blind study. Diabetes Care 21: 1288–1294
23. Hâncu N, Roman G (1999) Sindromul X metabolic. In N. Hâncu, IA Veresiu (eds) Diabetul zaharat, Nutriţia, Bolile metabolice. National, Bucharest, pp 477–489
24. Hâncu N, Roman G (1999) Obezitatea. In N. Hâncu, IA Veresiu (eds) Diabetul zaharat, Nutriţia, Bolile metabolice. National, Bucharest, pp 93–143
25. Hâncu N (coordinator) (2001) Recomandări pentru managementul obezităţii si supraponderii la adulţi. Jurnalul Român de Diabet, Nutriţie şi Boli metabolice, 2 suppl. 1
26. Hâncu N, Roman G, Cif A, Vereşiu IA, Cerghizan A, Cernea S (2001) Obesity and cardiovascular risk in persons with newly diagnosed diabetes mellitus ("EPIDIAB" study in Romania-2000). International Journal of Obesity and related disorders, 25, supl. 2: S 86 (abstract)
27. Hâncu N, Vereşiu IA, Roman G (2001) Romanian diabetes epidemics programme ("EPIDIAB"). First year results. Diabetologia, Clinical and Experimental Diabetes and Metabolism, suppl. 1 (abstract)
28. Heymsfield SB., Segal KR., Hauptman J. et al (2000) Changes in effects of weight loss with orlistat on glucose tolerance and progression to type 2 diabetes in obese adults. Arch. Intern. Med.:1361-1369
29. Hollander PA, Elbein SC, Hirsch IB, Kelley D, McGill J, Taylor T, Weiss SR, Crockett SE, Kaplan RA, Comstock J, Lucas CP, Lodewick PA, Canovatchel W, Chung J, Hauptman J (1998) Role of orlistat in the treatment of obese patients with type 2 diabetes: a 1-tear randomized double-blind study. Diabetes Care 21: 1288–1294
30. Isomaa B, Almgren P, Tuomi T, Forsen B, Lahti K, Nissen M, Taskinen MR, Groop L (2001) Cardiovascular morbidity and mortality associated with the metabolic syndrome. Diabetes Care 24: 683–689
31. Juhan-Vague I, Alessi MC, Vague P (1991) Increased plasma plasminogen activator inhibitor 1 levels: a possible link between insulin resistance and atherothrombosis. Diabetologia 34:457–462
32. Laakso M, Leato S (1997) Epidemiology of macrovascular disease in diabetes. Diabetes Rev 5: 294–315
33. Lean M.(1998) Clinical handbook of weight management. Martin Dunitz (ed), London
34. Leyva F., Godsland IF, Ghatei M, Proudler AJ, Aldis S, Walton C, Bloom S, Stevenson JC (1998) Hyperleptinemia as a Component of a Metabolic Syndrome of Cardiovascular Risk. Arteriosclerosis, Thrombosis, and Vascular Biology 18(6): 928–933

35. Marchesini G, Brizi M, Bianchi G, Tomassetti S, Bugianesi E, Lenzi M, McCullough AJ, natale S, Forlani G, Melchionda N (2001) Nonalcoholic Fatty Liver Disease-A Feature of the Metabolic Syndrome. Diabetes 50: 1844–1850
36. Mattfeldt-Beman MK, Corrigan SA, Stevens VJ, Sugars CP, Dalcin AT, Givi MJ et al. (1999) Participants' evaluation of a weight-loss program. J Am Diet Assoc, 99: 66–71
37. National Institutes of Health, National Heart Lung and Blood Institute (1998). Clinical Guidelines for the Identification, Evaluation and Treatment of Overweight and Obesity in Adults: The Evidence Report. Bethesda: US Department of Health and Human Services, Public Health Service, NIH, NHLBI
38. Ruderman N, Chisholm D, Pi-Sunier X, Schneider S (1998) The Metabolically Obese, Norma-Weight Individual Revisited. Diabetes 47: 699–713
39. Reaven G (1998) Role of insulin resistance in human disease. Diabetes 37:1595–1607
40. Serrano-Rios M (1998) Relationship between obesity and the increased risk of major complications in non-insulin-dependent diabetes mellitus. Eur J Clin Invest 28:14–18
41. Shick SM, Wing RR, lem ML, McGuire MT, Seagle H (1998) Persons successful at long-term weight loss and maintenance continue to consume a low-energy, low-fat diet. J Am Diet Assoc, 98: 408–413
42. Sjöström S (2000). Obesity, diabetes and other cardiovascular risk factors. Int J Obes, 24: S7
43. Sjostrom I., Rissanen A., Andersen I. et al. (1998) Randomised placebo-controlled trial of orlistat for weight loss and prevention of weight regain in obese patients. Lancet, 352: 167-172.
44. Sowers JR, Sowers PS, Peuler JD (1994) Role of insulin resistance and hyperinsulinemia in development of hypertension and atherosclerosis. J Lab Clin Med 123: 647–652
45. Valantine H, Rickenbacker P, Kemna M, Hunt S, Chen YD, Reaven G, Stinson EB (2001) Metabolic abnormalities characteristic of dysmetabolic syndrome predict the development of transplant coronary artery disease: a prospective study. Circulation 103 (17): 2144–2152
46. Wilding J, Williams G (1998) Diabetes and Obesity. In: Kopelman PG, Stock MJ (eds) Clinical obesity. Blackwell Science, pp 308–350
47. Williams G (1999) Obesity and type 2 diabetes: a conflict of interests?. International Journal of Obesity 23, suppl 7: S2-S4
48. Williamson DF, Thompson TJ, Michael T, Flanders D, Pamuk E, Byers T (2000) Intensional weight loss and mortality among overweight individuals with diabetes. Diabetes Care, 23: 1499–1504
49. Wing RR (2001) Weight loss in the management of Type 2 Diabetes. In: Gerstein HC, Haynes RB (eds) Evidence-Based Diabetes Care. BC Decker Inc, Hamilton, London, pp 252–277

CHAPTER 11

The Hypertriglyceridemic Waist Concept: Implication for Evaluation and Management of Cardiovascular Disease Risk in Type 2 Diabetes

I. Lemieux, J.-P. Després

Obesity Versus Body Fat Distribution

Obesity has long been recognized as a major risk factor for chronic disorders such as coronary heart disease (CHD) and Type 2 diabetes [1, 2]. Its increasing prevalence has led the World Health Organization to claim that increased adiposity is the major factor for the development of Type 2 diabetes [3]. However, despite this well established contribution of obesity in the etiology of diabetes, it is also more and more recognized that not every obese individual will develop this disease. In this regard, the regional distribution of body fat is a relevant factor playing a role in the modulation of the health hazards of obesity. The importance of body fat distribution as a determinant of various metabolic disorders has been initially emphasized by Vague who was the first to observe that android obesity was more closely associated with diabetes, atherosclerosis and gout than gynoid obesity [4]. Android obesity has also been referred to as upper body obesity, central obesity or abdominal obesity. This condi-

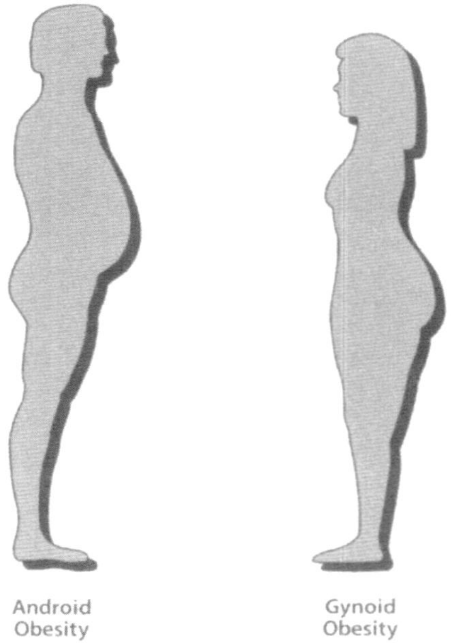

Fig. 11.1. Android and gynoid types of obesity as first defined by Vague (Vague, 1947), with preferential accumulation of adipose tissue respectively in the abdominal and gluteo-femoral regions. The android pattern of adipose tissue distribution is closely associated with the metabolic complications of obesity

tion is obviously more frequently observed in men than in women. Gynoid obesity, also referred to as lower body obesity or peripheral obesity, is the typical body fat distribution pattern observed in women (Fig. 11.1).

Influence of Gender, Age and Menopause Status on Regional Body Fat Distribution
Sexual Dimorphism

It is well recognized that there are gender differences in body fat distribution. Men are prone to accumulate upper body and abdominal fat, whereas women preferentially accumulate body fat in the gluteo-femoral region [5 – 7]. Furthermore, a striking gender evidence has been found in visceral adipose tissue accumulation which can be assessed by imaging techniques such as computed tomography [8, 9]. Visceral adipose tissue was found to represent on average 21% of the total body fat mass in men whereas in women only 8% of the body fat mass was located in the visceral depot [9]. Lemieux et al. [8] have examined the associations between amount of abdominal adipose tissue, measured by computed tomography, and the amount of total body fat in a sample of men and premenopausal women. Cross-sectional areas of abdominal adipose tissue were highly associated with total body fat mass in both men and women [8]. However, despite the fact that they had lower amounts of total body fat than did women, it was quite obvious that for any given total body fat mass, men had about twice the amount of abdominal visceral fat than that noted in premenopausal women [8] (Fig. 11.2). On the other hand, the accumulation of abdominal subcutaneous adipose tissue and its relationship to total body fatness was found to be essentially similar in both men and women [8]. In addition, an increase in total body fat was associated with a greater increase in visceral adipose tissue volume in men than in women,

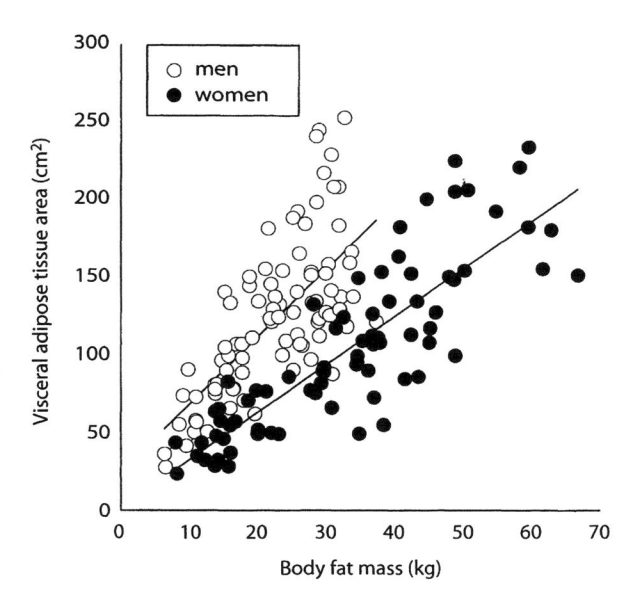

Fig. 11.2. Relationships between cross-sectional area of visceral adipose tissue measured by computed tomography and body fat mass in men and women ($r=0.71$, $p<0.0001$ in men and $r=0.76$, $p<0.0001$ in women). (Adapted from Lemieux et al. Am. J. Clin. Nutr., 1993)

suggesting that the greater health hazards generally associated with obesity in men than women could be explained by the fact that premenopausal women "can afford" to accumulate more body fat before reaching the levels of visceral adipose tissue found in men [8].

It is well known that the prevalence of cardiovascular diseases is greater in men than in women particularly before the onset of menopause and the reasons for this difference are not completely understood [10, 11]. Since the regional distribution of body fat is a distinct feature of sexual differentiation, it has been suggested that gender differences in body fat distribution could explain, at least to a certain extent, differences in cardiovascular disease risk factors noted between men and women [12–14]. In this regard, it was reported by Freedman and co-workers [12] that gender differences in the lipoprotein-lipid profile were attenuated after adjustment for the waist-to-hip ratio (WHR), a widely used index of body fat distribution. Accordingly, Larsson et al. [13] reported that after adjustment for the WHR, the gender difference in the incidence of CHD almost disappeared. Furthermore, the contribution of the gender difference in visceral fat accumulation measured by computed tomography to the sex dimorphism found in cardiovascular disease risk factors has also been investigated by Lemieux and colleagues [15]. It was found that after adjustment for body fat mass and levels of visceral adipose tissue, most gender differences in the lipoprotein-lipid variables and in indices of plasma glucose-insulin homeostasis disappeared with the exception of plasma HDL cholesterol concentrations, which remained higher in women than in men [15]. Whereas premenopausal women must accumulate more body fat mass than men before showing a deterioration in glucose tolerance which would be similar to men, a given excess of visceral adipose tissue appears to be associated with a similar deterioration in glucose tolerance in both men and women [15].

Age

The potential determinants of abdominal fat accumulation have not been fully elucidated. In recent years, several reports have described the relationship between age and body fat distribution [16–27]. Indeed, it was demonstrated in several studies that WHR increases with age in both men and in women [16–19]. Moreover, in both genders, the visceral adipose tissue accumulation has been shown to increase with age [22–28]. In this regard, Kotani and co-workers [28] reported that this age-related increase was approximately 2.6 times higher in men than in women. Enzi et al. [23] have shown that in young subjects, fat tissue is mainly located in the subcutaneous region, especially in women. They noted that the ratio of subcutaneous fat to visceral fat areas decreased with age in both genders [23]. These results were confirmed by our group as we also reported that age *per se* was associated with a preferential accumulation of fat in the abdominal cavity in women, even before the onset of menopause [24]. At least two longitudinal studies have examined changes in body fatness and visceral adipose tissue over time [25, 27]. During the 7-year follow-up period, it was found that women showed a selective deposition of abdominal fat, supporting the notion that visceral adipose tissue deposition generally increases with age [25, 27].

There is also with age an overall deterioration in the metabolic risk profile as an increase in the prevalence of impaired glucose tolerance and Type 2 diabetes is found [29–34]. Moreover, it has also been observed that insulin sensitivity decreases with age [35, 36]. As it has been shown that age is associated with a preferential accumulation of visceral adipose tissue [22–28], it was suggested that the deterioration in glucose tolerance and in plasma lipoprotein-lipid variables found with age could be explained, at least to a certain extent, by the concomitant increase in visceral adipose tissue. In this regard, we have recently reported in a sample of premenopausal women that the age-related increase in visceral adipose tissue was indeed an important correlate of some of the deterioration in the plasma lipoprotein-lipid profile and in plasma glucose homeostasis found with age [24]. Moreover, in a 7-year longitudinal study, we found that changes in visceral adipose tissue accumulation observed over that followup period were predictive of changes in glucose tolerance and plasma insulin levels [25]. Thus, women who lost visceral adipose tissue improved their indices of plasma glucose-insulin homeostasis whereas women with the greatest gain of visceral adipose tissue showed the most substantial deterioration in glucose tolerance and in plasma insulin levels [25].

Menopause

The menopause transition has been described as another potential determinant of regional body fat accumulation and several studies have documented this phenomenon [17, 28, 37–40]. As numerous studies had shown an age-related increase in the proportion of abdominal fat, more specifically in the visceral adipose depot [22–28], it is important to take into account the concomitant effect of age and of total body fat in the evaluation of the independent effect of menopause on body fat distribution and visceral adipose tissue accumulation. Results of cross-sectional studies on menopause and body fat distribution, in which WHR or waist circumference were used as a surrogate of visceral fat accumulation, failed to detect an effect of the menopause transition that was independent of age or of total body fatness as crudely estimated by the body mass index (BMI) [16, 19, 20, 41–45]. However, studies that measured visceral adipose tissue with imaging techniques found an effect of the menopause transition *per se* on body fat distribution which was independent of age, BMI or total body fatness [17, 28, 37–40]. Thus, more precise techniques to measure visceral adipose tissue indicate that the menopause transition is associated with an accelerated rate of selective deposition of visceral adipose tissue [17, 28, 37–40].

The menopause transition is also associated with an increased risk of cardiovascular diseases [46, 47], which has been partly attributed to the deleterious changes in the plasma lipoprotein-lipid profile and in plasma glucose-insulin homeostasis related to a state of relative estrogen deficiency [48–50]. The menopause-induced estrogen deficiency has also been suggested to be associated with an acceleration of visceral adipose tissue deposition [17, 28, 37–40]. Changes in the metabolic profile and in body fat distribution observed with the menopause transition may have been confounding factors in some studies, thereby contributing to the overestimation of the effect of menopause *per se* on the cardiovascular disease risk factors. The effect of body fat distribution on metabolic variables in pre- and postmenopausal women were examined in a cross-sectional study [40]. Whereas basal glucose concentrations, the response to the glucose load and cholesterol levels were higher in postmenopausal women, only cholesterol concentrations remained significantly higher in postmenopausal women after adjusting for group differences in visceral adipose tissue [40]. Moreover, in a stepwise multiple regression model, visceral abdominal adipose tissue proved to be the most powerful variable predicting metabolic risk variables in pre- and post-menopausal women [40].

Therefore, there is an obvious sexual dimorphism in the accumulation of body fat [5-7]. The selective accumulation of abdominal fat observed with age has been found to be largely due to a preferential fat deposition in the abdominal cavity [22-28]. This progressive increase in visceral adipose tissue mass during adulthood is about 2.6 times greater in men than in women until women reach menopause [28]. Then, the accumulation of visceral fat is markedly accelerated during the menopause transition [17, 28, 37-40]. After menopause there is no longer a gender difference in the rate of visceral adipose tissue accumulation [28].

Effects of Weight Loss on Regional Fat Distribution and the Metabolic Risk Profile

Weight loss is advocated in order to improve insulin sensitivity and variables of the metabolic risk profile [51-60]. Whether these favorable effects are explained by the loss of total body fat or of abdominal visceral adipose tissue have been investigated. It has also been clearly demonstrated that a high level of visceral adipose tissue is predictive of a preferential mobilization of this depot after dietary-induced weight loss [58, 59, 61-63]. For instance, in a weight loss study performed by Goodpaster et al. [56], substantial changes were found in visceral adipose tissue, which decreased by 40% as compared to 30% for subcutaneous adipose tissue. These results are in agreement with other observations in which the visceral fat depot was preferentially mobilized after weight loss in both men and women [64, 65]. Thus, these observations provide further support to the notion that the visceral adipose depot is more readily depleted during a weight loss program than subcutaneous adipose tissue.

This selective reduction in visceral adipose tissue in response to weight loss has been shown to be associated with metabolic improvements, which include improved glucose tolerance, reduced plasma insulin levels and a more favorable plasma lipoprotein-lipid profile [57, 59, 61, 66, 67]. The respective contributions of losses of total body fat and of visceral adipose tissue to the improvement of in vivo insulin sensitivity were explored in a weight loss study conducted by Goodpaster et al. [56]. At the end of the weight loss program, insulin sensitivity improved markedly by 25% and was mostly due to the enhancement of nonoxidative glucose disposal [56]. Furthermore, the level of insulin sensitivity achieved in reduced obese men after weight loss was identical to lean control men whereas reduced obese women remained more insulin resistant than lean women [56]. Although both obese men and women lost visceral adipose tissue with weight loss, reduced obese women still had higher levels of visceral adipose tissue than lean women and this residual difference explained the remaining difference in insulin sensitivity [56]. However, despite the fact that they were still overweight after weight loss, reduced obese men normalized their insulin sensitivity compared to lean control men and this lack of difference was explained by the normalization of their level of visceral adipose tissue [56]. Furthermore, relative changes in visceral adipose tissue correlated significantly with changes in insulin sensitivity whereas no association was found between relative changes in subcutaneous abdominal fat and changes in insulin sensitivity [56]. Thus, this simple weight loss study clearly showed that the normalization of the visceral adipose tissue mass can substantially improve insulin sensitivity and that normalization of body weight is not necessary to achieve this important therapeutic objective.

Obesity and Disturbances in the Lipoprotein–Lipid Profile and Glucose–Insulin Homeostasis: Importance of Body Fat Distribution

It is now well accepted that obesity represents an heterogeneous condition from a metabolic standpoint. Several prospective studies have shown that a high accumulation of upper body fat is associated with an increased risk of developing Type 2 diabetes [68–73]. Indeed, with the help of simple anthropometric measurements such as the waist and hip circumferences to evaluate the distribution of adipose tissue, it has been shown that a preferential accumulation of body fat in the abdominal region was associated with an increased risk of developing Type 2 diabetes and CHD [68–73]. Furthermore, a high deposition of abdominal fat has been associated with insulin resistance, hyperinsulinemia, glucose intolerance, dyslipoproteinemias and hypertension [2, 58, 74–78].

Although the WHR has been widely used as an anthropometric variable in order to estimate the proportion of abdominal fat, this measurement does not allow to distinguish subcutaneous fat from visceral adipose tissue. Furthermore, the WHR is an index of the relative accumulation of abdominal fat, not of the total amount of abdominal adipose tissue. With the development of imaging techniques, such as computed tomography, it has become possible to measure precisely cross-sectional areas of subcutaneous and visceral adipose tissue. Measurements performed with this imaging technique have allowed to document a strong association between visceral adipose tissue deposition and metabolic complications [79–81].

Abdominal Obesity and Plasma Glucose–Insulin Homeostasis

In the first study that we performed on the topic, we measured body fat distribution by computed tomography and plasma glucose and insulin levels both in the fasting state and after an oral glucose tolerance test in a sample of premenopausal women [82]. We found that the absolute amount of fat located in the abdominal cavity, the so-called visceral adipose tissue, is an important correlate of glucose tolerance and of plasma insulin levels [82]. Indeed, the level of visceral adipose tissue was the body fat distribution variable that showed the highest association with the area under the curve of the plasma glucose concentrations measured during the oral glucose tolerance test [82]. After control for total adipose tissue mass, the accumulation of visceral adipose tissue remained significantly associated with glucose tolerance [82]. To further dissociate the contribution of obesity vs visceral adipose tissue to disturbances in plasma glucose-insulin homeostasis, obese women matched for age and percentage of body fat, but with either low or elevated amounts of visceral adipose tissue, were compared to lean controls [83]. Whereas obese women characterized by low levels of visceral fat showed normal glucose tolerance but moderate increases in plasma insulin concentrations as compared to lean controls, a marked deterioration in glucose tolerance was noted among women characterized by elevated levels of visceral adipose tissue [83].

Additional studies from our laboratory conducted in men have yielded essentially similar results [84] (Fig. 11.3). Indeed, when we compared obese men matched for their percentage of body fat but having either high or low levels of visceral adipose tissue to a group of lean controls, obese subjects with a low accumulation of visceral adipose tissue had a glucose tolerance which was similar to what was measured in lean men [84]. However, obese men with high levels of visceral adipose tissue showed a substantially elevated glycemic response compared to obese men with low levels of visceral adipose tissue or to lean men [84]. Moreover, men with visceral obesity showed a marked increase in fasting and postglucose load plasma insulin concentrations compared with the group of obese men with low levels of visceral adipose tissue

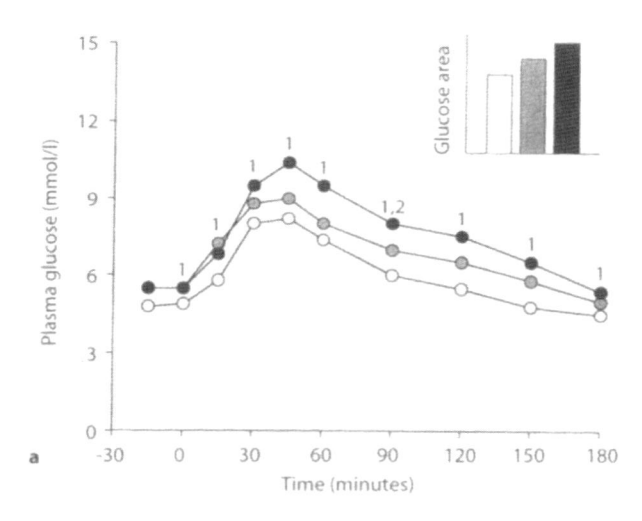

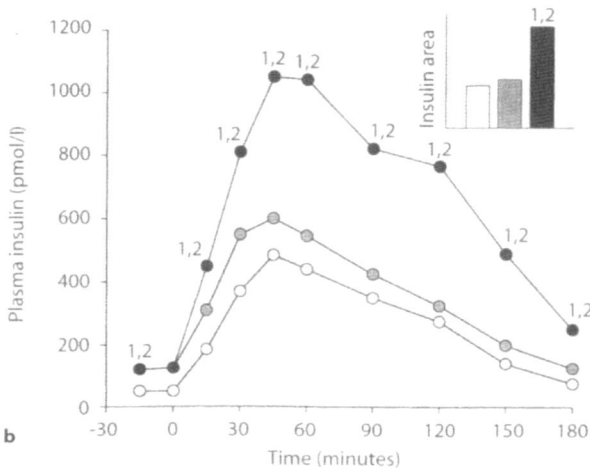

Fig. 11.3. Plasma glucose (*a*) and insulin (*b*) levels during a 75-g oral glucose tolerance test in lean men (*white circle*) and in obese men with either low (*gray circle*) or high (*black circle*) levels of visceral adipose tissue. Bar charts show plasma glucose (mmol/l/min) × 10^{-3} and insulin area (pmol/l/min) × 10^{-3}. [1] Significantly different from the lean control group. [2] Significantly different from the group of obese men with low levels of visceral adipose tissue. (Adapted from Pouliot et al. Diabetes, 1992)

[84]. These results further suggest that, among obese men, the amount of visceral adipose tissue is predictive of fasting plasma insulin concentrations and of insulin-glucose responses to an oral glucose load, independently of the degree of obesity [84].

In accordance with these previous results, many studies with computed tomography have provided evidences for an important role of the abdominal visceral fat depot in the etiology of the disturbances in carbohydrate metabolism that are often found in obese patients [66, 84–89]. For instance, Fujioka et al. [66] have reported that the proportion of visceral adipose tissue was correlated with the plasma glucose area under the curve after an oral glucose load. Sparrow et al. [85] also reported that abdominal visceral fat accumulation was significantly associated with plasma glucose levels measured 2 hours following glucose ingestion. They also found that Type 2 diabetic patients had significantly higher levels of visceral adipose tissue than normal glucose tolerant subjects even after adjustment for BMI and age [85]. Moreover, Park et al. [89] showed that, irrespective of the BMI, an increased deposition of visceral adipose tissue was associated with a reduced insulin sensitivity as determined by the euglycemic-hyperinsulinemic glucose clamp. Finally, a prospective study has also shown that visceral obesity was associated with an increased risk of developing Type 2 diabetes mellitus [90]. Thus, there is solid evidence to suggest that among obese patients, the most severe disturbances in indices of plasma glucose-insulin homeostasis resulting from an insulin resistant state are observed in patients with a high accumulation of visceral adipose tissue.

The Atherogenic Dyslipidemia of Abdominal Obesity

A preferential deposition of adipose tissue in the abdominal cavity has also been associated with a deteriorated lipoprotein-lipid profile, predictive of an increased risk of CHD. Early studies had reported that excess upper body fat was associated with elevated plasma triglyceride concentrations [91–95]. It has also been reported that an excessive accumulation of abdominal body fat was associated with marked reductions in plasma HDL cholesterol levels [95–99]. Studies that have assessed the number of LDL particles or studied the composition and density of LDL particles have reported that a high proportion of abdominal fat, as crudely assessed by an elevated WHR, was associated with an increased proportion of small, dense LDL particles [100–102].

Furthermore, studies in which abdominal fat accumulation was directly measured by computed tomography have shown that a high accumulation of visceral adipose tissue is associated with an altered plasma lipoprotein-lipid profile in both genders [58, 66, 77, 82, 84, 103, 104]. For instance, we have previously reported that abdominal obesity is associated with increased plasma triglyceride levels and reduced HDL cholesterol concentrations, the latter alteration being mostly attributable to a decrease in the HDL_2 fraction [105]. These associations appeared to be independent from the concomitant variation in the level of total body fat [105]. In these analyses, the 2 groups of obese subjects studied were matched for their percentage of body fat but were characterized by either low or high levels of visceral adipose tissue and also compared to a group of lean controls [105]. While obese subjects characterized by low levels of visceral adipose tissue had essentially a normal plasma lipoprotein-lipid profile, obese women with high levels of visceral adipose tissue showed a marked deterioration in their plasma lipoprotein-lipid profile [105]. Furthermore, obese patients with a high accumulation of visceral fat showed a marked increase in apo B concentration [106]. Visceral adipose tissue accumulation was also associated with alterations in the size of LDL particles as viscerally obese men were characterized by an increased proportion of small, dense LDL particles despite the lack of difference in LDL cholesterol levels between men with either low or high levels of visceral adipose tissue [104]. Although there was an association between the small, dense LDL phenotype and the amount of visceral adipose tissue, visceral obesity was not an independent predictor of an increased proportion of small, dense LDL particles as this phenomenon was mostly explained by the hypertriglyceridemic state.

Abdominal Obesity as an Important Component of the Insulin Resistance Syndrome

It therefore appears that abdominal visceral obesity is related to in vivo insulin resistance and to an atherogenic dyslipidemia (Fig. 11.4). Reaven was the first in 1988 to suggest the term "insulin resistance syndrome" to describe a cluster of metabolic abnormalities that includes increased triglyceride and insulin concentrations, low HDL cholesterol levels as well as elevated blood pressure [107]. Recently, atherogenic small, dense LDL particles and elevated apo B levels have also been suggested as additional elements of this syndrome [108]. Reaven also estimated the prevalence of insulin resistance to reach about 25% of the adult sedentary population even among non-diabetic sujects [107]. This insulin resistant state would be compatible with the pres-

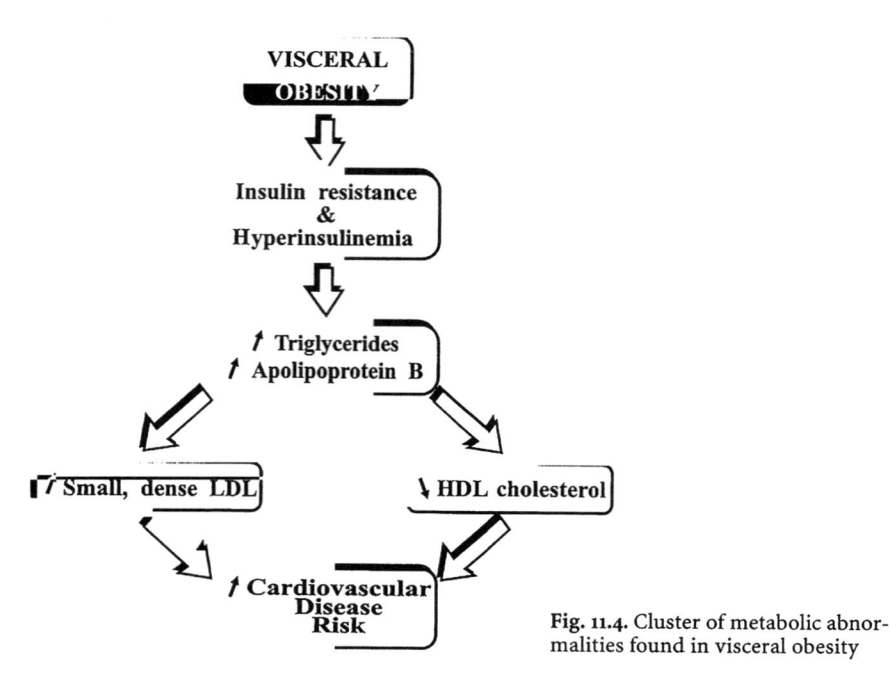

Fig. 11.4. Cluster of metabolic abnormalities found in visceral obesity

ence of a dyslipidemia which also increases the risk of CHD. As visceral adipose tissue accumulation is associated with this cluster of metabolic disturbances leading to an increased risk of Type 2 diabetes and CHD, we have proposed that abdominal visceral obesity is another important component of the insulin resistance syndrome and a major cause of CHD [75, 108]. However, there is limited information on visceral obesity as an independent risk factor for CHD.

Are There Simple Tools to Adequately Estimate Visceral Adipose Tissue Accumulation?

Computed tomography is a very precise technique to measure the cross-sectional area of visceral adipose tissue, but this technique is very expensive and not accessible to most health professionals. Anthropometry has often been used to estimate the amount of total body fat and the proportion of abdominal adipose tissue.

Several studies have examined the correlations between various anthropometric measurements and visceral adipose tissue deposition [80, 109–111]. In this regard, the WHR has been the most widely used anthropometric index. Indeed, the WHR has been shown to be correlated, although moderately, with visceral obesity and predictive of CHD or Type 2 diabetes incidence in prospective studies [68–73]. However, it has been reported that the waist circumference alone was generally more closely associated with the levels of visceral adipose tissue than the WHR [26, 80, 110, 112]. Indeed, the shared variance between visceral obesity and waist girth has been generally found to be higher than with the WHR [110]. Moreover, the association between the WHR and total body fat mass is substantially weaker than with waist girth, while a fairly strong association between waist girth and total body fat mass in both sexes has been found [110, 111]. As an example of the potentially misleading information produced by the WHR, lean and obese persons may have similar WHR values but totally differing levels of visceral adipose tissue. Furthermore, we found that men and women with similar waist girth values tend to have comparable levels of visceral adipose tissue, suggesting that a single critical circumference value in both genders could be considered [110, 111]. Finally, since the correlation between height and waist girth has been shown to be weak or even nonsignificant, it appears that there is no need to adjust waist circumference for height in the estimation of the absolute amount of visceral adipose tissue.

Are There Critical Values of Waist Circumference Associated with the Cluster of Metabolic Abnormalities of Visceral Obesity?

As visceral obesity is a major health hazard, we were also interested in the identification of the critical level of visceral adipose tissue which would be predictive of finding atherogenic and diabetogenic metabolic abnormalities. In order to explore this issue, men and premenopausal women were divided into quintiles of cross-sectional areas of visceral adipose tissue [113]. According to these analyses, a cross-sectional area below 100 cm^2 was associated with a low prevalence of metabolic abnormalities [113]. However, subjects characterized by cross-sectional areas of visceral adipose tissue above 130 cm^2 had a substantially deteriorated metabolic profile predictive of an increased risk of Type 2 diabetes and CHD [113]. Similar analyses were performed with the use of the waist circumference as a screening tool [77, 110]. We found that for men and women below 40 years of age, a waist circumference of 100 cm and above was associated with a deteriorated metabolic risk profile [77, 110]. This "critical" waist girth value also corresponded to a visceral adipose tissue accumulation of about 130 cm^2 [111], a finding consistent with the presence of a deteriorated risk factor profile.

Critical Waist Values: Importance of Considering Age

There is, with age, a well documented selective deposition of visceral adipose tissue [22–28]. Thus, for any given waist girth, older individuals are characterized by a higher accumulation of visceral adipose tissue than young adults. We therefore proposed that age had to be taken into account in the prediction of visceral adipose tissue accumulation from anthropometry [25, 27, 114]. For instance, we found that a waist girth above 100 cm was associated with a greater probability of finding an excessive visceral fat accumulation in men and women before 40 years of age, whereas this threshold had to be reduced to 90 cm in subjects aged between 40 and 60 years [111].

Evidence for the Importance of Measuring Waist Circumference: Prospective Studies

The waist circumference measurement may be useful for clinicians not only in the estimation of risk but also as a therapeutic target as it could allow to monitor changes in visceral adipose tissue over time. These changes could occur even in absence of any variation in weight or in total body fatness [25, 27]. In a 7-year longitudinal study that we conducted in women, we found a 30% increase in the cross-sectional area of visceral adipose tissue in the absence of any change in weight, BMI or total body fat mass [27]. These changes in visceral adipose tissue were predicted by changes in waist girth (which increased by about 4 cm) but not appropriately by changes in the WHR [27]. Thus, only weighing the patient over time could provide misleading information in the follow-up of patients.

None of the above anthropometric measurements alone can adequately distinguish between visceral and subcutaneous abdominal adipose tissue although they show correlations with risk factors for diabetes and CHD. However, after considering age, the waist circumference appears to represent the best anthropometric measurement of the cumulative amount of abdominal fat which can be used by health professionals. Furthermore, we found that waist girth was a particularly suitable measurement to appreciate changes in visceral adipose tissue over the years [25, 27]. Thus, from a clinical perspective, a change in waist circumference over time is predictive of a modification in the amount of visceral adipose tissue. Thus, the "tape measurement" can be considered as a simple and inexpensive therapeutic target.

The Dyslipidemic Profile of Abdominal Obesity: Influence on CHD Risk

Several papers from our laboratory have documented the metabolic complications associated with an excessive deposition of visceral adipose tissue [75, 76, 84, 86, 104, 108, 115, 116]. Overall, we found visceral abdominal obesity to be associated, even in nondiabetic subjects, with all the features of the insulin resistance syndrome such as hyperinsulinemia, a greater glycemic response to an oral glucose load, elevated triglyceride and apo B concentrations, reduced HDL cholesterol levels, an increased cholesterol/HDL cholesterol ratio and a increased proportion of smaller, cholesterylester depleted LDL particles [75, 76, 84, 86, 104, 108, 115, 116]. This cluster of metabolic disturbances is of course also found in Type 2 diabetic patients who are most of the time characterized by insulin resistance and abdominal obesity.

These components of the insulin resistance syndrome have been shown in the cohort of middle-aged men of the Québec Cardiovascular Study to be associated with a substantial increase in the risk of CHD [117–119]. For instance, we found that apo B concentration was a strong predictor of CHD over the 5-year follow-up of the study [117]. We have then examined the CHD risk associated with elevated fasting insulin levels among subjects of the Québec Cardiovascular Study [119]. For that purpose, men who developed CHD during the follow-up were matched with CHD-event-free controls for age, BMI, smoking habits and alcohol consumption. We found that fasting insulin concentrations were elevated at baseline among men who developed CHD [119]. Multivariate analyses revealed that hyperinsulinemia was an independent predictor of CHD in these men [119]. Finally, a high proportion of small, dense LDL particles was another condition associated with an increased risk of CHD in the Québec Cardiovascular Study [118].

We were then interested to investigate whether our ability to discriminate individuals at high risk for CHD could be improved by measuring 3 nontraditional metabolic risk factors (hyperapoB, hyperinsulinemia and small, dense LDL particles) beyond what can be achieved using more traditional lipid risk factors (elevated triglyceride and LDL cholesterol concentrations and reduced HDL cholesterol levels) [120]. We found that being simultaneously above the median of the distribution for LDL cholesterol and triglyceride concentrations and below the median of the distribution for HDL cholesterol levels was associated with a 4.5-fold increase in the risk of CHD over the 5-year follow-up period of the study [120]. However, being simultaneously above the median of the distribution for apo B and insulin levels and below the median for LDL peak particle size was associated with 20-fold increase risk of CHD and adjustment for the traditional lipid triad failed to significantly alter this ratio suggesting that this cluster of new metabolic markers could improve our ability to identify individuals at high risk for CHD [120].

Hypertriglyceridemic Waist as a Screening Tool for the Presence of the Atherogenic Metabolic Triad and of the Insulin Resistance Dyslipidemic Syndrome of Visceral Obesity

As most general physicians do not have access to insulin, apo B and LDL particle size measurements, we were interested in developing a simple algorithm which could be used in daily clinical practice to identify at low cost, high risk individuals who would likely be carriers of this atherogenic metabolic triad [121].

The working model that we have used to identify carriers of the non traditional atherogenic metabolic triad included waist girth (which was considered as a proxi variable for insulin and apo B levels) and fasting triglyceride concentration (which was used to screen for the presence of small, dense LDL particles). Since we have suggested that waist girth could be used as a crude index of abdominal visceral adipose tissue accumulation [110], we consider that a simple anthropometric variable such as the waist circumference may contribute to refine the assessment of cardiovascular risk. In this regard, we have demonstrated that apo B and fasting insulin levels are very sensitive to an increase in waist circumference probably resulting from an accumulation of abdominal visceral fat [121]. Indeed, we found that men with an elevated waist circumference ($\geq$ 90 cm) were characterized by fasting hyperinsulinemia and increased apo B levels (Fig. 11.5). Furthermore, fasting triglyceride concentration has been found to be the best predictor of LDL size [104, 122, 123]. In accordance with these previous results, our results showed that men with hypertriglyceridemia ($\geq$ 2.0 mmol/l) were characterized by smaller and denser LDL particles compared to normotriglyceridemic men (Fig. 11.5).

We therefore proposed that this "hypertriglyceridemic waist" concept may useful to screen for the presence of the new metabolic triad of risk factors (Fig. 11.6). After having divided our cohort of men according to triglyceride levels (< 2.0 mmol/l; $\geq$ 2.0 mmol/l) and waist girth (< 90 cm ; 90 – 100 cm ; $\geq$ 100 cm), we found that only 12 % and 53 % of men with a moderate or a high waist girth, in the absence of elevated triglyceride levels, were characterized by the atherogenic triad [121] (Table 11.1). However, a high proportion of men with simultaneous elevations in waist girth and triglyceride concentrations (more than 80 %) were characterized by the new metabolic triad of risk factors (Table 11.1). It is also important to point out that these subjects were also characterized by substantial elevations in the cholesterol/HDL cholesterol ratio (a well accepted predictor of CHD risk) [124, 125]. We then performed a validation study by testing our simple waist-triglyceride algorithm in a sample of male patients who underwent an angiographic exam. The relative odds of being affected by coronary artery disease were only significantly increased (by 3.6-fold) among men with both elevated waist girth and triglyceride concentrations [121].

There is also additional evidence supporting the notion that waist circumference and triglyceride concentrations could be used as effective screening tools. Recent

Table 11.1. Prevalence of men with the atherogenic metabolic triad (hyperinsulinemia, elevated apo B, small, dense LDL) among subgroups of men classified on the basis of waist girth and triglyceride levels (adapted from Lemieux et al. Circulation 2000)

Screening tools		Carriers (%)
Waist girth (cm) < 90:	Triglycerides (mmol/l):< 2.0	10 %
Waist girth (cm) 90 – 100:	Triglycerides (mmol/l): < 2.0	12 %
	$\geq$ 2.0	83 %
Waist girth (cm) $\geq$ 100:	Triglycerides (mmol/l): < 2.0	53 %
	$\geq$ 2.0	84 %

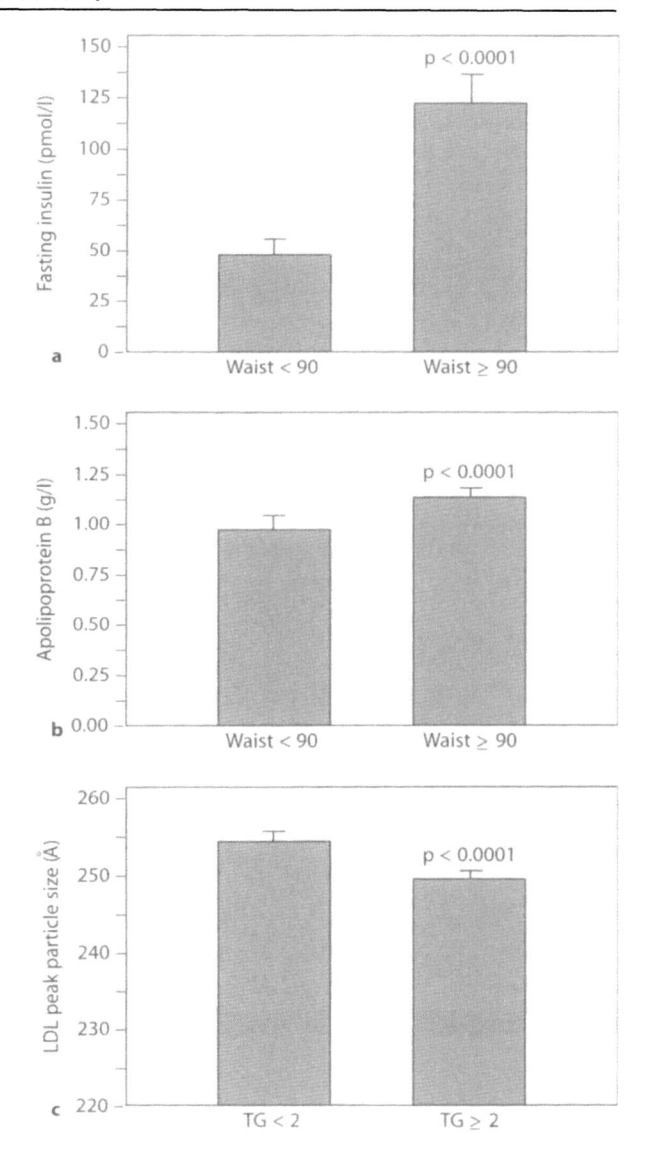

Fig. 11.5. Fasting insulin (*a*) and apo B (*b*) concentrations according to a low waist girth (<90 cm) or high waist girth (≥90 cm). The LDL peak particle size (*c*) among subgroups divided on the basis of fasting triglyceride levels (<2.0 mmol/l or ≥2.0 mmol/l)

analyses from the Québec Health Survey revealed that about 50% of men are characterized by low triglyceride levels and low waist girth values [126]. However, 20% of Quebecers had simultaneous elevations in waist circumference and triglyceride levels [126]. In women, 76% of them presented a low waist girth and were characterized by low levels of triglycerides, whereas only 5% were characterized by simultaneous elevations in waist girth and triglyceride concentrations [126]. In this population-based study of men living in the province of Québec, we also quantified the prevalence of an

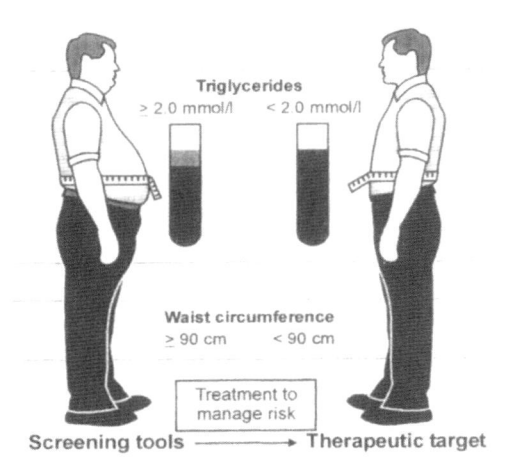

Fig. 11.6. Illustration of how waist circumference and fasting triglyceride levels could be used both for the screening of high risk patients and as therapeutic targets

elevated cholesterol/HDL cholesterol ratio (as defined by a value greater or equal to 6) among men classified on the basis of waist girth and triglyceride concentrations [126]. Whereas only 3% of men with low waist girth and low triglyceride concentrations had an elevated cholesterol/HDL cholesterol ratio, almost 50% of subjects with a high waist circumference and high triglyceride levels were characterized by the presence of an elevated cholesterol/HDL cholesterol ratio [126]. Finally, in a subgroup of apparently healthy men, when the subjects' characteristics were examined across waist girth and triglyceride groups, it was interesting to note that marked differences were observed in the cholesterol/HDL cholesterol ratio in the absence of any difference in BMI and WHR [126]. Thus, substantial variation in the cholesterol/HDL cholesterol ratio was noted as a function of combined waist and triglyceride values. For instance, abdominally obese men with triglyceride levels above 2 mmol/l had a cholesterol/HDL cholesterol ratio of about 1 and a half units greater than men with triglyceride concentrations below 2 mmol/l and with waist girth below 90 cm [126]. Thus, the combined interpretation of waist circumference and fasting triglyceride levels may be superior to the WHR and BMI as screening tools to identify abdominally obese men with the atherogenic dyslipidemia of insulin resistance.

Implications for Prevention and Treatment

As the insulin resistance syndrome is a highly prevalent condition with considerable public health implications, there is a need to develop simple and inexpensive screening markers for the identification of individuals at increased risk of developing Type 2 diabetes and CHD before the occurrence of the disease. However, as the majority of abdominally obese men at high risk for CHD may never develop Type 2 diabetes, it is of paramount importance to use early markers of the insulin resistance syndrome in order to implement primary prevention strategies focussing on high risk abdominally obese patients. On that basis, it has been suggested that fasting hyperinsulinemia could be the simplest and best marker of early insulin resistance in nondiabetic and euglycemic individuals [127, 128]. However, measuring fasting insulin concentration is not a routine procedure in most clinical biochemistry laboratories as the assay is not standardized. Meanwhile, a high proportion of nondiabetic individuals with abdominal obesity, who had never smoked and who may never be affected by hypercholesterolemia and hypertension, are characterized by a cluster of metabolic complications substantially increasing the risk of CHD and Type 2 diabetes.

Therefore, we would like to propose that the simultaneous measurement and interpretation of waist circumference and fasting triglyceride levels could be a very useful screening procedure to crudely assess the CHD risk resulting from the atherogenic dyslipidemia of insulin resistance and abdominal obesity. Unfortunately, the validity of our simple model cannot be extended to women and to other ethnic groups than caucasians. It is hoped that further studies will be conducted to identify critical waist and triglyceride values in both genders and in every ethnic population.

Acknowledgments. Studies conducted by the authors discussed in this review have benefited from the support of the Canadian Institutes of Health Research (pp 14014 and MGC-15187), the Canadian Diabetes Association and the Heart and Stroke Foundation of Canada. Isabelle Lemieux is the recipient of a research studentship from the Heart and Stroke Foundation of Canada whereas Jean-Pierre Després is chair professor of nutrition, lipidology and prevention of cardiovascular disease supported by Provigo and Pfizer Canada.

References

1. Bray GA. Complications of obesity. Ann Intern Med. 1985;103:1052–62.
2. Kissebah AH, Freedman DS, Peiris AN. Health risk of obesity. Med Clin North Am. 1989;1989:111–138.
3. WHO Expert Committee on Diabetes Mellitus. Second report. WHO Tech Rep Ser, no 646. Geneva: World Health Organization; 1980.
4. Vague J. The degree of masculine differentiation of obesities: a factor determining predisposition to diabetes, atherosclerosis, gout and ulric calculous disease. Am J Clin Nutr. 1956;4:20–34.
5. Vague J. Sexual differentiation, a factor affecting the forms of obesity. Presse Méd. 1947; 30:339–340.
6. Kvist H, Chowdhury B, Grangard U, Tylen U, Ströström L. Total and visceral adipose-tissue volumes derived from measurements with computed tomography in adult men and women: predictive equations. Am J Clin Nutr. 1988;48:1351–61.
7. Sjöström L, Kvist H. Regional body fat measurements with CT-scan and evaluation of anthropometric predictions. Acta Med Scand Suppl. 1988;723:169–77.
8. Lemieux S, Prud'homme D, Bouchard C, Tremblay A, Després JP. Sex differences in the relation of visceral adipose tissue accumulation to total body fatness. Am J Clin Nutr. 1993;58: 463–7.
9. Kvist H, Ströström L, Tylen U. Adipose tissue volume determinations in women by computed tomography: technical considerations. Int J Obes. 1986;10:53–67.
10. Lerner DJ, Kannel WB. Patterns of coronary heart disease morbidity and mortality in the sexes: a 26-year follow-up of the Framingham population. Am Heart J. 1986;111:383–90.
11. Wingard DL, Suarez L, Barrett-Connor E. The sex differential in mortality from all causes and ischemic heart disease. Am J Epidemiol. 1983;117:165–72.
12. Freedman DS, Jacobsen SJ, Barboriak JJ, Sobocinski KA, Anderson AJ, Kissebah AH, Sasse EA, Gruchow HW. Body fat distribution and male/female differences in lipids and lipoproteins. Circulation. 1990;81:1498–506.

13. Larsson B, Bengtsson C, Bjorntorp P, Lapidus L, Ströström L, Svardsudd K, Tibblin G, Wedel H, Welin L, Wilhelmsen L. Is abdominal body fat distribution a major explanation for the sex difference in the incidence of myocardial infarction? The study of men born in 1913 and the study of women, Goteborg, Sweden. Am J Epidemiol. 1992;135:266-73.
14. Seidell JC, Cigolini M, Charzewska J, Ellsinger BM, Bjorntorp P, Hautvast JG, Szostak W. Fat distribution and gender differences in serum lipids in men and women from four European communities. Atherosclerosis. 1991;87:203-10.
15. Lemieux S, Després JP, Moorjani S, Nadeau A, Thériault G, Prud'homme D, Tremblay A, Bouchard C, Lupien PJ. Are gender differences in cardiovascular disease risk factors explained by the level of visceral adipose tissue? Diabetologia. 1994;37:757-64.
16. Lanska DJ, Lanska MJ, Hartz AJ, Rimm AA. Factors influencing anatomic location of fat tissue in 52,953 women. Int J Obes. 1985;9:29-38.
17. Shimokata H, Tobin JD, Muller DC, Elahi D, Coon PJ, Andres R. Studies in the distribution of body fat: I. Effects of age, sex, and obesity. J Gerontol. 1989;44:M66-73.
18. Shimokata H, Andres R, Coon PJ, Elahi D, Muller DC, Tobin JD. Studies in the distribution of body fat. II. Longitudinal effects of change in weight. Int J Obes. 1989;13:455-64.
19. Tonkelaar ID, Seidell JC, van Noord PA, Baanders-van Halewijn EA, Jacobus JH, Bruning PF. Factors influencing waist/hip ratio in randomly selected pre- and post- menopausal women in the DOM-project (preliminary results). Int J Obes. 1989;13:817-24.
20. Tonkelaar I, Seidell JC, van Noord PA, Baanders-van Halewijn EA, Ouwehand IJ. Fat distribution in relation to age, degree of obesity, smoking habits, parity and estrogen use: a cross-sectional study in 11,825 Dutch women participating in the DOM-project. Int J Obes. 1990;14:753-61.
21. Borkan GA, Hults DE, Gerzof SG, Robbins AH, Silbert CK. Age changes in body composition revealed by computed tomography. J Gerontol. 1983;38:673-7.
22. Schwartz RS, Shuman WP, Bradbury VL, Cain KC, Fellingham GW, Beard JC, Kahn SE, Stratton JR, Cerqueira MD, Abrass IB. Body fat distribution in healthy young and older men. J. Gerontol. 1990;45:M181-M185.
23. Enzi G, Gasparo M, Biondetti PR, Fiore D, Semisa M, Zurlo F. Subcutaneous and visceral fat distribution according to sex, age, and overweight, evaluated by computed tomography. Am J Clin Nutr. 1986;44:739-46.
24. Pascot A, Lemieux S, Lemieux I, Prud'homme D, Tremblay A, Bouchard C, Nadeau A, Couillard C, Tchernof A, Bergeron J, Després JP. Age-related increase in visceral adipose tissue and body fat and the metabolic risk profile of premenopausal women. Diabetes Care. 1999;22:1471-8.
25. Lemieux S, Prud'homme D, Nadeau A, Tremblay A, Bouchard C, Després JP. Seven-year changes in body fat and visceral adipose tissue in women. Association with indexes of plasma glucose-insulin homeostasis. Diabetes Care. 1996;19:983-91.
26. Seidell JC, Oosterlee A, Deurenberg P, Hautvast JGAJ, Ruijs JHJ. Abdominal fat depots measured with computed tomography: effects of degree of obesity, sex, and age. Eur J Clin Nutr. 1988;42:805-815.
27. Lemieux S, Prud'homme D, Tremblay A, Bouchard C, Després JP. Anthropometric correlates of changes in visceral adipose tissue over 7 years in women. Int J Obes Relat Metab Disord. 1996;20:618-624.
28. Kotani K, Tokunaga K, Fujioka S, Kobatake T, Keno Y, Yoshida S, Shimomura I, Tarui S, Matsuzawa Y. Sexual dimorphism of age-related changes in whole-body fat distribution in the obese. Int J Obes Relat Metab Disord. 1994;18:207-2.
29. Abbott RD, Garrison RJ, Wilson PW, Epstein FH, Castelli WP, Feinleib M, LaRue C. Joint distribution of lipoprotein cholesterol classes. The Framingham study. Arteriosclerosis. 1983;3:260-72.
30. Dedonder-Decoopman E, Fievet-Desreumaux C, Campos E, Moulin S, Dewailly P, Sezille G, Jaillard J. Plasma levels of VLDL- and LDL-cholesterol, HDL-cholesterol, triglycerides and apoproteins B and A-I in a healthy population- influence of several risk factors. Atherosclerosis. 1980;37:559-68.
31. Rifkind BM, Segal P. Lipid Research Clinics Program reference values for hyperlipidemia and hypolipidemia. JAMA. 1983;250:1869-72.
32. Williams P, Robinson D, Bailey A. High-density lipoprotein and coronary risk factors in normal men. Lancet. 1979;1:72-5.

33. Grundy SM, Vega GL, Bilheimer DW. Kinetic mechanisms determining variability in low density lipoprotein levels and rise with age. Arteriosclerosis. 1985;5:623–30.
34. Harris MI, Hadden WC, Knowler WC, Bennett PH. Prevalence of diabetes and impaired glucose tolerance and plasma glucose levels in U.S. population aged 20–74 yr. Diabetes. 1987;36:523–34.
35. Chen M, Bergman RN, Pacini G, Porte D, Jr. Pathogenesis of age-related glucose intolerance in man: insulin resistance and decreased beta-cell function. J Clin Endocrinol Metab. 1985;60:13–20.
36. Jackson RA, Hawa MI, Roshania RD, Sim BM, DiSilvio L, Jaspan JB. Influence of aging on hepatic and peripheral glucose metabolism in humans. Diabetes. 1988;37:119–29.
37. Ley CJ, Lees B, Stevenson JC. Sex- and menopause-associated changes in body-fat distribution. Am J Clin Nutr. 1992;55:950–4.
38. Tremollieres FA, Pouilles JM, Ribot CA. Relative influence of age and menopause on total and regional body composition changes in postmenopausal women. Am J Obstet Gynecol. 1996;175:1594–600.
39. Panotopoulos G, Ruiz JC, Raison J, Guy-Grand B, Basdevant A. Menopause, fat and lean distribution in obese women. Maturitas. 1996;25:11–9.
40. Zamboni M, Armellini F, Milani MP, De Marchi M, Todesco T, Robbi R, Bergamo-Andreis IA, Bosello O. Body fat distribution in pre- and post-menopausal women: metabolic and anthropometric variables and their inter-relationships. Int J Obes Relat Metab Disord. 1992;16:495–504.
41. Pasquali R, Casimirri F, Labate AM, Tortelli O, Pascal G, Anconetani B, Gatto MR, Flamia R, Capelli M, Barbara L. Body weight, fat distribution and the menopausal status in women. Int J Obes Relat Metab Disord. 1994;18:614–21.
42. Pasquali R, Vicennati V, Bertazzo D, Casimirri F, Pascal G, Tortelli O, Labate AM. Determinants of sex hormone-binding globulin blood concentrations in premenopausal and postmenopausal women with different estrogen status. Metabolism. 1997;46:5–9.
43. Razay G, Bolton CH. Coronary heart disease risk factors in relation to the menopause. Q J Med. 1992;85:307–308.
44. Poehlman ET, Toth MJ, Bunyard LB, Gardner AW, Donaldson KE, Colman E, Fonong T, Ades PA. Physiological predictors of increasing total and central adiposity in aging men and women. Arch Intern Med. 1995;155:2443–8.
45. Troisi RJ, Wolf AM, Mason JE, Klingler KM, Colditz GA. Relation of body fat distribution to reproductive factors in pre- and postmenopausal women. Obes Res. 1995;3:143–51.
46. Gordon T, Kannel WB, Hjortland MC, McNamara PM. Menopause and coronary heart disease. The Framingham Study. Ann Intern Med. 1978;89:157–61.
47. Kannel WB. Metabolic risk factors for coronary heart disease in women: perspective from the Framingham Study. Am Heart J. 1987;114:413–9.
48. Guetta V, Cannon RO, 3rd. Cardiovascular effects of estrogen and lipid-lowering therapies in postmenopausal women. Circulation. 1996;93:1928–37.
49. Nabulsi AA, Folsom AR, White A, Patsch W, Heiss G, Wu KK, Szklo M. Association of hormone-replacement therapy with various cardiovascular risk factors in postmenopausal women. The Atherosclerosis Risk in Communities Study Investigators. N Engl J Med. 1993;328:1069–75.
50. Manson JE. Postmenopausal hormone therapy and atherosclerotic disease. Am Heart J. 1994;128:1337–43.
51. Golay A, Felber JP, Dusmet M, Gomez F, Curchod B, Jequier E. Effect of weight loss on glucose disposal in obese and obese diabetic patients. Int J Obes. 1985;9:181–91.
52. Dengel DR, Pratley RE, Hagberg JM, Rogus EM, Goldberg AP. Distinct effects of aerobic exercise training and weight loss on glucose homeostasis in obese sedentary men. J Appl Physiol. 1996;81:318–25.
53. Bryson JM, King SE, Burns CM, Baur LA, Swaraj S, Caterson ID. Changes in glucose and lipid metabolism following weight loss produced by a very low calorie diet in obese subjects. Int J Obes Relat Metab Disord. 1996;20:338–45.
54. Niskanen L, Uusitupa M, Sarlund H, Siitonen O, Paljarvi L, Laakso M. The effects of weight loss on insulin sensitivity, skeletal muscle composition and capillary density in obese non-diabetic subjects. Int J Obes Relat Metab Disord. 1996;20:154–60.
55. Webber J, Donaldson M, Allison SP, Fukagawa NK, Macdonald IA. The effects of weight loss

in obese subjects on the thermogenic, metabolic and haemodynamic responses to the glucose clamp. Int J Obes Relat Metab Disord. 1994;18:725-30.
56. Goodpaster BH, Kelly DE, Wing RR, Meier A, Thaete FL. Effects of weight loss on regional fat distribution and insulin sensitivity in obesity. Diabetes. 1999;48:839-847.
57. Bouchard C, Després JP, Tremblay A. Exercise and obesity. Obes Res. 1993;1:40-54.
58. Després JP. Obesity and lipoprotein metabolism: relevance of body fat distribution. Curr Opin Lipidol. 1991;2:5-15.
59. Després JP, Lamarche B. Effects of diet and physical activity on adiposity and body fat distribution: implications for the prevention of cardiovascular disease. Nutr Res Rev. 1993;6:137-159.
60. Goldstein DJ. Beneficial health effects of modest weight loss. Int J Obes. 1992;16:397-415.
61. Fujioka S, Matsuzawa Y, Tokunaga K, Yoshiaki K, Takashi K, Seiichiro T. Treatment of visceral obesity. Int J Obes. 1991;15:59-65.
62. Leenen R, van der Kooy K, Deurenberg P, Seidell JC, Weststrate JA, Schouten FJM, Hautvast JGAJ. Visceral fat accumulation in obese subjects: relation to energy expenditure and response to weight loss. Am J Physiol. 1992;263:E913-E919.
63. Schwartz RS, Shuman WP, Larson V, Cain KC, Fellingham MD, Abrass IB. The effect of intensive endurance exercise training on body fat distribution on young and older men. Metabolism. 1991;40:545-551.
64. Zamboni M, Armellini F, Turcato E, Todesco T, Bissoli L, Bergamo-Andreis IA, Bosello O. Effect of weight loss on regional body fat distribution in premenopausal women. Am J Clin Nutr. 1993;58:29-34.
65. van der Kooy K, Leenen R, Seidell JC, Deurenberg P, Droop A, Bakker CJ. Waist-hip ratio is a poor predictor of changes in visceral fat. Am J Clin Nutr. 1993;57:327-33.
66. Fujioka S, Matsuzawa Y, Tokunaga K, Tarui S. Contribution of intra-abdominal fat accumulation to the impairment of glucose and lipid metabolism in human obesity. Metabolism. 1987;36:54-9.
67. Leenen R, van der Kooy K, Droop A, Seidell JC, Deurenberg P, Weststrate JA, Hautvast JG. Visceral fat loss measured by magnetic resonance imaging in relation to changes in serum lipid levels of obese men and women. Arterioscler Thromb. 1993;13:487-94.
68. Ohlson LO, Larsson B, Svardsudd K, Welin L, Eriksson H, Wilhelmsen L, Bjorntorp P, Tibblin G. The influence of body fat distribution on the incidence of diabetes mellitus. 13.5 years of follow-up of the participants in the study of men born in 1913. Diabetes. 1985;34:1055-8.
69. Haffner SM, Stern MP, Mitchell BD, Hazuda HP, Patterson JK. Incidence of type II diabetes in Mexican Americans predicted by fasting insulin and glucose levels, obesity, and body-fat distribution. Diabetes. 1990;39:283-8.
70. Lapidus L, Bengtsson C, Larsson B, Pennert K, Rybo E, Sjöström L. Distribution of adipose tissue and risk of cardiovascular disease and death: a 12 year follow up of participants in the population study of women in Gotenburg, Sweden. Br J Nutr. 1984;289:1261-1263.
71. Larsson B, Svardsudd K, Welin L, Wilhelmsen L, Björntorp P, Tibblin G. Abdominal adipose tissue distribution, obesity, and risk of cardiovascular disease and death: 13 year follow-up of participants in the study of men born in 1913. Br Med J. 1984;288:1401-1404.
72. Ducimetiere P, Richard J, Cambien F. The pattern of subcutaneous fat distribution in middle-aged men and the risk of coronary heart disease: the Paris Prospective Study. Int J Obes. 1986;10:229-40.
73. Donahue RP, Abbott RD, Bloom E, Reed DM, Yano K. Central obesity and coronary heart disease in men. Lancet. 1987;1:821-4.
74. Björntorp P. Abdominal obesity and the development of non-insulin dependent diabetes mellitus. Diabetes Metab Rev. 1988;4:615-622.
75. Després JP. Visceral obesity: A component of the insulin resistance-dyslipidemic syndrome. Can J Cardiol. 1994;10:17B-22B.
76. Després JP, Lemieux I, Pned'homme O. Treatment of obesity: need to focus on high risk abdominally obese patients. BMJ. 2001; 322: 716-20.
77. Després JP. Lipoprotein metabolism in visceral obesity. Int J Obes. 1991;15 Suppl 2:45-52.
78. Kissebah AH, Krakower GR. Regional adiposity and morbidity. Am J Physiol. 1994;74:761-811.
79. Sjöström L, Kvist H, Cederblad A, Tylen U. Determination of total adipose tissue and body fat in women by computed tomography, 40 K, and tritium. Am J Physiol. 1986;250:E736-E745.

80. Ferland M, Després JP, Tremblay A, Pinault S, Nadeau A, Moorjani S, Lupien PJ, Thériault G, Bouchard C. Assessment of adipose tissue distribution by computed axial tomography in obese women: association with body density and anthropometric measurements. Br J Nutr. 1989;61:139–48.
81. Després JP, Prud'homme D, Pouliot MC, Tremblay A, Bouchard C. Estimation of deep abdominal fat accumulation from simple anthropometric measurements in men. Am J Clin Nutr. 1991;54:471–477.
82. Després JP, Nadeau A, Tremblay A, Ferland M, Moorjani S, Lupien PJ, Thériault G, Pinault S, Bouchard C. Role of deep abdominal fat in the association between regional adipose tissue distribution and glucose tolerance in obese women. Diabetes. 1989;38:304–9.
83. Després JP. Visceral obesity, insulin resistance, and related dyslipoproteinemias. In: Rifkin H, Colwell JA, Taylor SI, eds. Amsterdam: Elsevier; 1991:95–99.
84. Pouliot MC, Després JP, Nadeau A, Moorjani S, Prud'homme D, Lupien PJ, Tremblay A, Bouchard C. Visceral obesity in men. Associations with glucose tolerance, plasma insulin, and lipoprotein levels. Diabetes. 1992;41:826–34.
85. Sparrow D, Borkan GA, Gerzof SG, Wisniewski C, Silbert CK. Relationship of fat distribution to glucose tolerance. Results of computed tomography in male participants of the Normative Aging Study. Diabetes. 1986;35:411–5.
86. Després JP, Ferland M, Moorjani S, Nadeau A, Tremblay A, Lupien PJ. Role of hepatic-triglyceride lipase activity in the association between intra-abdominal fat and plasma HDL cholesterol in obese women. Arterioscler Thromb Vasc Biol. 1989;9:485–492.
87. Peiris AN, Sothmann MS, Hennes MI, Lee MB, Wilson CR, Gustafson AB, Kissebah AH. Relative contribution of obesity and body fat distribution to alterations in glucose insulin homeostasis: predictive values of selected indices in premenopausal women. Am J Clin Nutr. 1989;49:758–64.
88. Seidell JC, Bjorntorp P, Ströström L, Kvist H, Sannerstedt R. Visceral fat accumulation in men is positively associated with insulin, glucose, and C-peptide levels, but negatively with testosterone levels. Metabolism. 1990;39:897–901.
89. Park KS, Rhee BD, Lee KU, Kim SY, Lee HK, Koh CS, Min HK. Intra-abdominal fat is associated with decreased insulin sensitivity in healthy young men. Metabolism. 1991;40:600–3.
90. Bergstrom RW, Newell-Morris LL, Leonetti DL, Shuman WP, Wahl PW, Fujimoto WY. Association of elevated fasting C-peptide level and increased intra-abdominal fat distribution with development of NIDDM in Japanese-American men. Diabetes. 1990;39:104–11.
91. Kissebah AH, Vydelingum N, Murray R, Evans DJ, Hartz AJ, Kalkhoff RK, Adams PW. Relation of body fat distribution to metabolic complications of obesity. J Clin Endocrinol Metab. 1982;54:254–60.
92. Kalkhoff RK, Hartz AH, Rupley D, Kissebah AH, Kelber S. Relationship of body fat distribution to blood pressure, carbohydrate tolerance, and plasma lipids in healthy obese women. J Lab Clin Med. 1983;102:621–7.
93. Krotkiewski M, Björntorp P, Sjöström L, Smith U. Impact of obesity on metabolism in men and women. Importance of regional adipose tissue distribution. J Clin Invest. 1983;72:1150–1162.
94. Evans DJ, Hoffman RG, Kalkhoff RK, Kissebah AH. Relationship of body fat topography to insulin sensitivity and metabolic profiles in premenopausal women. Metabolism. 1984;33:68–75.
95. Després JP, Allard C, Tremblay A, Talbot J, Bouchard C. Evidence for a regional component of body fatness in the association with serum lipids in men and women. Metabolism. 1985;34:967–973.
96. Foster CJ, Weinsier RL, Birch R, Norris DJ, Bernstein RS, Wang J, Pierson RN, Van Itallie TB. Obesity and serum lipids: an evaluation of the relative contribution of body fat and fat distribution to lipid levels. Int J Obes. 1987;11:151–61.
97. Kissebah AH, Evans DJ, Peiris A, Wilson CR. Endocrine characteristics in regional obesities: role of sex steroids. In: Metabolic complications of human obesities. Vague J, Björntorp P, Guy-Grand B, Rebuffe-Scrive M, Vague P, eds. Amsterdam: Elsevier; 1985:115–130.
98. Haffner SM, Stern MP, Hazuda HP, Pugh J, Patterson JK. Do upper-body and centralized adiposity measure different aspects of regional body-fat distribution? Relationship to non-insulin-dependent diabetes mellitus, lipids, and lipoproteins. Diabetes. 1987;36:43–51.

99. Anderson AJ, Sobocinski KA, Freedman DS, Barboriak JJ, Rimm AA, Gruchow HW. Body fat distribution, plasma lipids and lipoproteins. Arterioscler Thromb Vasc Biol. 1988;8:88–94.
100. Terry RB, Wood PD, Haskell WL, Stefanick ML, Krauss RM. Regional adiposity patterns in relation to lipids, lipoprotein cholesterol, and lipoprotein subfraction mass in men. J Clin Endocrinol Metab. 1989;68:191–9.
101. Peeples LH, Carpenter JW, Israel RG, Barakat HA. Alterations in low-density lipoproteins in subjects with abdominal adiposity. Metabolism. 1989;38:1029–36.
102. Katzel LI, Krauss RM, Goldberg AP. Relations of plasma TG and HDL-C concentrations to body composition and plasma insulin levels are altered in men with small LDL particles. Arterioscler Thromb. 1994;14:1121–8.
103. Peiris AN, Sothmann MS, Hoffmann RG, Hennes MI, Wilson CR, Gustafson AB, Kissebah AH. Adiposity, fat distribution, and cardiovascular risk. Ann Intern Med. 1989;110:867–72.
104. Tchernof A, Lamarche B, Prud'homme D, Nadeau A, Moorjani S, Labrie F, Lupien PJ, Després JP. The dense LDL phenotype. Association with plasma lipoprotein levels, visceral obesity, and hyperinsulinemia in men. Diabetes Care. 1996;19:629–37.
105. Després JP. Dyslipidaemia and obesity. Bailliere's Clin Endocrinol Metab. 1994;8:629–60.
106. Lemieux S, Després JP. Metabolic complications of visceral obesity: contribution to the aetiology of type 2 diabetes and implications for prevention and treatment. Diabete Metab. 1994;20:375–93.
107. Reaven GM. Banting lecture 1988. Role of insulin resistance in human disease. Diabetes. 1988;37:1595–607.
108. Després JP, Marette A. Relation of components of insulin resistance syndrome to coronary disease risk. Curr Opin Lipidol. 1994;5:274–89.
109. Seidell JC, Oosterlee A, Thijssen MAO, Burema J, Deurenberg P, Hautvast JGAJ, Ruijs JHJ. Assessment of intra-abdominal and subcutaneous abdominal fat: relation between anthropometry and computed tomography. Am J Clin Nutr. 1987;45:7–13.
110. Pouliot MC, Després JP, Lemieux S, Moorjani S, Bouchard C, Tremblay A, Nadeau A, Lupien PJ. Waist circumference and abdominal sagittal diameter: best simple anthropometric indexes of abdominal visceral adipose tissue accumulation and related cardiovascular risk in men and women. Am J Cardiol. 1994;73:460–8.
111. Lemieux S, Prud'homme D, Bouchard C, Tremblay A, Després JP. A single threshold value of waist girth identifies normal-weight and overweight subjects with excess visceral adipose tissue. Am J Clin Nutr. 1996;64:685–693.
112. Borkan GA, Hults DE, Gerzof SG, Burrows BA, Robbins AH. Relationships between computed tomography tissue areas, thicknesses and total body composition. Ann Hum Biol. 1983;10:537–45.
113. Després JP. Abdominal obesity as important component of insulin-resistance syndrome. Nutrition. 1993;9:452–9.
114. Lemieux S, Prud'homme D, Moorjani S, Tremblay A, Bouchard C, Lupien PJ, Després JP. Do elevated levels of abdominal visceral adipose tissue contribute to age-related differences in plasma lipoprotein concentrations in men ? Atherosclerosis. 1995;118:155–164.
115. Després JP, Moorjani S, Lupien PJ, Tremblay A, Nadeau A, Bouchard C. Regional distribution of body fat, plasma lipoproteins, and cardiovascular disease. Arteriosclerosis. 1990;10: 497–511.
116. Després JP, Moorjani S, Ferland M, Tremblay A, Lupien PJ, Nadeau A, Pinault S, Thériault G, Bouchard C. Adipose tissue distribution and plasma lipoprotein levels in obese women. Importance of intra-abdominal fat. Arteriosclerosis. 1989;9:203–10.
117. Lamarche B, Moorjani S, Lupien P-J, Cantin B, Bernard P-M, Dagenais GR, Després JP. Apolipoprotein A-I and B levels and the risk of ischemic heart disease during a five-year follow-up of men in the Québec cardiovascular study. Circulation. 1996;94:273–278.
118. Lamarche B, Tchernof A, Moorjani S, Cantin B, Dagenais GR, Lupien P-J, Després JP. Small, dense low-density lipoprotein particles as a predictor of the risk of ischemic heart disease in men. Prospective results from the Québec Cardiovascular Study. Circulation. 1997;95:69–75.
119. Després JP, Lamarche B, Mauriège P, Cantin B, Dagenais GR, Moorjani S, Lupien P-J. Hyperinsulinemia as an independent risk factor for ischemic heart disease. N Engl J Med. 1996;334:952–957.
120. Lamarche B, Tchernof A, Mauriège P, Cantin B, Dagenais GR, Lupien PJ, Després JP. Fasting

insulin and apolipoprotein B levels and low-density lipoprotein particle size as risk factors for ischemic heart disease. JAMA. 1998;279:1955–1961.
121. Lemieux I, Pascot A, Couillard C, Lamarche B, Tchernof A, Alméras N, Bergeron J, Gaudet D., Tremblay G., Prud'homme D, Nadeau A, Després JP. Hypertriglyceridemic waist: a marker of the atherogenic metabolic triad (hyperinsulinemia, hyperapoB, small, dense LDL) in men? Circulation. 2000; 102:179–184.
122. Lemieux I, Pascot A, Tchernof A, Bergeron J, Prud'homme D, Bouchard C, Després JP. Visceral adipose tissue and low-density lipoprotein particle size in middle-aged versus young men. Metabolism. 1999;48:1322–7.
123. McNamara JR, Jenner JL, Li Z, Wilson PW, Schaefer EJ. Change in LDL particle size is associated with change in plasma triglyceride concentration. Arterioscler Thromb Vasc Biol. 1992;12:1284–1290.
124. Manninen V, Tenkanen L, Koshinen P, Huttunen JK, Mänttäri M, Heinonen OP, Frick MH. Joint effects of serum triglyceride and LDL cholesterol and HDL cholesterol concentrations on coronary heart disease risk in the Helsinki Heart Study: implications for treatment. Circulation. 1992;85:37–45.
125. Stampfer MJ, Sacks FM, Salvini S, Willett WC, Hennekens CH. A prospective study of cholesterol, apolipoproteins, and the risk of myocardial infarction. N Engl J Med. 1991;325:373–381.
126. Lemieux I, Alméras N, Mauriège P, Blanchet C, Sauvé L, Dewailly E, Després JP, Bergeron J. Waist circumference and triglyceride levels as screening tools for the evaluation of IHD risk in men. Obes Res. 1999;7:60 S.
127. Ferrannini E, Haffner SM, Mitchell BD, Stern MP. Hyperinsulinaemia: the key feature of a cardiovascular and metabolic syndrome. Diabetologia. 1991;34:416–22.
128. Laakso M. How good a marker is insulin level for insulin resistance? Am J Epidemiol. 1993;137:959–965.

CHAPTER 12

Oxidative Stress and Cardiovascular Risk in Type 2 Diabetes

A. Ceriello

Abstract. Accelerated atherosclerotic vascular disease is the leading cause of mortality in patients with diabetes mellitus. Endothelium-derived nitric oxide (NO) is a potent endogenous nitrovasodilator and plays a major role in modulation of vascular tone. Selective impairment of endothelium-dependent relaxation has been demonstrated in aortas of both nondiabetic animals exposed to elevated concentrations of glucose in vitro and insulin-dependent diabetic animals. The impaired NO release in experimentally induced diabetes may be prevented by a number of antioxidants. It has been hypothesized that oxygen-derived free radicals (OFR) generated during both glucose autoxidation and formation of advanced glycosylation end products may interfere with NO action and attenuate its vasodilatory activity. The oxidative injury may also be increased in diabetes mellitus because of a weakened defense due to reduced endogenous antioxidants (vitamin E, reduced glutathione [GSH]). A defective endothelium-dependent vascular relaxation has been found in animal models of hypertension and in hypertensive patients. An imbalance due to reduced production of NO or increased production of free radicals, mainly superoxide anion, may facilitate the development of an arterial functional spasm. Treatment with different antioxidants increases blood flow in the forearm and decreases blood pressure and viscosity in normal humans; vitamin E inhibits nonenzymatic glycosylation, oxidative stress, and red blood cell microviscosity in diabetic patients. Long-term randomized clinical trials of adequate size in secondary and primary prevention could support the free-radical hypothesis for diabetic vascular complications and the use of antioxidants to reduce the risk of coronary heart disease.

Type 2 diabetes is associated with an excessive incidence of cardiovascular disease and a reduction in life-expectancy of 5–10 years (Panzram 1987). This is mainly due to a clustering of established risk factors such as hypertension, hyperlipidemia, smoking (Stamler et al. 1993) and activation of thrombosis (Ceriello 1993), being hyperglycemia, a typical feature of diabetes, also an important contributing factor (Laasko 1999).

Recently, the possibility that oxidative stress may play a central role in the poor cardiovascular outlook of the diabetic patient has been suggested (Giugliano et al. 1996). This article will focus on the evidence supporting this hypothesis.

Oxidative Stress in Diabetes: The Role of Hyperglycemia

Hyperglycemia as the Source of Free Radicals

Hyperglycemia is the distinguishing feature of diabetes. One possible source of oxygen free radicals in diabetes is autoxidation of glucose (Hunt et al. 1988). Glucose can oxidize, which generates free radicals, hydrogen peroxide, and reactive ketoaldehydes. These last compounds may largely partecipate in the formation of glycated proteins, which are themselves a source of oxygen free radicals (Gillery et al. 1988, Sakurai and Tsuchiya 1988). The term "glycoxidation products" has been coined by

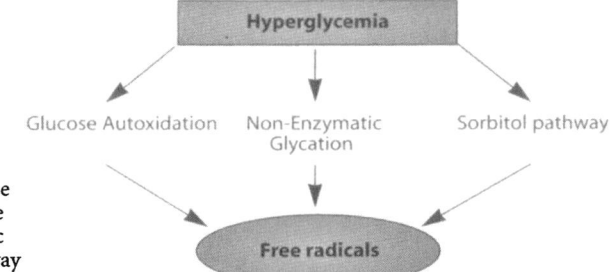

Fig. 12.1. Glucose can produce free radicals through glucose autoxidation, non-enzymatic glycation and sorbitol pathway activation

Baynes (Baynes 1991) to indicate autoxidation products, such as carboxymethyllysine and pentosidine, to stress the obligatory role of oxygen in the formation from Amadori products. Increased flux of glucose through the polyol pathway, which is hyperactive in hyperglycemia (Greene et al. 1987), may deplete NADPH which is required for generation of NO from arginine (Moncada and Higgs 1993). Furthermore, increased oxidation of sorbitol to fructose increases the ratio of cytosolic NADH/NAD$^+$. This redox imbalance, also referred to as hyperglycemic pseudohypoxia, augments production of superoxide anion (O_2^-) via reduction of PGG$_2$ to PGH$_2$ by prostaglandin hydroperoxidases that use NADH as a reducing cosubstrate (Williamson et al. 1993). Figure 12.1 summarizes these hypotheses.

The possibility that oxygen free radicals play a role in the pathogenesis of vascular complications of diabetes is suggested by studies that have shown that antioxidants such as vitamin E, SOD, catalase, GSH, and ascorbic acid are all decreased in diabetic tissues and blood (Oberley 1988, Asayama et al 1993, Ceriello et al. 1997). Moreover, elevated levels of oxygen free radical products in diabetic patients have been reported (Collier et al. 1990, Ceriello et al. 1991, Paolisso et al. 1993). In one study, the plasma concentration of O_2^- is increased in patients with IDDM, but showed a trend to normalization after strict metabolic control (Ceriello et al. 1991). There was a strong correlation between plasma glucose and O_2^- concentrations in both normal subjects and diabetic patients over a wide range of glucose concentrations.

Diabetic patients show reduced plasma levels of antioxidant power (Ceriello et al. 1997). The role of hyperglycemia in producing this situation is supported by the evidence that during an OGTT there is an increase of plasma malondialdehyde and a reduction of circulating antioxidants both in diabetic and normal subjects (Ceriello et al. 1998). This finding is consistent with the evidence that in diabetic patients meals are accompanied by a significant decrease of antioxidant defenses (Ceriello et al. 1998) (Fig. 12.2), proportional to the level of hyperglycemia (Ceriello et al. 1999). It seems true that the lower antioxidant power of plasma may favour the susceptibility of LDL to oxidation (Ceriello et al. 1999), which has been shown, in vitro, to be affected by hyperglycemia via superoxide-generation (Kawamura et al. 1994).

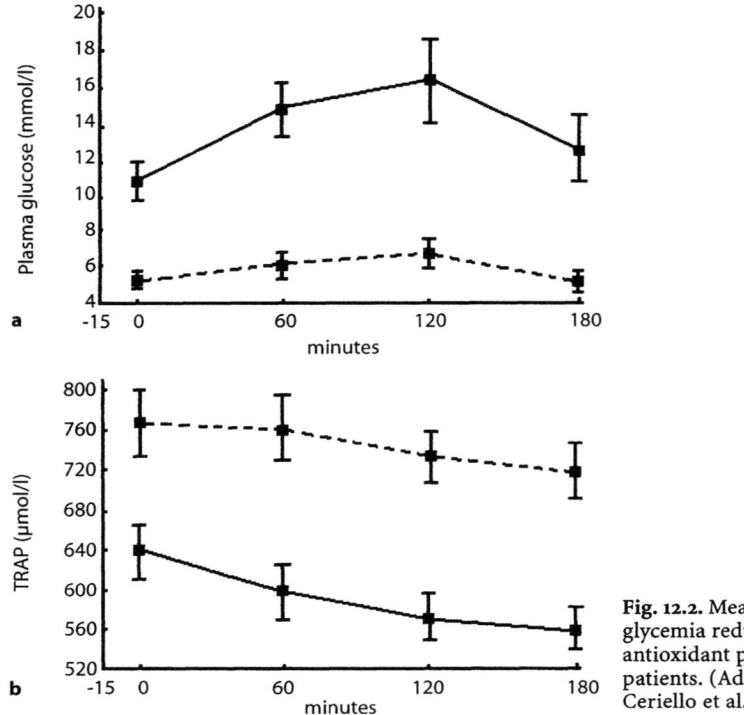

Fig. 12.2. Meal-induced hyperglycemia reduces plasma antioxidant power in diabetic patients. (Adapted from Ceriello et al. 1998)

Oxidative Stress and Endothelium in Diabetes

The endothelium has been shown to release a substance that induces smooth muscle relaxation by increasing the production of cyclic guanosine monophosphate. This factor is called endothelium-derived relaxing factor, and NO is believed to be one such factor (Palmer et al. 1987). The strongest evidence for a physiologic role of NO in humans lies in the results of intravenous injection of NG-monomethyl-L-arginine, an inhibitor of NO formation from L-arginine, into the forearm. Such injections cause substantial vasoconstriction that lasts for 45 to 60 minutes unless it is reversed by L-arginine (Vallance et al. 1989). Moreover, local forearm infusion of acetylcholine (ACh) causes vasodilation that is primarily due to stimulation of NO synthesis. Thus, vessels of healthy humans are continuously dilated by NO released from endothelial cells. Exposure to elevated concentrations of glucose in vitro causes selective impairment of endothelium-dependent relaxation (Tesfamarian and Cohen 1992). Oxidative stress induced by hyperglycemia is implicated as a source of altered endothelium relaxation in diabetes. Tesfamariam and Cohen (1992) have shown, for example, that elevated glucose concentrations impair ACh-stimulated endothelium relaxation in vitro and that this impairment can be reversed by antioxidants, which include superoxide dismutase (SOD) and catalase. Similarly, in diabetic animals impairment of ACh relaxation in aortas was restored to normal by SOD. Others have recently reported that the transient endothelium-dependent relaxation in the aorta of streptozotocin-induced diabetic rats was due to accumulation of O_2^- (Hattory et al. 1991) which confirms previous reports that oxygen-derived free radicals inactivate endothelium-derived releasing factors (Gryglewski et al 1986) and selectively attenuate endothelium-dependent relaxation (Pieper and Gross 1988, Rubanyi and Vanhoutte 1986).

The inhibition of Na^+-K^+ adenosine triphosphatase activity seen in endothelium-intact aortas from severely diabetic rabbits, as well as in aortic rings from normal rabbits incubated in high-glucose medium, may be due to a decrease in basal release of NO (Gupta et al. 1992). High glucose concentrations have been reported to lengthen cell proliferation time and slightly increase cell death in cultured human endothelial cells derived from the umbilical vein (Lorenzi et al. 1985). Curcio and Ceriello (1992) have shown that a hyperglycemia-induced delay in cell replication time that occurs in cultured human endothelial cells may be reversed by a number of antioxidants with different mechanisms of action, such as SOD, catalase, and reduced glutathione (GSH). A pathophysiologic link between hyperglycemia and development of endothelium dysfunctions through increased synthesis and/or release of oxygen free radicals thus may be hypothesized. This hypothesis is strongly supported by the evidence that exposure of endothelial cells to hyperglycemia is followed by an increase of intracellular antioxidant enzymes (Ceriello et al. 1996).

With this in mind, one would expect disturbed endothelium-dependent vascular relaxation in diabetes mellitus. Many (de Tejada et al. 1989, Calver et al. 1992, Mc Veigh et al. 1992, Elliott et al. 1993, Johnstone et al. 1993) but not all (Halkin et al. 1991) recent studies have shown that endothelium-dependent vasodilation is abnormal in diabetic patients (both IDDM and NIDDM) and that this abnormality is caused by decreased release or activity of NO. Moreover, several properties of NO (inhibition of platelet aggregation, monocyte adhesion to endothelial cells, and smooth muscle cell proliferation) suggest that if its biosynthesis were reduced, this could predispose to atheroma (Moncada et al. 1991). Studies on effects of antioxidants in human diabetes are scanty. Pharmacologic vitamin E supplementation (900 mg/d for 4 months) in patients with NIDDM improves insulin action (nonoxidative glucose metabolism, mainly synthesis of glycogen), reduces oxidative stress (GSSG/GSH ratio decreased by 47%), and ameliorates red blood cell microviscosity (Paolisso et al. 1993). These results confirm and extend previous studies that found that daily oral vitamin E supplementation (600 or 1,200 mg) to IDDM subjects for 2 months reduced oxidative stress and protein glycation (Ceriello et al. 1991). An indirect mechanism by which vitamin E may reduce the unfavorable effects of oxygen free radicals on endothelial function is through an increased production of the vasodilating prostaglandin PGI_2, as demonstrated in cultured bovine aortic endothelial cells, where specific binding sites for D-alpha-tocopherol have also been found (Kunisaki et al. 1993). Interestingly enough and perhaps relevant to the vascular toxicity of hyperglycemia in human diabetes is the finding that high concentrations of glucose (16.8 or 22.4 mmol/l) reduce D-alpha-tocopherol binding through oxidative stress (Kunisaki et al. 1993).

Oxidative Stress as Pathogenetic Factor of Hypertension in Diabetes

Endothelium-dependent relaxation has been found to be impaired in animal models of hypertension (Auch-Schwalk et al. 1989). Moreover, the frequency of endothelial cell death and associated endothelial permeability is significantly increased in the aorta of spontaneously hypertensive rats (Wu et al. 1990). The response of forearm blood flow to ACh but not to sodium nitroprusside, an agent that produces vasodilation by direct activation of guanylate cyclase in vascular smooth muscle cells (Schultz et al. 1977) was significantly reduced in 18 middle-aged hypertensive patients (Panza et al. 1990). Since ACh only produces an endothelium-mediated vasodilator response, a defect in endothelium-dependent vascular relaxation has been hypothesized. An acute antihypertensive effect of three structurally unrelated antioxidant agents, such as vitamin C, thiopronine (a substrate for glutathione synthesis), and glutathione, has been reported in hypertensive subjects, regardless of whether they are diabetic (Ceriello et al. 1991). An imbalance due to reduced production of NO, as demon-

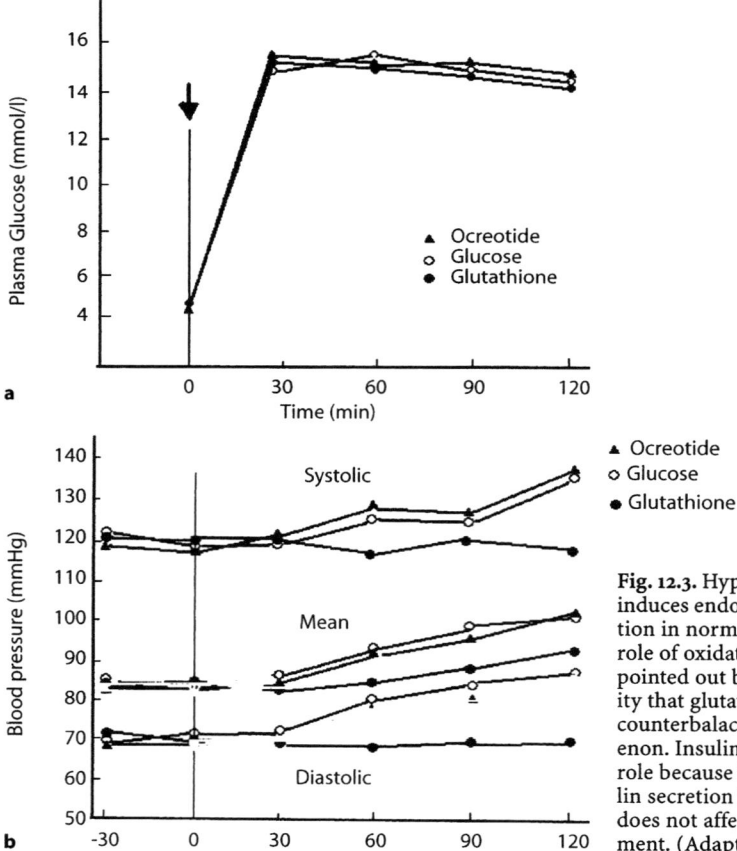

Fig. 12.3. Hyperglycemia induces endothelial dysfunction in normal subjects. The role of oxidative stress in pointed out by the possibility that glutathione infusion counterbalaces this phenomenon. Insulin does not play a role because inhibiting insulin secretion by ocreotide does not affect the experiment. (Adapted from Marfella et al. 1995)

strated in spontaneously hypertensive rats (Auch-Schwalk et al. 1989) or increased destruction by a relative or absolute increase in O_2^- may facilitate the development of an arterial functional spasm. A physiologic role for O_2^- is suggested by results of intravenous infusions of the three different antioxidants that have a vasodilating action in the skeletal muscle of the forearm in normal humans (Ceriello et al. 1991). Thus, it seems likely that a continuous production of O_2^- offsets the vasodilatory action of NO, which allows the maintenance of a proper vascular tone. Several studies report that free radicals may be the mediators of the effects of acute hyperglycaemia. In vivo studies demonstrate that in diabetic patients as well as normal subjects acute hyperglycaemia increases blood pressure values, an effect reversed by antioxidant administration (Ceriello et al. 1997, Marfella et al. 1995) (Fig. 12.3).

Oxidative Stress and Aging

The prevalence of diabetes (up to 12% after 65 years) and hypertension (up to 30% after 70 years) increases with age. Therefore, age may be a common factor that amplifies the association between diabetes and hypertension. Paolisso et al. (1993) found significant increments of serum O_2^- with age associated with increases in both membrane viscosity and the GSSG/GSH ratio, as well as a reduction of total-body glucose disposal evaluated during euglycemic glucose clamp (1 mU/kg/min) with simultaneous D-^{3}H-glucose infusion and indirect calorimetry. In the multivariate analysis, only O_2^- displayed an independent relationship with total-body glucose disposal and nonoxidative glucose metabolism. Elderly NIDDM patients who took vitamin E (900 mg/d) for 3 months demonstrated significant benefits on many parameters of both glucose (glycemia and hemoglobin A_{1c}) and lipid (triglycerides, low-densitylipoprotein [LDL] cholesterol, and apoprotein A) metabolism (Paolisso et al. 1993). Moreover, plasma O_2^- production and the GSSG/GSH ratio significantly decreased after vitamin E therapy. In another study, elderly atherosclerotic patients showed decreased blood viscosity and improved blood filterability in response to exogenous glutathione (600 mg/d as intravenous infusion per 7 days) (Coppola et al. 1992).

Pathogenetic Implications

Treatment with different antioxidants improves many metabolic abnormalities reported to occur in diabetic subjects. Vitamin E and glutathione ameliorate insulin sensitivty mainly by stimulation of nonoxidative glucose metabolism (Paolisso et al. 1992); short-term administrations of vitamin C, thiopronine, and GSH all increase resting blood flow in the forearm of normal and diabetic patients irrespective of the presence of hypertension, which suggests that a continuous basal production of O_2^- offsets the vasodilatory action of NO by quenching it (Ceriello et al. 1993); GSH ameliorates hemorrheologic parameters in diabetic patients, atherosclerotic subjects, and normal people (Coppola et al. 1992). Thus, an increased production of oxygen free radicals may be a cause of the increased cardiovascular morbidity and mortality found in diabetes mellitus.

It is known that free radicals are capable of activating coagulation (Barrowcliffe et al. 1987) and direct evidence already exists to indicate that oxidative stress is accompanied by hemostatic alterations in diabetic patients (Collier et al. 1992).

Reduced levels of vitamin E are reported in the platelets of diabetic subjects, accompanied by hyperaggregation (Wanatabe et al. 1984). Treatment with vitamin E improves this situation (Wanatabe et al. 1984).

The hypothesis that oxidative stress may be involved in the thrombin activation by hyperglycemia has been confirmed by a study showing that during oral glucose tolerance test glutathione administration normalized prothrombin fragment 1 + 2 increase in both diabetic and normal subjects (Ceriello et al. 1995). Glutathione administered alone significantly decreased prothrombin fragment 1 + 2 in diabetic patients while no effect was observed in the normal subjects (Ceriello et al. 1995). These data suggest that hyperglycemia may induce thrombin activation possibly inducing an oxidative stress, and that antioxidant glutathione may counterbalance this effect.

Abnormalities of the NO/O_2^- pathway have been demonstrated in humans with diabetes mellitus and essential hypertension (Ceriello et al. 1993) and hyperlipidemia (Creager et al. 1990). A dysfunction of the NO/O_2^- system may be a common mechanism by which such apparently diverse conditions result in similar chronic vascular complications. A diminished basal production or effect of NO, as well as an increased concentration or effect of O_2^- would tip the balance in favor of vasoconstriction and blood hyperviscosity and thus favor the development of vaso-occlusive disorders at the level of coronary, cerebral, and peripheral vessels.

This hypothesisi is strongly supported by the finding that exposure of endothelial cells to high glucose increases NO release, wich, however, is associated with a more marked concomitant increase of O_2^- production, favouring a O_2^- prevalence (Cosentino et al. 1997).

Completing this gloomy scenario, oxygen free radicals are capable of activation of coagulation and oxidation of LDL, and both hemostatic alterations (Ceriello et al. 1993) and increased levels of plasma and tissue oxidized lipids (Lyons 1991) are found in diabetic patients. Hyperlipidemia may alter the redox state of vascular smooth muscle (Yla-Herttuala et al. 1989) and thereby reduce the responsiveness of the vessel wall to nitrovasodilators. In fact, there are sulfhydryl groups associated with guanylate cyclase, the oxidation of which inactivates the enzyme (Craven et al. 1978). In humans, the susceptibility of LDL to oxidation correlated with the severity of coronary stenosis in 35 male survivors of myocardial infarction (Regnström et al. 1992), and LDL from volunteers treated with alpha-tocopherol supplements (200 mg for 6 months) showed increased resistance to oxidation (Abbey et al. 1993). Although the antioxidant hypothesis of atherosclerosis is supported by experimental and epidemiologic data, it has not yet attained the status of a clinically validated hypothesis (Steinberg 1993). More than one third of NIDDM patients and half of IDDM patients remain free of hypertension throughout their lives; the suggested chain of events that links high blood glucose to hypertension may only occur in patients who also have other risk factors for hypertension, e.g., a family history or increased Na^+-Li^+ countertransport (1993). Moreover, diabetic patients with hypertension seem more susceptible than diabetic subjects without hypertension to the blood pressure-increasing effects of oxygen frre radicals generated by glucose (Ceriello et al. 1993). On the other hand, alterations of blood rheology, blood-flow response to ACh, coagulative parameters, and lipidemic pattern may be present in the majority of diabetic patients. Recent epidemiologic and clinical evidence supports a role for hyperglycemia in the increased cardiovascular morbidity and mortality found in human diabetes (Laasko

1999). Increased plasma and tissue glucose levels may be one important source of the increased oxidative stress seen in diabetic patients. Although more than one factor may be involved, as the beneficial effects of vitamin E on vasculature unrelated to its antioxidant capability seem to suggest (Kunisaki et al. 1993) the evidence that oxygen free radicals are implicated in the endothelial dysfunction of diabetic patients is growing and may offer novel therapeutic approaches.

References

Abbey M, Nestel PJ, Baghurst PA (1993) Antioxidant vitamins and low density-lipoprotein oxidation. Am J Clin Nutr 58:525-532
Asayama K, Uchida N, Nakane T et al. (1993) Antioxidants in the serum of children with insulin-dependent diabetes mellitus. Free Rad Biol Med 15: 597-602 1. Panzram G (1987) Mortality and survival in type 2 (non-insulin-dependent) diabetes mellitus. Diabetologia 30: 123-131
Auch-Schwalk W, Katusic ZS, Vanhoutte PM (1989) Contractions to oxygen-derived free radicals are augmented in aorta of the spontaneously hypertensive rat. Hypertension 13:859-862
Baynes JW (1991) Role of oxidative stress in development of oxidative complications in diabetes. Diabetes 40:405-412
Barrowcliffe TW, Gutteridge JM, Gray E (1987) Oxygen radicals, lipid peroxidation and the coagulation system. Agent Actions 22: 347-348
Calver AC, Collier JG, Vallance PJT (1992) Inhibition and stimulation of nitric oxide synthesis in the human forearm arterial bed of patients with insulin-dependent diabetes. J Clin Invest 90:2548-2554
Ceriello A, Quatraro A, Caretta F et al. (1990) Evidence for a possible role of oxygen free radicals in the abnormal functional arterial vasomotion in insulin dependent diabetes. Diabete Metab 16:318-322
Ceriello A, Giugliano D, Quatraro A et al. (1991) Metabolic control may influence the increased superoxide generation in diabetic serum. Diabetic Med 8:540-542
Ceriello A, Giugliano D, Quatraro A et al. (1991) Vitamin E reduction of protein glycosylation in diabetics: New prospect for prevention of diabetic complications. Diabetes Care 14:68-72
Ceriello A, Giugliano D, Quatraro A et al. (1991) Antioxidants show an anti-hypertensive effect in diabetic and hypertensive subjects. Clin Sci 81:739-742
Ceriello A (1993) Coagulation activation in diabetes mellitus: the role of hyperglycaemia and therapeutic prospects. Diabetologia 36: 1119-1125
Ceriello A (1993) Coagulation activation in diabetes mellitus: The role of hyperglycaemia and therapeutic prospects. Diabetologia 36:1119-1125
Ceriello A, Quatraro A, Giugliano D (1993) Diabetes mellitus and hypertension: the possible role of hyperglycemia through oxidative stress. Diabetologia 36:265-266
Ceriello A, Giacomello R, Stel G et al. (1995) Hyperglycaemia-induced thrombin formation in diabetes: the possible role of oxidative stress. Diabetes 44: 924-928
Ceriello A, Dello Russo P, Amstad P, Cerutti P (1996) High glucose induces antioxidant defence in endothelial cell in culture. Evidence linking hyperglycemia and oxidative stress. Diabetes 45: 471-477
Ceriello A, Bortolotti N, Falleti E et al. (1997) Total radical-trapping antioxidant parameter in non-insulin dependent diabetic patients. Diabetes Care 20: 194-197
Ceriello A, Motz E, Cavarape A et al. (1997) Hyperglycemia counterbalances the anti-hypertensive effect of glutathione in diabetic patients. Evidence linking hypertension and glycemia through the oxidative stress in diabetes mellitus. J Diab Compl 11: 250-255
Ceriello A, Bortolotti N, Crescentini A et al. (1998) Antioxidant defenses are reduced during oral glucose tolerance test in normal and non-insulin dependent diabetic subjects. Eur J Clin Invest 28: 329-333
Ceriello A, Bortolotti N, Motz E et al. (1998) Meal-generated oxidative stress in type 2 diabetic patients. Diabetes Care 21: 1529-1533
Ceriello A, Bortolotti N, Motz E et al. (1999) Meal-induced oxidative stress and LDL oxidation in diabetes: the possible role of hyperglycemia. Metabolism 48: 1503-1508

Consensus Statement: Treatment of hypertension in diabetes (1993) Diabetes Care 16:1394–1401
Collier A, Rumley AG, Paterson JR et al. (1992) Free radical activity and hemostatic factor in NIDDM patients with and without microalbuminuria. Diabetes 41: 909–913
Collier A, Wilson R, Bradley H et al. (1990) Free radical activity in type-2 diabetes. Diabetic Med 7:27–30
Coppola L, Grassia A, Giunta R et al. (1992) Glutathione (GSH) improves haemostatic and haemorrheological parameters in atherosclerotic subjects. Drugs Exp Clin Res 18:493–498
Cosentino F, Hishikawa K, Katusie ZS, Lüscher TF (1997) High glucose increases nitric oxide synthase expression and superoxide anion generation in human aortic endothelial cells. Circulation 96: 25–28
Craven PA, DeRubertis FR (1978) Restoration of the responsiveness of purified guanylate cyclase to nitrosoguanidine, nitric oxide and related activators by heme and heme proteins. J Biol Chem 253:8433–8443
Creager MA, Cooke JP, Mendelsohn SJ et al. (1990) Impaired vasodilation of forearm resistance vessels in hypercholesterolemic humans. J Clin Invest 86:228–234
Curcio F, Ceriello A (1992) Decreased cultured endothelial cell proliferation in high glucose medium is reversed by antioxidants: new insights on the pathophysiological mechanisms of diabetic vascular complications. In Vitro Cell Dev Biol 28A:787–790
de Tejada S, Goldstein I, Azadzoi K et al. (1989) Impaired neurogenic and endothelium-mediated relaxation of penile smooth muscle from diabetic men with impotence. N Engl J Med 320:1025–1030
Elliott TG, Cockcroft JR, Groop P-H et al. (1993) Inhibition of nitric oxide synthesis in forearm vasculature of insulin-dependent diabetic patients: Blunted vasoconstriction in patients with micro-albuminuria. Clin Sci 85:687–693
Gillery P, Monboisse JC, Maquat FX et al. (1988) Glycation of proteins as a source of superoxide. Diabete Metab 14:25–30
Giugliano D, Ceriello A, Paolisso G (1996) Oxidative stress and diabetic vascular complications. Diabetes Care 19: 257–267
Greene DA, Lattimer SA, Sima AF (1987) Sorbitol, phosphoinositides and sodium-potassium-ATPase in the pathogenesis of diabetic complications. N Engl J Med 316:599–606
Gryglewski RJ, Palmer RMJ, Moncada S (1986) Superoxide anion is involved in the breakdown of endothelium-derived relaxing factor. Nature 320:454–456
Gupta S, Sussman I, McArthur CS, et al. (1992) Endothelium-dependent inhibition of Na^+-K^+ ATPase activity in rabbit aorta by hyperglycemia. Possible role of endothelium-derived nitric oxide. J Clin Invest 90:727–732
Halkin A, Bejamin N, Doktor HS, et al. (1991) Vascular responsiveness and cation exchange in insulin-dependent diabetes. Clin Sci 81:223–232
Hattori Y, Kawasaki H, Abe K, et al. (1991) Superoxide dismutase recovers altered endothelium dependent relaxation in diabetic rat aorta. Am J Physiol 261:H1086-H1094
Hunt JV, Dean RT, Wolff SP (1988) Hydroxyl radical production and autoxidative glycosylation. Glucose autoxidation as the cause of protein damage in the experimental glycation model of diabetes mellitus and aging. Biochem J 256:205–212
Laakso M (1999) Hyperglycemia and cardiovascular disease in type 2 diabetes. Diabetes 48: 937–942
Lorenzi M, Cagliero E, Toledo S (1985) Glucose toxicity for human endothelial cells in culture. Diabetes 34:621–627
Johnstone MT, Creager SJ, Scales KM, et al. (1993) Impaired endothelium-dependent vasodilation in patients with insulin-dependent diabetes mellitus. Circulation 88:2510–2516
Kawamura M, Heinecke JW, Chait A (1994) Pathophysiological concentrations of glucose promote oxidative modification of low density lipoprotein by a superoxide-dependent pathway. J Clin Invest 94: 771–778
Kunisaki M, Umeda F, Yamauchi T et al. (1993) High glucose reduces specific binding for D-alpha-tocopherol in cultured aortic endothelial cells. Diabetes 42:1138–1146
Lyons TJ (1991) Oxidized low density lipoproteins: A role in the pathogenesis of atherosclerosis in diabetes. Diabetic Med 8:414–419
Marfella R, Verrazzo G, Acampora R et al. (1995) Glutathione reverses systemic hemodynamic changes by acute hyperglycemia in healthy subjects. Am J Physiol 268: E1167-E1173

12 Oxidative Stress and Cardiovascular Risk in Type 2 Diabetes

McVeigh GE, Brennan GM, Johnston GD, et al. (1992) Impaired endothelium-dependent and -independent vasodilation in patients with type-2 (non-insulin-dependent) diabetes mellitus. Diabetologia 35:771-776
Moncada S, Higgs A (1993) Mechanisms of disease: The L-arginine-nitric oxide pathway. N Engl J Med 329:2002-2012
Moncada S, Palmer RMJ, Higgs EA (1991) Nitric oxide: Physiology, pathophysiology and pharmacology. Pharmacol Rev 43:109-142
Oberley LW (1988) Free radicals and diabetes. Free Rad Biol Med 5: 113-124
Palmer RM, Ferrige AG, Moncada S (1987) Nitric oxide release accounts for the biological activity of endothelium-derived relaxing factor. Nature 327:524-526
Panza JA, Arshed AQ, Brush JE et al. (1990) Abnormal endothelium-dependent vascular relaxation in patients with essential hypertension. N Engl J Med 323:22-27
Paolisso G, D'Amore A, Di Maro G et al. (1993) Evidence for a relationship between free radicals and insulin action in the elderly. Metabolism 42:659-663
Paolisso G, D'Amore A, Galzerano D et al. (1993) Daily vitamin E supplements improve metabolic control but not insulin secretion in elderly type II diabetic patients. Diabetes Care 16:1433-1437
Paolisso G, D'Amore A, Giugliano D et al. (1993) Pharmacological doses of vitamin E improve insulin action in healthy subjects and non-insulin-dependent diabetic patients. Am J Clin Nutr 57:650-656
Paolisso G, Di Maro G, Pizza G et al. (1992) Plasma GSH/GSSG affects glucose homeostasis in healthy subjects and non-insulin-dependent diabetics. Am J Physiol 263:E435-E440
Pieper GM, Gross G (1988) Oxygen free radicals abolish endothelium-dependent relaxation in diabetic rat aorta. Am J Physiol 255:H825-H833
Regnström J, Nilsson J, Tornvall P et al. (1992) Susceptibility to low-density lipoprotein oxidation and coronary atherosclerosis in man. Lancet 339:1183-1186
Rubanyi GM, Vanhoutte PM (1986) Oxygen-derived free radicals, endothelium, and responsiveness of vascular smooth muscle. Am J Physiol 250:H815-H821
Sakurai T, Tsuchiya S (1988) Superoxide production from non-enzymatically glycated proteins. FEBS Lett 236:406-410
Schultz K, Schultz K, Schultz G (1977) Sodium nitroprusside and other smooth muscle relaxants increase cyclic GMP levels in rat ductus deferens. Nature 265:750-751
Stamler J, Vaccaro O, Neaton JD, Wentworth D, for the Multiple Risk Factor Intervention Trial Research Group (1993) Diabetes, other risk factors, and 12-yr cardiovascular mortality for men screened in the multiple risk factor intervention trial. Diabetes Care 16: 434-444
Steinberg D (1993) Antioxidant vitamins and coronary heart disease. N Engl J Med 328:1487-1489
Tesfamarian B, Brown ML, Deykin D, et al. (1990) Elevated glucose promotes generation of endothelium-dependent vasoconstrictor prostanoids in rabbit aorta. J Clin Invest 85:929-932
Tesfamarian B, Cohen RA (1992) Free radicals mediate endothelial cell dysfunction caused by elevated glucose. Am J Physiol 263:H321-H326
Vallance P, Collier J, Moncada S (1989) Effects of endothelium-derived nitric oxide on peripheral arteriolar tone in man. Lancet 2:997-1000
Wanatabe J, Umeda F, Wakasugi H, Ibayashi H (1984) Effect of vitamin E on platelet aggregation in diabetes mellitus. Thromb Haemostas 51:313-316
Williamson JR, Chang K, Frangos M, et al. (1993) Hyperglycemic pseudohypoxia and diabetic complications. Diabetes 42:801-813
Wu CH, Chi JC, Jenig JS et al. (1990) Transendothelial macromolecular transport in the aorta of spontaneously hypertensive rats. Hypertension 16:154-161
Yla-Herttuala S, Palinski W, Rosenfeld ME et al. (1989) Evidence for the presence of oxidatively modified LDL in human atherosclerotic lesions. Circulation 80(suppl 2):145-160

CHAPTER 13

Lifestyle and Cardiovascular Risk in Type 2 Diabetes

M.W. Conard, W.S. Carlos Poston

Abstract. Type 2 diabetes is diagnosed with ever increasing frequency in the U.S. among both adults and children. Type 2 diabetes accounts for 17.2% of all deaths primarily related to cardiovascular disease (CVD) mortality. Various CVD risk factors that result from the effects of type 2 diabetes have been discovered including hyperglycemia, insulin resistance, hypertension, and dyslipidemia. Research has uncovered numerous lifestyle influences that affect the development of type 2 diabetes and these CVD risk factors include diet, physical inactivity, obesity, socioeconomic status, and acculturation. Alterations in lifestyle have been shown to reduce the impact of type 2 diabetes on CVD risk. The most effective lifestyle modification appears to be when individuals with type 2 diabetes lower their weight by eating a diet high in fruits, vegetables, and low-fat diary foods combined with regular, moderate exercise to reduce hypertension, hyperglycemia, and regain lipid balance.

Prevalence of Type 2 Diabetes

Type 2 diabetes, which also is known as non-insulin-dependent diabetes, can be diagnosed by the presence of the classical signs and symptoms of diabetes together with unequivocally elevated blood glucose levels (Harris 2000). Typically, type 2 diabetes is preceded by a period of asymptomatic impaired glucose tolerance (Laakso 1999; Nathan et al. 1997). Type 2 diabetes develops after the insulin resistance associated with the impaired glucose tolerance is compounded by failing insulin secretion along with functionally compromised pancreatic beta cells (Nathan et al. 1997).

Of the 7.8 million people in the United States diagnosed with diabetes in 1993, approximately 90%–95% were diagnosed with type 2 diabetes (Harris 2000). In addition, there are approximately seven million undiagnosed cases of type 2 diabetes in the United States (Harris 2000). This increasing prevalence is linked to the current obesity epidemic and the high levels of sedentary activity in the U.S. and it is predicted to continue to increase sharply as the population ages (Crespo et al. 1996; Flegal et al. 1998; MMWR 2000; Seidell 2000). The direct medical costs associated with diabetes in 1997 totaled $44.1 billion, with $11.8 billion due to excess prevalence of related chronic complications and $24.6 billion due to excess prevalence of general medical conditions (American Diabetes Association 1998).

While there are no gender differences in the prevalence rates of type 2 diabetes in the U.S., type 2 diabetes is more common in African-Americans, Mexican-Americans, Japanese-Americans, and Native Americans than in non-Hispanic whites and it is increasingly more common in children (Harris 2000; Libman and Arslanian 1999). In addition, it is substantially more common among overweight individuals over 40 and this trend is emerging in most developed and developing nations (Nathan et al. 1997; Seidell 2000). Type 2 diabetes-related mortality is estimated to account for 17.2 % of all deaths in the United States for those age twenty-five years or older (Harris 2000). The leading cause of death for type 2 diabetics (approximately 50 %) is cardiovascular disease (CVD; e.g., coronary heart disease, stroke, and peripheral vascular disease); the risk of CVD-related mortality is approximately two to four times higher for type 2 diabetes than nondiabetitic persons (Harris 2000). Costs of the increased risk of CVD have found that the greatest savings for the population would come from preventing major cardiovascular events (Brown et al. 1999).

Cardiovascular Risk Factors and Type 2 Diabetes

Among the many complications that result from type 2 diabetes, CVD appears to be a major cause of morbidity and mortality in the United States (Harris 2000; Marks and Raskin 2000) with a mortality rate of approximately 80 % (O'Keefe et al. 1999). CVD is more common in persons with type 2 diabetes than in non-diabetic persons (Laakso 1999). It is important to note that diabetes has a multiplicative effect on CVD risk in the presence of other CVD risk factors, so it is difficult to separate the individual roles of CVD risk factors in the context of diabetes (Clark Jr. and Perry 1999). For example, both hypertension and dyslipidemia coexist and are common in persons with diabetes, thus synergistically increasing the risk of CVD (Barbery 1999). Also, the majority of persons with type 2 diabetes also are insulin resistant (the primary mechanism contributing to type 2 diabetes), which usually precedes the actual development of type 2 diabetes (Lebovitz 1999; Marks and Raskin 2000).

Insulin resistance also has been independently associated with hypertension and dyslipidemia (Barbery 1999). The resulting metabolic abnormalities in type 2 diabetes and their coexistence with hyperglycemia and hyperinsulinemia appear to create risk factors that can lead to CVD (Barbery 1999; Marks and Raskin 2000; Sowers and Lester 1999; Ryden 2000). However, the coexistence of several metabolic disorders and cardiovascular problems have led some researchers to indicate that cardiovascular complications may already be evident when type 2 diabetes is eventually diagnosed. Thus, correcting one cardiovascular risk factor may not be enough of a treatment or preventative measure to lower the risk of CVD in persons with type 2 diabetes (Laakso 1999).

One associated risk factor for increased CVD is hyperglycemia. Laakso (1999) reviewed several prospective studies that indicated glycemic control is important for reducing CVD risk. Laakso (1999) concluded that hyperglycemia and poor glycemic control were associated with increased risk for CVD in type 2 diabetes. Marks and Raskin (2000) reviewed several observational studies indicating that associations exist between glycemic levels and cardiovascular risk. These studies suggest that higher levels of glucose are associated with higher rates of CVD, as well as indicating that hyperglycemia is an independent predictor of CVD.

Insulin resistance and the resulting hyperinsulinemia have been documented as another possible risk factor for CVD. Insulin resistance interferes with the cellular absorption of glucose, mainly into skeletal muscle tissue, leading to hyperinsulinemia and sometimes evolving into type 2 diabetes (O'Keefe et al. 1999). However, it is unclear exactly through what mechanisms hyperinsulinemia increases CVD risk. It is believed that the effects of hyperinsulinemia are mediated through chemical receptors, either directly by these chemicals or indirectly by high concentrations of insulin (Sowers and Lester 1999). Much research has been done on the associations between hyperinsulinemia and CVD risk with positive results, yet some researchers believe the association is actually between insulin resistance and CVD, with hyperinsulinemia being a compensatory physiologic response to insulin resistance (Marks and Raskin 2000). Past research suggests that insulin resistance was the leading candidate for explaining CVD risk; however recent studies investigating its link to CVD risk have been unable to confirm this association in men and none have found an association in women (Wingard and Barrett-Connor 2000). Some investigators have suggested that insulin resistance in many persons with type 2 diabetes is a result of visceral obesity (Lebovitz 1999). Type 2 diabetes has been associated as well with hypertension, left ventricular hypertrophy, sedentary lifestyle, impaired fibrinolysis, and atherogenic dyslipidemia and each of these are independently associated with progressive atherosclerosis and CVD (O'Keefe et al. 1999).

Increased risk for CVD is associated with hypertension. This relationship is believed by some to be mediated through shared causal factors with type 2 diabetes such as insulin resistance, obesity, sedentary lifestyle, and diet (O'Keefe et al. 1999). Barbery (1999) noted that when hypertension is associated with diabetes mellitus, there is acceleration of atherosclerosis, diabetic nephropathy, and diabetic retinopathy. However, hypertension is part of the metabolic syndrome, i.e., a majority of those with type 2 diabetes are hypertensive (Ryden 2000). Likewise, those with hypertension, but not diagnosed with type 2 diabetes, are more prone to type 2 diabetes than individuals with normal blood pressure (Barbery 1999). Several studies have demonstrated this link between hypertension and type 2 diabetes by investigating the effects of controlling hypertension on incidents of CVD in persons diagnosed with type 2 diabetes (Marks and Raskin 2000; Ryden 2000). The results from these studies indicate that lowering blood pressure in persons diagnosed with type 2 diabetes significantly lowers the risk of CVD.

Dyslipidemia is an additional risk factor for CVD. Research has shown that there is a distinct difference in lipid patterns between persons with type 2 diabetes and non-diabetic persons with type 2 diabetes, which is characterized by low concentrations of high-density lipoproteins, high concentrations of triglycerides, and a lower rate of raised low-density lipoprotein (Ryden 2000). Numerous studies have indicated that dyslipidemia is an independent risk factor for CVD in persons with diabetes. For example, Marks and Raskin (2000) evaluated three international studies that demonstrated lowering of CVD risk when dyslipidemia was successfully treated. However, Ryden (2000) noted that these studies should be viewed with caution because the subjects were not very representative of the diabetic population.

Lifestyle Factors

Numerous population studies, as well as ecological data and observational studies, provide evidence for environmental and lifestyle influences affecting the development of type 2 diabetes (Goldberg 1998; Rewers and Hamman 2000). These environmental and lifestyle factors include diet, physical inactivity, obesity, thinness at birth, socioeconomic status, urbanization, acculturation, and the interactions between genetic and environmental factors (Rewers and Hamman 2000).

Diet has long been discussed as a possible cause of diabetes, with caloric intake, carbohydrates, and fats considered leading components of diet affecting diabetes (Rewers and Hamman 2000). Historical studies that examined food shortages during wars showed that diabetes-related mortality and morbidity declined abruptly during these times (Rewers and Hamman 2000). With a regard to dietary carbohydrate and fiber intake, Rewers and Hamman (2000) found that studies provided inconsistent results, with several studies not finding significant relationships between carbohydrate or fiber intake and type 2 diabetes, yet one study did find a positive association between development of glucose intolerance and carbohydrate intake (Feskens et al. 1991). Dietary fat has been investigated as well as a possible environmental factor in the incidence of type 2 diabetes. Similar to carbohydrate and fiber intake studies, a review of studies on high-fat, low-carbohydrate diets and incidence of type 2 diabetes also found inconsistent results (Rewers and Hamman 2000). A high-fat diet was associated with the occurrence of type 2 diabetes, however Rewers and Hamman (2000) noted that diets high in omega-3 fatty acids appears to protect people from developing type 2 diabetes by lowering serum lipids, lipoprotein, platelet aggregation, blood pressure, and insulin resistance.

Alcohol consumption is a possible independent risk factor for type 2 diabetes, either through its effects on the pancreas and liver, or due to its additional calories and the resulting increases in weight and adipose tissue. Rewers and Hamman (2000) also pointed to several studies that found a positive association between alcohol use and increased incidence of type 2 diabetes. However, more research needs to be conducted in order to clarify this issue further.

Physical inactivity is another behavioral influence on the occurrence of type 2 diabetes. Most studies in this area examined the effects of differing levels of physical activity on increased incidence of type 2 diabetes and found that increased levels of physical activity are associated with lower incidence of type 2 diabetes diagnosis (Rewers and Hamman 2000). This protective effect results from the prevention of insulin resistance, but some studies suggest that this protective effect differs depending on the level of insulin that was present when the physical activity was initiated (Rewers and Hamman 2000). The overall results from these studies suggest that increased physical activity decreases the risk of type 2 diabetes.

Closely linked to physical inactivity is obesity, a longstanding risk factor associated with diabetes. With regards to type 2 diabetes, the association between the two is less clear and somewhat controversial because there are some non-obese persons who develop type 2 diabetes and there are obese persons who do not develop type 2 diabetes (Rewers and Hamman 2000). Numerous studies have shown higher incidence and prevalence of type 2 diabetes among various ethnic populations. Studies also have shown that duration of obesity was a predictor of increased incidence of type 2 diabetes (Rewers and Hamman 2000). Visceral adiposity also has been shown to be another risk factor for type 2 diabetes, independent of the presence of obesity (Rewers and Hamman 2000).

Recent studies on socioeconomic status demonstrate that lower income, education, and social class are associated with increased prevalence of type 2 diabetes

(Rewers and Hamman 2000). In addition, urban residents have higher rates of type 2 diabetes than those in rural areas (Rewers and Hamman 2000). Some researchers hypothesized that stress is a potential risk factor for type 2 diabetes, but there appears to be little epidemiologic support for this association (Rewers and Hamman 2000). Connected to socioeconomic status is a belief that acculturation to western lifestyles affects incidence of type 2 diabetes, but studies examining this link have yielded inconsistent results (Rewers and Hamman 2000). Other theories about this association contend that acculturation occurs more easily among individuals that appear less different than the dominant culture (e.g., lighter skinned African-Americans and Hispanics in the United States). Studies have shown that those that are the most acculturated and lighter skinned also have lowered risk of type 2 diabetes as compared to the least acculturated and darker skinned (Rewers and Hamman 2000), yet the difficulty in separating out the confounding between acculturation and genetics is great and requires more clarification in future studies. Studies examining migrant groups have found consistently high prevalence rates of type 2 diabetes with westernization, usually accompanied by increases in obesity, decreases in physical activity, and increases in fat and caloric intake (Rewers and Hamman 2000).

A final possible environmental/behavioral influence on type 2 diabetes comes from a little studied area of genetic-environmental interactions. The lack of work in this area comes from too few candidate genetic markers, incorrect family histories of diabetes, and a need for large samples. Rewers and Hamman (2000) reviewed the literature in this area and found that, not surprisingly due to their complexity, studies have yielded inconsistent results. For example, when examining family history, studies have found both a positive association between a family history for type 2 diabetes and physical activity, as well as obesity, but no association between family history and fat intake. Rewers and Hamman (2000) remarked that more studies looking at genetic markers need to be conducted to further understand the interactions between these variables and environmental factors.

Review of Lifestyle Interventions That Lower Risk for CVD

Both lifestyle modification (Barbery 1999; Foreyt and Poston 1999; Goldberg 1998) and various pharmacologic interventions (Goldberg 1998; Flemmer and Vinik 2000; Marks and Raskin 2000) are effective in lowering the risk of CVD in persons with type 2 diabetes. Lifestyle interventions can include dietary alterations, increased physical activity, and weight reduction. Several of these lifestyle interventions can be accomplished through behavior modification techniques that have been consistently found to useful including: self-monitoring, stimulus control, cognitive-behavior therapy interventions, and social support (Foreyt and Poston 1999). Pharmacologic interventions include treating hypertension, hyperinsulinemia, hyperglycemia, and dyslipidemia.

Altering one's diet has been found to be effective in reducing risk of type 2 diabetes and subsequent CVD risk and is a cornerstone in treating type 2 diabetes. Barbery (1999) reviewed several studies in which symptoms of type 2 diabetes were lowered when patients ate diets high in fiber and complex carbohydrates, but diets high in excessive refined carbohydrates increased risk for type 2 diabetes and CVD. In addi-

13 Lifestyle and Cardiovascular Risk in Type 2 Diabetes

tion to lowering the amount of refined carbohydrates, it was found lowering total dietary fat (especially saturated fat) and modifying caloric intake reduces CVD risk in obese diabetic persons (Foreyt and Poston 1999). Researchers also have investigated the effects of dietary monounsaturated dietary fatty acids on the risk factors for type 2 diabetes, finding that diets rich in monounsaturated fatty acids or rich in carbohydrates seem to have similar effects on CVD risk factors in persons at high risk for developing type 2 diabetes (Thomsen et al. 1999).

Physical activity has been reported to significantly improve insulin sensitivity and glycemic control in persons with type 2 diabetes reducing CVD risk (Barbery 1999; Foreyt and Poston 1999; Goldberg 1998). Goldberg (1998) noted several studies that linked increased physical activity with lowered incidence and risk of type 2 diabetes. Likewise, a more recent review of the literature observed that increased levels of physical activity were associated with lower incidence of type 2 diabetes diagnosis (Rewers and Hamman 2000). Goldberg (1998) concluded that this connection occurs through increasing the number and sensitivity of insulin sensitive glucose GLUT 4 glucose transporters in skeletal muscle along with increasing muscle glycogen synthase activity. A recent study found a similar inverse relationship between physical activity and CVD risk in type 2 diabetics, however it appeared to be unclear exactly what was the mechanism of action (Wannamethee et al. 2000). Shahid and Schneider (2000) have found that even a moderate increase in regular activity can begin to reduce the risks of CVD and symptoms related to type 2 diabetes.

Weight reduction is another method of reducing CVD risk and is associated with dietary modification and increased physical activity. While the association between type 2 diabetes and obesity is unclear and controversial, several studies found health benefits associated with weight reduction in persons with type 2 diabetes (Foreyt and Poston 1999; Metz et al. 2000; O'Keefe et al. 1999). A study investigating the effects of weight loss with a prepared meal plan found that significant weight loss was connected to an improved cardiovascular risk in persons with type 2 diabetes (Metz et al. 2000). Foreyt and Poston (1999) noted that weight loss, in conjunction with lifestyle modification programs, significantly lowered the risk of CVD in persons with type 2 diabetes.

More recently, a comprehensive intervention trial was conducted comparing a lifestyle modification program and a diabetic drug (metformin) in reducing the incidence of type 2 diabetes (Diabetes Prevention Program Research Group 2002). The lifestyle modification program consisted of a 16-lesson curriculum covering diet, exercise, and behavior modification that was designed to teach the participants to eat a healthy low-fat, low-calorie diet and to engage in moderate physical activity. The metformin group took an initial dose of 850 mg orally once daily; at one month, the dose was increased to 850 mg twice daily unless gastrointestinal side effects warranted a slower titration period.

Both groups demonstrated reductions in the incidence of type 2 diabetes; however, the results for the lifestyle modification group were much more pronounced than for the metformin group. At follow-up, the incidence of type 2 diabetes was 4.8 cases per 100 person-years as compared to 7.8 cases per 100 person-years for the metformin group. The investigators reported that the lifestyle modification intervention reduced the incidence by 58% compared to 31% in the metformin group. When comparing treatments across various subgroups (sex, gender, age, ethnicity, BMI, and plasma glucose), the lifestyle modification program was highly effective in all subgroups. The lifestyle intervention was particularly advantageous for older individuals and those who had lower BMI when compared to younger persons and those with a higher BMI. Thus, the investigators concluded the lifestyle modification program was more effective than metformin in reducing the risk of type 2 diabetes (Diabetes Prevention Program Research Group, 2002).

Given the high prevalence of hypertension (40% – 75%) among type 2 diabetics, it is integral to control blood pressure in order to reduce the risk of CVD (Flemmer and Vinik 2000). There appears to be a lack of consensus in the medical community about what drugs are preferable in treating hypertension in this population, however Flemmer and Vinik (2000) suggested that the choice of drug is not as important as reaching a target blood pressure level (which they believe is close to 120/80 mm Hg) in maximizing the reduction of CVD risk. They concluded that combination drug therapy occurs is common and it is important to take into account any comorbid conditions if they exist (Flemmer and Vinik 2000). However, Barbery (1999) noted that many commonly used antihypertensives specifically diuretics and beta-blockers have a negative effect on insulin resistance, LDL and total cholesterol, triglycerides, and glucose, so they are not as effective in reducing CVD risk, but it was noted that angiotensin converting enzyme (ACE) inhibitors and calcium channel blockers do have a positive effect on controlling hypertension in diabetes.

In light of the questions surrounding the use of anti-hypertensives, alterations in lifestyle also have been shown to be another possible method in controlling hypertension. Kokkinos and Papademetriou (2000) found that mild to moderate exercise appeared to be effective in significantly lowering blood pressure in individuals that have essential hypertension. Blumenthal et al. (2000) also found that exercise alone was effective in reducing blood pressure but discovered that combining exercise with a weight reduction program improved this effect as well as significantly lowering fasting glucose and insulin levels more than other participants. A recent review of controlled trials in hypertensives found the use of supplemental potassium, fiber, omega-3 fatty acids, and diets rich in fruit and vegetables as well as low in saturated fats lowered blood pressure and the effects of type 2 diabetes (Beilen et al. 1999). The Dietary Approaches to Stop Hypertension (DASH) study examined the impact of dietary patterns on blood pressure, finding that a combination diet rich in fruits, vegetables, and low-fat dairy foods significantly lowered blood pressure as compared to a typical American diet (Harsha et al. 1999). Moore et al. (1999) investigated the round-the-clock effectiveness of the DASH combination diet on blood pressure and found that it provided a significant 24-hour decrease in blood pressure. Recent literature reviews examining hypertension reduction found that modest weight loss and diets similar to the DASH combination diet were effective in reducing blood pressure as well (Hermansen 2000; Landsberg 1999).

Conclusion

The rates of persons diagnosed with type 2 diabetes are increasing at alarming rates and are expected to escalate as the population ages. This increasing prevalence has been linked to the epidemic in America of obesity and sedentary lifestyle. The central characteristics of individuals diagnosed with type 2 diabetes are increasing age, overweight, and ethnic minority-status, however recent data show that the rates for children are on the rise. Several of the resulting effects of type 2 diabetes have been found to be associated with an increased risk for cardiovascular disease (CVD). These effects include hyperglycemia, insulin resistance and resulting hyperinsulinemia, hypertension, and dyslipidemia. It is important to note that diabetes has been found to have a multiplicative effect on the risk for CVD when some CVD risk factors are already present so the effects of these present CVD risk factors may increase the risk for CVD in the presence of diabetes.

Several lifestyle and environmental factors that affect the development of type 2 diabetes and contribute to the increased risk for developing CVD. Diet, physical inactivity, obesity, socioeconomic status, and acculturation appear to have a significant impact on the incidence of type 2 diabetes and increased risk for CVD. Modifying one's lifestyle has been shown to reduce the risk of developing CVD in individual's with type 2 diabetes. These modifications include altering one's diet, engaging in increased physical activity, and subsequent reduction in weight. It appears that the most effective lifestyle modification method for reducing an individual's risk of CVD with type 2 diabetes is a combination of increased exercise, eating a diet rich in fruits, vegetables, and low-fat diary products, and lowering one's weight. These modification have been shown to successfully lower blood pressure in individuals with hypertension as well as lower glucose and triglyceride levels, all key factors in the risk for CVD. With the increasing prevalence of type 2 diabetes, it is essential that individuals with this diagnosis learn methods that they can utilize and implement them in order to reduce the risk of CVD and live healthier lives.

References

American Diabetes Association (1998) Economic consequences of diabetes mellitus in the U.S. in 1997. Diabetes Care 21:296:309
Barbery CM (1999) Managing cardiovascular risk in noninsulin dependent diabetes mellitus. Journal of American Academy of Nurse Practitioners 11:261–265
Beilin LJ, Puddey IB, Burke V (1999) Lifestyle and hypertension. Amer J Hypertens 12:934–945
Blumenthal JA, Sherwood A, Gullette ECD, Babyak M, Waugh R, Georgiades A, Craighead L, Tweedy D, Feinglos M, Applebaum M, Hayano J, Hinderliter A (2000) Exercise and weight loss reduce blood pressure in men and women with mild hypertension: effects on cardiovascular, metabolic, and hemodynamic functioning. Arch Intern Med 160:1947–1958
Brown JB, Pedula KL, Bakst AW (1999) The progressive cost of complications in type 2 diabetes mellitus. Arch Intern Med 159:1873–1880
Clark Jr CM, Perry RC (1999) Type 2 diabetes and macrovascular disease: epidemiology and etiology. Am Heart J 138:S330-S333
Crespo CJ, Keteyian SJ, Heath GW, Sempos CT (1996) Leisure-time physical activity among US adults. Arch Intern Med 156:93–98
Diabetes Prevention Program Research Group (2002) Reduction in the incidence of type 2 diabetes with lifestyle intervention or metformin. New Engl J Med 348:393–403
Feskens EJ, Bowles CH, Kromhout D (1991) Carbohydrate intake and body mass index in relation to the risk of glucose intolerance in an elderly population. Am J Clin Nutr 54:136–140
Flegal KM, Carroll MD, Kuczmarski RJ, Johnson CL (1998) Overweight and obesity in the United States: Prevalence and trends, 1960–1994. Int J Obes Relat Metab Disord 22:39–47
Flemmer MC, Vinik AI (2000) Evidence-based therapy for type 2 diabetes. Postgrad Med 107:27–47

Foreyt JP, Poston WSC (1999) The challenge of diet, exercise and lifestyle modification in the management of the obese diabetic patient. International Journal of Obesity 23:S5-S11

Goldberg RB (1998) Prevention of type 2 diabetes. In: Skyler JS (ed) The Medical Clinics of North America: Prevention and Treatment of Diabetes and Its Complications. W.B. Saunders Company, Philadelphia, pp 805-821

Harris MI (2000) Summary. In: Harris MI, Cowie CC, Stern MP, Boyko EJ, Reiber GE, Bennett PH (eds) Diabetes in America, 2nd Ed. National Diabetes and Digestive and Kidney Diseases, National Institutes of Health, pp 1-13

Harsha DW, Lin P, Obarzanek E, Karanja NM, Moore TJ, Caballero B (1999) Dietary Approaches to Stop Hypertension: a summary of study results. Journal of the American Dietetic Association 99:S35-S39

Hermansen K (2000) Diet, blood pressure and hypertension. Br J Nutr 83:S113-S119

Kokkinos PF, Papademetriou, V (2000) Exercise and hypertension. Coron Artery Dis 11:99-102

Laakso M (1999) Hyperglycemia and cardiovascular disease in type 2 diabetes. Diabetes 18:937-942

Landsberg L (1999) Weight reduction and obesity. Clin Exp Hypertens 21:763-768

Lebovitz HE (1999) Type 2 diabetes: an overview. Clin Chem 45:1339-1345

Libman I, Arslanian SA (1999) Type II diabetes mellitus: no longer just adults. Pediatr Ann 28:589-593

MMWR. Prevalence of leisure-time and occupational physical activity among employed adults- United States, 1990. MMWR 49:420-424

Marks JB, Raskin P (2000) Cardiovascular risk in diabetes a brief review. J Diabetes Complications 14:108-115

Metz JA, Stern JS, Kris-Etherton P, Reusser ME, Morris CD, Hatton DC, Oparil S, Haynes RB, Resnick LM, Pi-Sunyer, FX, Clark S, Chester L, McMahon M, Snyder GW, McCarron DA (2000) A randomized trial of improved weight loss with a prepared meal plan in overweight and obese patients: impact on cardiovascular risk reduction. Arch Intern Med 160:2150-2158

Moore TJ, Vollmer WM, Appel LJ, Sacks FM, Svetkey LP, Vogt TM, Conlin PR, Simons-Morton DG, Carter-Edwards L, Harsha DW (1999) Effects of dietary patterns on ambulatory blood pressure: results from the Dietary Approaches to Stop Hypertension (DASH) Trial. Hypertension 34: 472-7

Nathan DM, Meigs J, Singer DE (1997) The epidemiology of cardiovascular disease in type 2 diabetes mellitus: how sweet it is ... or is it? Lancet 350(Suppl 1):4-9

O'Keefe JH, Miles JM, Harris WH, Moe RM, McCallister BD (1999) Improving the adverse cardiovascular prognosis of type 2 diabetes. Mayo Clin Proc 74:171-180

Rewers M, Hamman RF (2000) Risk factors for non-insulin-dependent diabetes. In: Harris MI, Cowie CC, Stern MP, Boyko EJ, Reiber GE, Bennett PH (eds) Diabetes in America, 2nd Ed. National Diabetes and Digestive and Kidney Diseases, National Institutes of Health, pp 179-196

Ryden L (2000) Managing cardiovascular risk in patients with diabetes. Heart 84:I23-I25

Seidell JC (2000) Obesity, insulin resistance and diabetes- a worldwide epidemic. Br J Nutr 83:S5-8

Shahid SK, Schneider SH (2000) Effects of exercise on insulin resistance syndrome. Coron Artery Dis 11:103-109

Sowers JR, Lester MA (1999) Diabetes and cardiovascular disease. Diabetes Care 22:C14-C20

Thomsen C, Rasmussen O, Christiansen C, Pedersen E, Vesterlund M, Storm H, Ingerslev J, Hermansen K (1999) Comparison of the effects of a monounsaturated fat diet and a high carbohydrate diet on cardiovascular risk factors in first degree relatives of type-2 diabetic patients. Eur J of Clin Nutr 52:818-823

Wannamethee SG, Shaper AG, Alberti KGMM (2000) Physical activity, metabolic factors, and the incidence of coronary heart disease and type 2 diabetes. Arch Intern Med 160:2108-2116

Wingard DL, Barrett-Connor E (2000) Heart disease and diabetes. In: Harris MI, Cowie CC, Stern MP, Boyko EJ, Reiber GE, Bennett PH (eds) Diabetes in America, 2nd Ed. National Diabetes and Digestive and Kidney Diseases, National Institutes of Health, pp 429-448

CHAPTER 14

The Prothrombotic Syndrome in Type 2 Diabetes: Assessment and Control

M. Cucuianu, M. Coca

Abstract. High plasma levels of fibrinogen, clotting factor VII, plasminogen activator inhibitor-1 as well as of endothelia-derived von Willebrand factor are increased in patients with type 2 diabetes and are considered to be predictive for the thrombotic complications of atherosclerosis. Circumstantial evidence suggests that a peculiar association of stimuli including hyperinsulinism and the release into the portal circulation of excess free fatty acids and of proinflammatory cytokines, originating in the enlarged visceral adipose tissue, would enhance the synthesis of liver- derived hemostatic variables. Glycation of antithrombin may contribute to the abnormal hemostatic balance. It should be mentioned that association of cardiovascular disease with clotting factors and antifibrinolytic potential elevations illustrates correlations not causality. The above mentioned changes of hemostatic variables are therefore relevant only in context with hyperreactive platelets and endothelial lesions or dysfunction. Correction of overweight and the improved metabolic control would however diminish the pathologically increased plasma levels of protrombothic hemostatic variables and in association with an efficient antiplatlet therapy (clopidogrel) may reduce the thrombotic tendency.

Introduction

Vascular pathology is characterized by a shift of the thrombogenic/thrombolytic balance in favour of vascular lumen closure and fatal ischemic events. Life-threatening thrombotic events occuring in patients with type 2 diabetes are related to atherosclerotic lesions, more specifically with the rupture of a vulnerable atherosclerotic plaque and any reasonable approach to the control of these events would imply the unraveling of the involved pathogenic mechanisms.

Major Determinants of Thrombotic Events

It is considered that the major determinants for the development of a thrombotic response to plaque rupture are: (1) the character and extent of exposed thrombogenic materials; (2) the degree of stenosis and irregularities of the arterial wall causing local flow disturbances; (3) the thrombotic-thrombolytic equilibrum at the time of plaque rupture (Falk and Fernandez-Ortiz 1995).

Mechanisms Leading to Exposed Thrombogenic Materials

Only lipid rich plaques, provided with a rather thin fibrous cap are vulnerable and this vulnerability seems to be related to impaired generation of fibrous material and/or an enhanced degradation of collagen and of other matrix components of the fibrous cap. A smoldering inflammation within the atherosclerotic plaque could favour the aforementioned mechanisms leading to the weakening of the fibrous cap (Libby 1995). The soft atheromatous gruel expressed by plaque disruption and containing lipids, degraded extracellular matrix components and necrotic desintegrated cells (mainly foam cells) is rich in tissue factor and therefore highly thrombogenic. Noteworthy, tissue factor may be exposed at the surface of dysfunctional endothelia, a process mediated by various stimuli including cytokines, superoxide anions, oxidized LDL and persistent hyperlipidemia. Since widespread endothelial damage or dysfunction may occur rather early in type 2 diabetes (Tooke 1998), abnormal behaviour of endothelia might explain a certain degree of fibrin formation and intravascular deposition of thrombotic material, even in the absence of a detectable plaque disruption. Such endothelial dysfunction leading to an upregulation of the prothrombotic mechanisms associated with a down-regulation of the antithrombotic ones would be particularly relevant for vascular complications of diabetic patients.

Local Flow Disturbance

A normal blood flow would often disperse platelet aggregates and would wash off clotting factors activated at the site of lesioned or dysfunctional endothelia, so that such activated clotting factors may not reach the critical concentration required for clot formation. Not so in conditions of disturbed blood flow, when irregularities of the exposed surface lead to formation of vortices and changes in the rate or direction of blood flow. Because of high plasma levels of fibrinogen, lipoprotein and alfa-2 macroglobulin, as well as reduced erithrocyte deformability, diabetic patients display increased blood viscosity which would accentuate flow disturbances (McMillan et al. 1976 and 1978). Glycation of plasma proteins and membrane proteins may also contribute to the increased blood viscosity of diabetic patients (Ney et al. 1985).

Systemic Thrombotic Propensity

Necroptic investigations emphasized aspects of healed plaque rupture in individuals who had never experienced an acute coronary syndrome during their life-time, suggesting that plaque rupture with nonocclusive progression may be clinically silent. Repeated episodes of plaque rupture with local activation of clotting may nevertheless represent a major pathway for progression of atherosclerotic lesions. It is reasonable to presume that evolution of a ruptured plaque toward sealing and healing or towards extensive thrombosis may depend not only on the extension of the fissure and on the efficiency of local tissue repair mechanisms but also on the systemic thrombotic propensity at the time of rupture (Falk and Fernandez-Ortiz 1995, Libby 1995). It is also conceivable that an association of platelet hyperreactivity, enhanced fibrin formation and impaired fibrinolysis would favour the development of an occlusive thrombosis. The behaviour of hemostatic variables in patients with the metabolic syndrome with or without clinical diabetes has been extensively studied during the last decade and these aspects will be discussed in the following subsection.

Abnormalities of Hemostatic Variables in Diabetes

According to recent reviews a striking prothrombotic dysbalance may exist in the presence of diabetes, associating hyperreactive platelets, with enhanced coagulability and impaired fibrinolysis (Jokl and Colwell 1997, Schernthaner 1997). The main questions raised by such findings are pertaining to: (a) the mechanisms leading to a prothrombotic dysbalance in diabetic patients; (b) the mechanisms by wich such a dysbalance would promote thrombotic events. An answer to these questions would exceed a pure academic interest and would be relevant for the assessment and control of thrombotic propensity.

Type 2 diabetes has a strong association with upper body obesity, which makes the relative impact of obesity and diabetes difficult to ascertain and this difficulty is clearly illustrated by studies concerning the behaviour of the fibrinolytic sistem.

Impaired Fibrinolytic Activity in Type 2 Diabetes

As shown in Fig. 14.1 dilute blood clot lysis time is obviously more prolonged in overweight hypertriglyceridemic diabetic patients than in diabetics at or bellow the ideal body weight. Noteworthy clot lysis time in overweight diabetic patients did not significantly differ from values occuring in body-weight and serum triglyceride matched nondiabetic subjects. It may also be noted that clot lysis times became shorter in the presence of p-chlormercuribenzoate, an inhibitor of fibrinstabilizing plasma factor XIII and it was presumed that the delayed clot lysis recorded in overweight hyperlipidemic patients with or without diabetes could be at least partially explained by an increased plasma factor XIII level (Cucuianu et al. 1979, 1984). High plasma levels of this transglutaminase, positively correlated with serum triglyceride

Fig. 14.1. Dilute blood clot lysis time (*DBCLT*) in 76 normal-weight normolipidemic control subjects (*C*), in 28 lean diabetic patients (*LD*), in 28 overweight hypertriglyceridemic diabetic patients (*DO*), and in 42 overweight hypertriglyceridemic subjects without diabetes (*OHTsD*). Mean values ± SEM. *Filled columns*, DBCLT in the presence of 40 mM p-chlormercuribenzoate (*PCMB*), an inhibitor of fibrin stabilizing factor XIII. Statisical significance: C vs. LD, nonsignificant (NS); C or LD vs. OD or OHTsD, $p<0,01$; OD vs. OHTsD, NS. (Cucuianu et al. 1984)

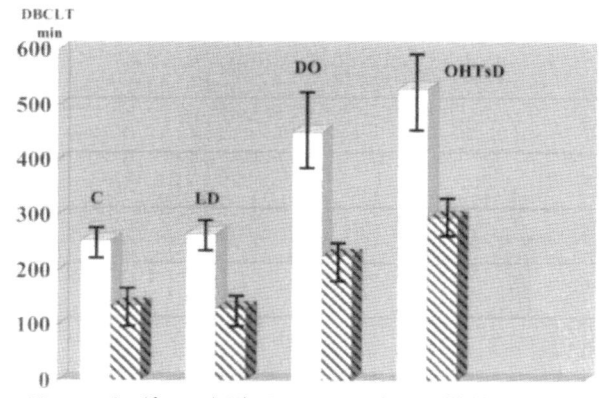

concentration and serum cholinesterase activity, a marker of hepatic protein syntesis, were actually reported in nondiabetic overweight hyperlipidemic subjects (Cucuianu et al. 1985). Noteworthy plasma factor XIII was found to catalyse the incorporation of alpha$_2$-antiplasmin into the fibrin network, thereby antagonising the plasmin generated within the clot (Sakata and Aoki 1980).

A greater importance is however attributed to increased plasma levels of plasminogen activator inhibitor (PAI-1) which were found to be correlated with relative bodyweight, insulinemia and serum triglyceride concentration (Juhan-Vague et al. 1987).

Experimental evidence was provided that insulin stimulates PAI-1 syntesis in the hepatocytes but not in endothelial cells (Alessi et al. 1995), while proinflammatory cytokines were found to enhance the production of this protease inhibitor in both the above mentioned cells (Dawson and Henney 1992). A possible role of adipocytes as a source of plasma PAI-1 was also reported (Loskutoff and Samad 1998). Evidence from both in vivo and in vitro experiments suggest there is a great deal of tissue specificity and synergism in the regulation of plasma PAI-1 level.

Data concerning the in vitro resistance of nonenzimatically glycosylated fibrin to degradation by plasmin are rather conflicting as both increased. (Brownlee et al. 1983) and decreased (Lütjens et al. 1988) resistance were reported. Although in vitro experiments emphasized that a glycation of plasminogen would render it less susceptible to t-PA induced activation (Geiger and Binder 1986), available data obtained by clinical and laboratory investigations sugest that impaired fibrinolysis in type 2 diabetes should rather be related to overweight, hyperlipidemia and possibly overloading of the liver with lipid, than to impaired glycemic control. We are lacking so far data about a possible glycation of plasma factor XIII resulting in impaired fibrincrosslinking activity.

Different rates of thrombin-induced activation of factor XIII, related to F.XIII Val34Leu polymorphism, may however influence the efficiency of this fibrin stabilizing factor (Wartiovaara 2000).

Hypercoagulable State

Increased concentration of plasma clotting factors, enhanced activation of these factors and impaired anticoagulant mechanisms may contribute to the development of such a state. Plasma levels of factor VII, factor VIII and fibrinogen were found to be increased in diabetic patients (Schernthaner 1997) yet mechanisms leading to their high plasma levels are still debatable.

Factor VII

Age, gender, body-mass index, oral contraceptives and menopausal status (Balleisen et al. 1985) as well as genetic polymorphism (Lane et al. 1992) were reported to influence the levels and the activity of factor VII, which are also related to plasma triglyceride (Constantino et al. 1977). As shown in Fig. 14.2, increased factor VII activity was however detected in type 2 diabetic patients who were neither obese, nor hyperlipidemic and this activity increased postprandially (Coca et al. 2000). Since addition of lipoproteins to plasma did not influence clotting assays (Constantino et al. 1977) and there was no correlation between the magnitude of postprandial increase of serum

Fig. 14.2. Behaviour of factor VII (*a*) as well as of factor VIII:c and the von Willebrand factor (*b*) in healthy normal-weight normolipidemic controls and in normal-weight normolipidemic diabetic patients without detectable cardiovascular disease or any acute conditions. Results are expressed as a percentage of normal coagulation control plasma percent of normal coagulation control plasma (*NCCP*). Mean ± SEM (Coca et al. 2000). (*a*) Factor VII clotting activity in 25 control subjects (*C*) and in 24 diabetic patients (*D*) preprandially (*white columns*) and postprandially (*filled columns*). Statistical significance: C vs. D, $p<0.01$; postprandial factor VII activity increased statistically significant ($p<0.01$) only in diabetic patients. (*b*) Factor VIIIc clotting activity and von Willebrand factor antigen (vWF:Ag) in 20 control subjects (*C*) and in diabetic patients with Hb.A1c less than 7% (group A, 15 patients) or higher than 7% (group B, 15 patients). Statistical significance: C vs. A or vs. B, $p<0.001$; A vs. B, $p<0.05$. The rather parallel behaviour of VIIIc and vWF:Ag is to be noted

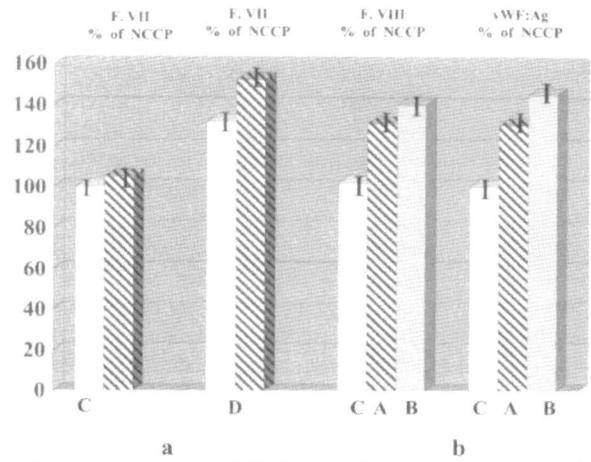

triglyceride and factor VII activity, it seems that the link between hyperlipidemia and increased clotting factor VII is more complicated and probably related to to the uptake of a lipid load by the liver. It was also reported that diabetic patients with retinopathy and/or proteinuria display higher factor VII levels and activity than diabetics without microangiopathy (Hirano et al. 1997). Such findings might suggest that a widespread endothelial dysfunction leading to an in vivo activation of coagulation could enhance the synthesis of factor VII.

Fibrinogen

Diabetic patients, especially those with proteinuria display significantly increased concentrations of this clotting factor (Ganda and Arkin 1998). Although in a population-based study plasma fibrinogen level was found to be correlated with fasting plasma insulin and it was considered to be a new marker of the metabolic syndrome (Imperatore et al. 1998), the mechanisms linking metabolic disorders to plasma fibrinogen are rather obscure, as insulin was reported to exert inhibitory rather than enhancing effects on hepatic fibrinogen synthesis (De Feo et al. 1993). Actually fibrinogen is not only the coagulation protein present in the highest concentration in human plasma, but also an acute phase reactant, its hepatic syntesis being stimulated by proinflammatory cytokines. A possible role of intraabdominal adipose tissue-derived cytokines was recently suggested (King and Wakasaki-1999, Yudkin 1999).

von Willebrand Factor and Factor VIIIc

Endothelia-derived von Willebrand factor (vWF), a high molecular weight glycoprotein mediating the adherence of platelets to subendothelial structures and consolidating platelet aggregates, was found to be significantly increased in diabetic patients and these changes were interpreted as a marker of endothelial lesions (Bensoussan et al. 1977). The vWF is also a component of the acute phase reaction and its levels were raported to be high in many disease states accompanied by this type of reaction (Cucuianu et al. 1980, Pottinger et al. 1989). According to a recent review, endothelial secretion of vWF may be triggered by mediators of hemostasis such as thrombin, fibrin, plasmin and adenine nucleotides as well as by mediators of inflammation like histamine, leukotrienes, superoxide anions, interleukin-1, tumor necrosis factor and activated complement components. The above mentionated data are highly suggestive that high vWF plasma levels may not necessarily reflect its leakage from injured endothelia but rather an endothelial response to stimuli and/or an endothelial dysfunction (Mannucci 1998).

Since vWF is also a carrier of plasma factor VIIIc, protecting this clotting factor from premature proteolysis, high vWF plasma levels are usually associated with increased factor VIIIc activity. High activities of this plasma clotting factor were actually reported in diabetic patients (Bern et al. 1980). Noteworthy the plasma factor VIII complex was found to be increased in diabetic children without vascular disease (Borkenstein and Muntean 1982). Also, as shown in Fig. 14.2, when compared to control subjects, slightly yet significantly higher values of both vWF:Ag levels and factor VIIIc activity were noted in normal-weight normolipidemic diabetic patients without detectable vascular disease and in the absence of any condition that might have triggered an acute phase reaction (Coca et al. 2000). Such findings would suggest that impaired glucose tolerance might lead to endothelial dysfunction although not necessarily endothelial damage. It was even claimed that an endotheliopathy may precede type 2 diabetes (Tooke 1998).

Anticoagulant Mechanisms

Both decreased (Ceriello et al. 1990) and increased (Grignani et al. 1981) plasma antithrombin III (ATIII) levels were reported in diabetic patients. Conflincting results could be due to different tehniques (immunologic or functional in the presence or absence heparin) or to the selection of the investigated patients (body weight, lipid pattern, glycemic control, proteinuria, vascular disease). Apparently the actual plasma ATIII activity may be the result of the balance between a possible cytokine-induced enhanced syntesis (Hoffman et al. 1986) and its inactivation by nonenzymatic glycosylation (Brownlee et al. 1984).

The behavior of the protein C system involved in the proteolytic degradation of activated factors V and VIII is highly dependent on the type of diabetes. Actually plasma levels of liver secreted protein C and of its cofactor protein S were found to be decreased in type 1 diabetes (Vukovich and Schernthaner 1986, Schernthaner 1997) while elevated or normal levels were reported in type 2 diabetic patients (Vigano et al. 1984, Saito et al. 1988). Plasma protein C antigen (PC:Ag) and activity are also increased in overweight and hypertriglyceridemic nondiabetic subjects and were

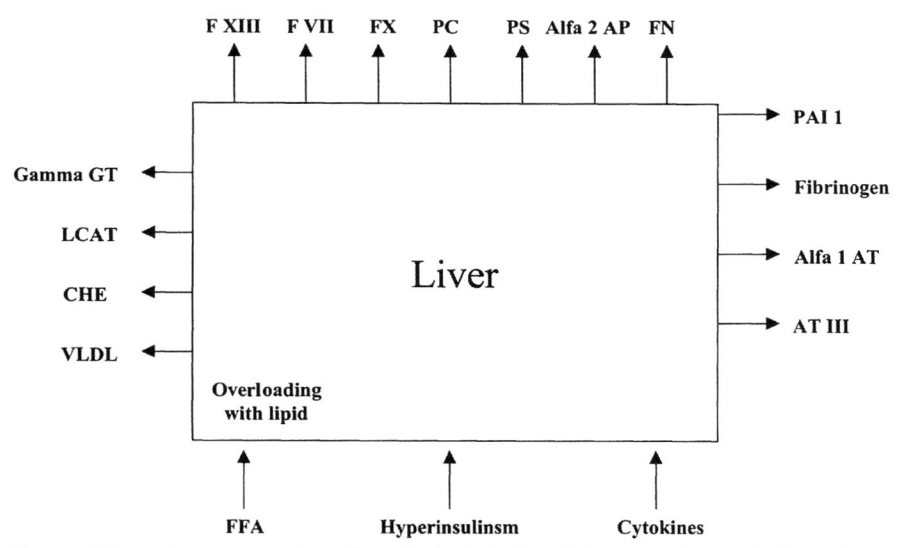

Fig. 14.3. Schematic representation of hypothetical relationship between the metabolic syndrome and enhanced hepatic secretion of VLDL and of several liver-derived enzymes and proteins including certain hemostatic variables. *FFA*, free fatty acid; *CHE*, serum cholinesterase; *LCAT*, lecithin cholesterol acyltransferase; γGT, glutamyltransferase; *PC*, protein C; *PS*, protein S; $\alpha_2 AP$, α_2 antiplasmin; *FN*, fibronectin; *PAI*, 1-plasminogen activator inhibitor-1; $\alpha_1 AT$, α_1 antitrypsin; *ATIII*, antithrombin III

correlated not only with serum cholesterol and triglyceride concentrations but also with serum cholinesterase activity (Knöbl et al. 1987, Cucuianu et al. 1993).

It should be noted that the liver is the main site of synthesis for not only procoagulant and antifibrinolytic proteins such as fibrinogen, vitamin K-dependent clotting factors, PAI-1, alfa-2 antiplasmin and presumably factor XIII, but also for certain anticoagulants like ATIII, protein C and protein S. Most of these hemostatic variables as well as other liver secreted enzymes and proteins, such as serum cholinesterase, lecithin-cholesterol acyltransferase (Cucuianu et al 1978), γ-glutamyltransferase (Perry et al. 1998), fibronectin (Cucuianu et al. 1985) are increased in patients with the metabolic syndrome. Apparenttly this pattern of hepatic protein synthesis is induced by a peculiar association of stimuli including hyperinsulinism and release into the portal circulation of excess free fatty acids and proinflammatory cytokines originating from the enlarged intraabdominal adipose tissue (Bjorntorp 1991, Yudkin 1999, King and Wakassaki 1999). A hypotesis about enhanced hepatic synthesis of certain enzymes and proteins is presented in Fig. 14.3.

Hyperreactive Platelets

By adhering to an injured site of the vascular wall and by aggregating, platelets provide a hemostatic plug, wich under abnormal conditions may evolve into a thrombus (Mustard and Pakham 1977). Evidence was provided that diabetes is associated with abnormal behaviour of blood platelets (Jokl and Colwell 1997). It is reasonable to presume that the previously mentioned increased vWF plasma levels would favour the adherence and spreading of platelets to subendothelial layers, and together with increased plasma fibrinogen would contribute to the stabilization of platelet aggregates. Noteworthy platelets of diabetic patients display an enhanced binding of fibrinogen, owing to an increased number of platelet surface receptors, the glycoprotein complex IIb/ IIIa (Tschöpe et al. 1991), and glycation of platelet membrane proteins would result in reduced membrane fluidity (Cohen et al. 1991, Winocour et al. 1991).It was also reported that hyperaggregability occuring in diabetic patients is associated with acccelerated arachidonic acid metabolism and enhanced production of thromboxane A_2 which may amplify the responsiveness of platelets to various stimuli (Halushka et al. 1981). By providing an activating surface for plasma clotting factors, platelets are also involved in coagulation, and an increased platelet-dependent thrombin generation was reported in hypercholesterolemic subjects (Aoki et al. 1997). Also platelets of diabetic patients display an increased inhibitory effect on fibrinolysis (Woods et al. 1994).

Assessment and Control of Prothrombotic Tendency in Diabetic Patients

In spite of progress achieved in the pathophysiology of hemostasis and trombosis, an accurate assessment of the prothrombotic state is rather difficult and submited to many uncertainties. The presence of overweight and hypertriglyceridemia in a patient with type 2 diabetes would be highly suggestive for the occurrence of the abnormalities shown in Fig. 14.3 as well as for increased endothelia-derived vWF levels and blood platelet hyperreactivity. Additionally, impaired glycemic control, an intercurrent inflammatory condition or a genetic polymorphism or deficit might distort the relationship between metabolic disturbances and the magnitude of prothrombotic changes affecting the hemostatic variables. A determination of all interacting factors would be highly desirable although expensive and time consuming. A moderately performant laboratory could however be able to assess plasma fibrinogen and vWF:Ag levels, factor VII activity, and also the unsophisticated evaluation of dilute blood clot lysis time.

Care should however be taken whenever interpreting changes of a hemostatic variable in terms of a thrombotic tendency. For example an enhanced factor XIII activity would increase resistance to thrombolysis (Reed-Houng 1999), while by promoting tissue repair (Beck et al. 1961), it would strengthen an atheroma's fibrous cap rendering it less vulnerable and would also presumably accelerate the sealing and healing of a fissured atheromatous plaque. It was also claimed that an activation of fibrinolysis and proteolysis within an atherosclerotic plaque could weaken its fibrous cap and favour plaque rupture (Libby 1995). Presumably an assessement of fibrinolytic activity in the circulating blood does not entirely encompass the complexity of the relationship between changes of the fibrinolytic system and vascular disease.

Increased plasma levels of clotting factors are relevant for thrombotic events only when their activation would occur in vivo. Recently developed technics allow the clinician to detect the various steps in the activation of clotting mechanisms. For exemple activation of prothrombin to thrombin is accompanied by the release of a measurable fragment (F1+ 2), while the iniation of fibrin formation leads to the release of

14 The Prothrombotic Syndrome in Type 2 Diabetes

fibrinopeptides (Fp A and Fp B) and the generation of fibrin monomers . The detection of D-dimer produced by lysis of stabilized fibrin provides information about the fibrinolytic response to crosslinked fibrin formation (Boisclair et al. 1990). Occurrence of activated clotting factors leads to complex formation with serine protease inhibitors such as antithrombin, while thrombin activated protein C is inactivated by complex formation with several inhibitors including alfa-1 antitrypsin (Pelzer et al. 1988, España et al. 1992).

Diabetic patients display elevated plasma levels of FpA not only when affected by documented vascular disease but also before the occurrence of vascular complications, expecially in conditions of inadequate metabolic control. Such observation are suggesting that activation of coagulation may contribute to rather than be the result of vascular complications (Rosove et al. 1984, Ford et al. 1990). Plasma F1+2 level may also be high in type 2 diabetic patients independently of $Hb.A_{1c}$ concentrations (Marongiu et al. 1995).

Since glycation of antithrombin would impair complex formation with activated clotting factors, the plasma levels of thrombin-antithrombin complexes (TAT) may be low in the presence of increased FpA levels (Ceriello et al. 1990). It should be stressed that an increase in the plasma concentration of certain markers for an intravascular activation of coagulation may not be constantly detected in hyperlipidemic and diabetic patients. According to a review on hyperlipidemia and in vivo hemostatic system activation, absence of significantly increased markers of an intravascular activation of clotting could be explained by their short half-life (only 3 – 5 min in the case of Fb.A). Intermitent bursts in the activation of clotting may therefore remain undetected by the laboratory, although they could be sufficient to cause fibrin formation and deposition (Owen et al. 1988). Such observations provide evidence for an episodic rather than an ongoing activation of coagulation. It was therefore claimed that urinary FpA excretion could better reflect the cumulative effect of thrombin on fibrinogen, than a single plasma Fp.A measurement wich only gives information on fibrinogen cleavage at the time of blood sampling (Gallino et al. 1985).

Markers for the detection of damaged or dysfunctional endothelia have also become available to the clinical laboratory. Beside the previously mentioned vWf, other markers such as thrombomodulin and E selectin fragments resulting from proteolytic cleavage of these endothelial proteins were found to be increased in a variety of systemic inflammatory conditions and in vascular disease including vascular complications of diabetes (Waine-Smith 1997).

A thorough investigation of platelet functions including adhesiveness, aggregability and secretion, related to platelet metabolic peculiarities, should be the task of more specific laboratories. It should however be mentioned that investigation of platelet responsivenes to stimuli in platelet rich plasma may be misleading because separation procedures could eliminate subpopulations of most reactive platelets. Mesurement of platelet reactivity in whole blood has therefore been recommended (Galvez et al. 1986). Particularly relevant for an in vivo activation of blood platelets in diabetic patients, are data emphasizing an increase of plasma beta-thrombomodulin released from activated platelets (Cella et al. 1979, Cho et al. 1992).

Since prothrombotic changes occuring in diabetic patients are mainly subsequent to metabolic disturbances, the most reasonable approach to control the thrombotic propensity of these patients would be a thorough correction of their metabolic disorders.

It was actually demonstrated that weight reduction is usually accompanied by a significant reduction of plasma PAI-1 levels (Sundell et al. 1989, Schernthaner 1997, Charles et al. 1998) while metformin had no significant additional effect on this inhibitor of fibrinolysis (Charles et al. 1998). It was also shown that the abnormally elevated plasma levels of fibrinogen, factor VIIIc and vWF, occuring in diabetic patients with inadequate glycometabolic control, returned to normal values after an intensified insulin therapy (Banga and Sixma 1986, Vukovich et al. 1989). Altough fibrates were reported to inhibit the syntesis of PAI-1, thereby reducing its plasma level, this effect was found to be independent of their triglyceride lowering activity (Arts et al. 1997).

A wide choice of antithrombotic remedies are now available. Discussing the pharmacology of this medication would however be beyond the purpose of the present chapter. Usually, anticoagulation is mainly used for secondary prevention according to well established criteria and under laboratory control (Aiach et al. 1991, Derlon and Fiessinger 1991).

Primary anticoagulant prevention could however be attempted in a diabetic patient, when triggering agents (trauma, surgery) are associating to the thrombotic propensity, and low molecular weight heparin (Lovenox 20 mg/day) is considered to exert an efficient protection (Aiach et al. 1991).

Since platelets are involved not only in acute thrombotic events but also in the initial stages of atherogenesis, it seems reasonable to recommend an antiplatelet therapy to patients with type 2 diabetes. Data concerning the efficacy of aspirin (330 mg/day) in preventing the development of vascular complications in diabetic patients are controversial and anyway rather modest (Dechavanne and Wautier 1991). A new antiplatelet agent, clopidogrel was found to irreversibly inhibit ADP-induced platelet aggregation by preventing the binding of fibrinogen to platelet glycoprotein receptor GpIIb/IIIA (Herbert et al. 1998). It was also shown that 75 mg clopidogrel/day orally is more efficient than aspirin in reducing the combined risk of ischemic stroke, myocardial infarction or vascular death (CAPRIE steering committee 1996, Haberl and Dembrowski 1999).

One may expect that improved metabolic control, antihypertensive and antiplatelet therapies could have additive preventive effects. A multimodal treatement should therefore recommended to patients with type 2 diabetes.

References

Aiach M, Boneu B, Potron G (1991) Utilisation des heparines en pratique medicale courante. Sang Thrombose Vaisseaux. STV 3: 4–10
Alessi M, Anfosso F, Henry M, Peiretti F, Nalbone G, Juhan Vague (1995) Upregulation of PAI-1 syntesis by insulin and proinsulin in Hep G2 cells but not in endothelial cells. Fibrinolysis 9: 237–242
Aoki I, Aoki N, Kawano K, Shimoyama K, Maki A, Homori M, Yanagisawa A, Yamamoto M, Kawai Y, Ishikawa K (1997) Platelet-dependent thrombin generation in patients with hyperlipidemia. J Am Coll Cardiol 30: 91–96
Arts J, Kockx M, Princen MG, Kooistra T (1997) Studies on the mechanisms of fibrate-inhibited expression of plasminogen activator inhibitor-1 in cultured hepatocytes from cynomolgus monkey. Arterioscler Thromb Vasc Biol 17: 26–32
Balleisen L, Bailey J, Epping PH, Schulte H, van de Loo I (1985) Epidemiological study on factor VII, factor VIII and fibrinogen in an industrial population. Baseline data and the relation to

age, gender, body weight, smoking, alcohol, pill using and menopause. Thromb Haemostas 54: 475-479
Banga JD, Sixma JJ (1986) Diabetes mellitus, vascular disease and thrombosis. Clin Haematol 15: 465-469
Beck E, Duckert F, Ernst M (1961) The influence of fibrin stabilizing factor on the growth of fibroblasts in vitro and wound healing. Thromb Diathes Haemorrh 6: 485-491
Bensoussan D, Levy-Toledano S, Passa P, Caen J, Canivet J (1975) Platelet hyperaggregability and increased plasma level of von Willebrand factor in diabetics with retinopathy. Diabetologia 11: 307-312
Bern MM, Cassoni MP, Horton J, Rand L, Davis G (1980) Changes of fibrinolysis and factor VIII coagulant antigen and ristocetin cofactor in diabetes mellitus and atherosclerosis. Thromb Res 19: 831-839
Björntorp P (1991) Metabolic implications of fat distribution. Diabetes Care 14: 1132-1143
Boisclair MD, Ireland HI, Lane DE (1990) Assessment of hypercoagulable states by measurement of activation fragments and peptides. Blood Reviews 4: 25-40
Borkenstein M, Muntean W (1982) Elevated factor VIII activity in diabetic children without vascular disease. Diabetes 31: 1006-1009
Brownlee A, Vlassara H, Cerami A (1983) Nonenzymatic glycosylation reduces the susceptibility of fibrin to degradation by plasmin Diabetes 32: 680-684
Brownlee A, Vlassara H, Cerami A (1984) Inhibition of heparin-catalyzed human antithrombin activity by nonenzymatic glycosylation. Diabetes 33: 532-535
CAPRIE steering committee (1996) A randomized blinded, trial of clopidogrel versus aspirin in patients at risk of ischaemic evevts (CAPRIE). Lancet 348: 1329-1339
Cella G, Zahavi J, de Haas HA, Kakkar VV (1979) β-thrombomodulin, platelet production time and platelet function in vascular disease. Br J Haematol 43: 126-127
Ceriello A, Giuliano D, Quatrano A, Marchi E, Barbanti M, Lefebre P (1990) Evidence for a hyperglycemic-dependent decrease of antithrombin III-thrombin complex formation in humans. Diabetologia 33: 163-167
Charles MA, Morange P, Eschwege E, André P, Vague P, Juhan-Vague I (1998) Effect of weight change and metformin on fibrinolysis and the von Willebrand factor in obese nondiabetic subjects. Diabetes Care 21: 1967-1972
Coca M, Cucuianu M, Hâncu N (2000) Preprandial and postprandial evaluation of clotting factor VII and VIII in type 2 diabetes (in Romanian). Infomedica 7 (77): 38-40
Coca M, Cucuianu M, Hâncu N (2000) von Willebrand factor, clotting factor VIII and antithrombin III in type 2 diabetes (in Romanian). Infomedica 9 (79): 30-32
Cho NH, Becker DJ, Ellis D, Kuller LH, Drash AL, Orchard TY (1992) Spontaneous whole blood platelet aggregation, hematological variables and complications in insulin dependent diabetes mellitus; the Pittsburg epidemiology of diabetes complications study. J Diabetes Complications 6: 12-18
Cohen I, Burk DL, Fullerton R, Veiss A, Green D (1991) Nonenzymatic glycation of platelet proteins in diabetic patients. Semin thromb Hemost 17: 426-432
Constantino M, Merskey C, Kudzma DI, Zucker MB (1977) Increased activity of vitamin K-dependent clotting factors in human hyperlipoproteinemia. Association with cholesterol and triglyceride levels. Thromb Haemostas 38: 465-474
Cucuianu M, Opincaru A, Tapalagă D (1978) Similar behaviour of lecithin: cholesterol acyltransferase and pseudocholinesterase in liver disease and hyperlipoproteinemia. Clin Chim Acta 85: 73-79
Cucuianu M, Stef C, Zdrenghea D, Popescu O (1979) In vitro effect of p-chlormercuribenzoate upon dilute blood clot lysis time in hyperlipidemia. Thromb Haemostas 42: 929-949
Cucuianu M, Missits I, Olinic N, Roman S (1980) Increased ristocetin cofactor in acute myocardial infarction; a component of the acute phase reaction. Thromb Haemostas 43: 41-44
Cucuianu M, Fekete T, Mărcusu C, Mössler R, Dutu A (1984) Fibrinolysis in diabetes mellitus. Role of overweight and hypertriglyceridemia. Rev Roum Med Int 22: 171-175
Cucuianu M, Rus HG, Cristea A, Niculescu F, Bedeleanu D, Porutiu D, Roman S (1985) Clinical studies on plasma fibronectin and factor XIII: with special reference to hyperlipoproteinemia. Clin Chim Acta 147: 273-281
Cucuianu M, Brudască I, Trif I, Stancu A (1993) Clinical studies on plasma protein C. Correlation with serum cholinesterase Nouv Rev Fr Hematol 35: 481-486

Dawson S, Henney A (1992) The status of PAI-1 as a risk factor for arterial and thrombotic disease. A review. Arteriosclerosis 93: 105–117
Dechavanne M, Wautier JL (1991) Utilisation des médicaments antiplaquettaires en pratique medicale courante. Sang Thrombose Vaisseaux STV 3: 16–22
De Feo P, Volpi E, Lucidi P, Cruciani G, Reboldi G, Siepi D, Mannarino E, Santeusanio F, Brunetti P, Bolli G (1993) Physiological increments in plasma insulin concentrations have selective and different effects on syntesis of hepatic proteins in normal humans. Diabetes 42: 995–1002
Derlon A, Fiessinger TN (1991) Utilisation des antivitamines K en practique medicale courante. Sang Thromb Vaisseaux STV 3: 11–15
España F, Gilabert J, Vicente V, Estellés A, Vasquez L, Hendl S, Aznar J (1992) Activated protein C-α1 antitrypsin complex as marker for in vitro diagnosis in prethrombotic states. Thromb Res 66: 499–508
Falk E, Fernandez-Ortiz A (1995) Role of thrombosis in atherosclerosis and its complications. Am J Cardiol 75: 5B-11B
Ford I, Singh TP, Kitchens S, Makris M, Ward JD, Preston FE (1990) Activation of coagulation in diabetes mellitus in relation to the presence of vascular complications. Diabetes Med 8: 322–329
Gallino A, Haeberli A, Straub PW (1985) Fibrinopeptide A excretion in urine in patients with atherosclerotic artery disease. Thromb Res 38: 237–244
Galvez A, Badimon L, Badimon JJ, Fuster V (1986) Electrical aggregometry in whole blood from human, pig and rabbit. Thromb Haemostas 56: 128–132
Ganda PO, Arkin CF (1992) Hyperfibrinogenemia an important risk factor for vascular complications in diabetes. Diabetes Care 15: 1245–1250
Geiger M, Binder BR (1986) Nonenzymatic glycosylation as a contributing factor to defective fibrinolysis in diabetes mellitus. Haemostasis 16: 439–446
Grignani G, Gamba G, Geroldi D, Pacchiarini L, Solerte B, Ferrari E, Ascari E (1981) Enhanced antithrombotic mechanisms in patients with maturity-onset diabetes mellitus without thrombotic complications. Thromb Haemostas 46: 648–651
Halushka PV, Rogers RC, Loadholt CB, Colwell JA (1981) Increased platelet thromboxane syntesis in diabetes mellitus. J Lab Clin Lab 97: 87–96
Haberl RL, Dembrowski K (1999) Atherothrombosis: common factor in stroke, myocardial infarction and peripheral vascular disease. Eur Heart J Supplements 1 (Suppl A): A41-A44
Herbert JM, Savi P, Maffrand JP (1998) Biochemical and pharmacological properties of clopidogrel; a new ADP receptor antagonist. Eur Heart J Supplements 1 (Suppl A): 31–
Hirano T, Kashiwazaki K, Morimoto Y, Nagano S, Adachi M (1997) Albuminuria is directly associated with increased plasma PAI-1 and factor VII levels in NIDDM patients. Diabetes Research and Clinical Practice 36: 11–18
Hoffman M, Fuchs HE, Pizzo SV (1986) The macrophage-mediated regulation of hepatocyte syntesis of antithrombin III and α1-proteinase inhibitor. Thromb Res 41: 707–715
Imperatore G, Rivellese AA, Ricardi G, Vaccaro O, Iovne C (1998) Plasma fibrinogen: a new factor of metabolic syndrome. A population based study. Diabetes Care 21: 649–653
Jokl R, Colwell JA (1997) Arterial thrombosis and atherosclerosis in diabetes. Diabetes Reviews 5: 316–330
Juhan-Vague I, Vague P, Alessi MC, Badier C, Valadier J, Ailland MF, Atlan C (1987) Relationship between plasma insulin, triglyceride, body mass index and plasminogen activator inhibitor-1. Diab Metabol 13: 331–336
King GL, Wakasaki H (1999) Theoretical mechanisms by wich hyperglycemia and insulin resistence could cause cardiovascular disease in diabetes. Diabetes Care 22 (Suppl 3):C31-C37
Knöbl PN, Fischer P, Kaliman JF, Vukovich TC (1987) Plasma level of protein C and protein S in patients with vasculopathy. Thromb Res 45: 857–863
Lane A, Cruickshank JK, Mitchell J, Henderson A, Humphries S, Green F (1992) Genetic and enviromental determinants of factor VII coagulant activity in ethnic groups at differing risk of coronary heart disease. Atheroslerosis 94: 43–50
Libby P (1995) Molecular bases of acute coronary syndromes. Circulation 91: 2844–2850
Loskutoff DJ, Samad F (1998) The adipocyte and hemostatic balance in obesity. Studies of PAI-1. Arterial Thromb Vasc Biol 18: 1–6
Lütjens A, Jonkhoff-Slak TW, Sandkuijl C, van den Veen EA, van den Meer J (1988) Polymerisation and crosslinking of fibrin monomers in diabetes mellitus. Diabetologia 36: 825–836

Mannucci PM (1998) von Willebrand Factor. A marker of endothelial damage. Arterioscler Thromb Vasc Biol 18: 1359–1362
Marongiu F, Mascia F, Mameli G, Cirillo R, Balestrieri A (1995) Prothrombin fragment F1 + 2 levels are high in NIDDM patients independently of Hb.A1$_c$. Thromb Haemostas 74: 805–806
McMillan DE (1976) Plasma protein changes, blood viscosity and diabetic microangiopathy. Diabetes 25 (Suppl 2): 858–864
McMillan DE, Utterback NG, La Puma J (1978) Reduced erythocite deformability in diabetes. Diabetes 26 27: 895–901
Mustard JF, Pakham MA (1977) Normal and abnormal hemostasis. Br Med Bull 33:187–192
Ney KA, Pasqua JJ, Colley KJ, Guthrow CE, Pizzo SV (1985) In vitro preparation of nonenzymatically glycosylated human transferin, α-2 macroglobulin and fibrinogen with preservation of function. Diabetes 34: 462–470
Owen J, Grossman B, Palmer RH (1988) Hyperlipidemia and in vivo hemostasic system activation. Semin Thromb Hemost 14: 241–245
Peltzer H, Schwartz A, Heimburger N (1988) Determination of human thrombin-antithrombin III complex in plasma with an enzyme-linked immunoabsorbent assay. Thromb Haemostas 59: 101–106
Perry IJ, Wannamethee GS, Shaper GA (1998) Prospective study of serum γ-glutamyltransferase and risk of NIDDM. Diabetes Care 21: 732–737
Pottinger BE, Read BC, Paleolog EM, Higgins PE, Pearson JD (1989) The von Willebrand factor is an acute phase reactant in man. Thromb Res 53: 387–394
Reed GL, Houng AK (1998) The contribution of activated factor XIII to fibrinolytic resistance in experimental pulmonary embolism. Circulation 99: 299–304
Rosove MH, Frank HJL, Harwig SSL (1984) Plasma β-thromboglobulin, platelet factor 4, fibrinopeptide A and other hemostatic functions during improved short term glycemic control in diabetes mellitus. Diabetes Care 7: 174–179
Saito M, Kumabashiri J, Asakura H, Uotani Ch, Otsuka M, Hamada M, Tatsamura M, Morinaga K, Matsuda T (1988) The levels of protein C and protein S in plasma in patients with type 2 diabetes mellitus. Thromb Res 52: 479–486
Sakata Y, Aoki N (1980) Crosslinking of α-2 plasmin inhibitor to fibrin by fibrin stabilizing factor. J Clin Invest 65: 280–297
Schernthaner G (1997) Abnormal hemostasis in diabetes mellitus and metabolic syndrome: contributing factors and potential therapeutic interventions. In Hanefeld M, Leonhardt W (Eds) The metabolic syndrome. Gustav Fischer Verlag, Jena pp 194–216
Sundell IB, Dahlgren S, Ranby M, Lundin E, Stenling R, Nilsson TK (1989) Reduction of elevated plasminogen activator inhibitor levels during modest weight loss. Fibrinolysis 3: 51–53
Tooke JE (1998) Endotheliopathy precedes type 2 diabetes (Editorial). Diabetes Care 21: 2047–2049
Tschöpe D, Rösen P, Kaufmann L, Schauseil S, Kehrel B, Ostermann H, Gries FA (1980) Evidence for abnormal platelet glycoprotein expression in diabetes mellitus. Eur J Clin Invest 20: 166–170
Vigano S, Mannuci PM, D Angelo AD, Gelfi C, Gensini GF, Rostagno C, Neri Serneri GG (1984) Protein C antigen is not an acute phase reactant and is often high in ischemic heart disease and diabetes. Thromb Haemostas 52: 263–266
Vukovich T, Schernthaner G (1986) Decreased protein C levels in patients with insulin-dependent type 1 diabetes mellitus. Diabetes 35: 617–619
Vukovich T, Schernthaner G, Knöbl P, Hay U (1989) The effect of near- normoglycemic control on factor VIII, von Willebrand factor and fibrin degradation products in insulin-dependent diabetic patients. J Clin Endocrinol Metab 69: 84–89
Waine-Smith C (1997) Potential significance of circulating E-selectin (Editorial). Circulation 95: 1986–1988
Wartiovaara V, Mikkola H, Szöke G, Haramura G, Kárpáti L, Balogh I, Lassila R, Muszbek L, Palotie A.(2000) Effect of val34leu polymorphism on the activation of the coagulation factor XIII-A. Thromb Haemostas 84:595-600
Winocour PD, Watala C, Kinlough-Rathbone Rl (1991) Membrane fluidity is related to the extent of glycation of proteins, but not to alterations in the cholesterol to phospholipid molar ratio in isolated platelet membranes from diabetic and control subjects. Thromb Haemostas 67: 567–571

Woods AI, Santarelli MT, Lazzari MA (1994) The inhibitory effect of platelets on fibrinolysis in diabetic patients Thromb Res 76: 391-396

Yudkin JS (1999) Abnormalities of coagulation and fibrinolysis in insulin resistance. Diabetes Care 22 (Suppl 3): C25-C30

Addendum

Three months after having submitted the manuscript, relevant data relating insulin resistance to increased plasma factor XIII levels became known to me. Actually factor XIII A and B subunit antigen plasma levels were higher in patients with type 2 diabetes than in control subjects (Mansfield et al. 2000), and liver secreted B subunit was found to be significantly correlated with several markers of insulin resistance, such as waist:hip ratio, HbA1c, fasting triglycerides, total cholesterol and PAI-1 antigen (Warner et al. 2001). Noteworthy in patients on dimethylbiguanide therapy factor XIII antigen and activity levels in vivo were reduced over a 12-week period (Standeven et al. 2002).

Mansfield MW, Kohler HP, Ariëns RAS, Cormack LJ, Grant PJ (2000) Circulating levels of coagulation factor XIII in subjects with type 2 diabetes and in their first degree relatives. Diabetes Care 23: 703-705

Standeven KF, Ariëns RAS, Whitaker P, Ashcroft A, Weisel JW, Grant PJ (2002) The effect of dimethylbiguanide on thrombin activity, factor XIII activation, fibrin polymerization and fibrin clot formation. Diabetes 51: 189-197

Warner D, Mansfield MW, Grant PI (2001) Coagulation factor XIII and cardiovascular disease in UK Asian patients undergoing coronary angiography. Thromb Haemostas 85: 408-411

CHAPTER 15

Hyperhomocysteinemia as Cardiovascular Risk Factor in Type 2 Diabetes Mellitus

A. de Leiva

Abstract. Hyperhomocysteinemia has been associated to the development of cardiovascular disease, mainly premature atherosclerosis and thromboembolic disorders.
Experimental results indicate an involvement of hyperhomocysteinemia in endothelial dysfunction, lipid peroxidation, impaired synthesis of nitric oxide, and reduced expression of thrombomodulin.
Genetic defects leading to deficiencies of cystathionine beta synthase and methylene tetrahydrofolate reductase are responsible of increased plasma homocysteine in homozygotes.
Ageing, postmenopause, hypothyroidism, renal insufficiency, and reduction of plasma folate, account for non-genetic causes of hyperhomocysteinemia.
Increased plasma homocysteine have been recorded in both type 1 and type 2 diabetic subjects. Experimental evidence suggests that advanced glycation end products may act synergistically with homocysteine in the development of endothelial dysfunction. In general, diabetic patients with associated hyperhomocysteinemia showed higher levels of serum creatinine, and in type 2 diabetic subjects, multiple regression analysis has depicted albumin excretion rate as the parameter with strongest independent association with elevated plasma homocysteine. Patients with nephropathy and hyperhomocysteinemia were older and showed a more advanced stage of renal disease.
Succesful treatment of hyperhomocysteinemia is achieved with the oral administration of folate in association either to piridoxine, vitamin B_{12} and betaine. Higher doses of folate are required in patients with marked hyperhomocysteinemia and chronic renal failure.

Introduction

Homocysteine is a thiol-containing aminoacid originated from demethylation of methionine. Main metabolic transformations of homocysteine are, either remethylation to methionine, or transsulfuration to cysteine.

Genetic, biochemical, clinic and epidemiologic reports have indicated an involvement of hyperhomocysteinemia in the development of atherosclerotic and thrombotic disorders [1–3]. A causal relationship between hyperhomocysteinemia and cardiovascular disease (CVD) have been proposed by prospective studies [4–5]. Normal plasma homocysteine (Hcy) levels range between 5 and 15 mcmol/l. Hyperhomocysteinemia has been graded as moderate (15–30 mcmol/l), intermediate (30–100 mcmol/l), and severe (>100 mcmol/l) [6].

Homocystinuria is an inherited defect associated to elevated plasma levels of homocysteine (Hcy) and premature CVD, with marked risk for arterial thrombosis and atherosclerosis [1–3, 7].

Recent studies have suggested a relationship between accelerated CVD and mild/

moderate hyperhomocysteinemia in patients with diabetes mellitus, leading to the hypothesis that hyperhomocysteinemia may represent an important cardiovascular risk factor in the population with diabetes mellitus [8].

Various publications have established a positive association between increased plasma hcy levels and increased albumin excretion among diabetic and non diabetic people [9–14]. Presence of diabetes increases the risk of CVD [15], and the association of nephropathy increases this risk even further.

Homocysteine Metabolism

Methionine (Me) is converted to Hcy after two consecutive reactions. The first one involves the activity of the enzyme L-Me-adenosyltransferase and the donation of methyl-groups to Me, generating S-adenosyl-Me (SAM). This metabolite provides methyl-groups to various metabolic pathways, leading to S-adenosyl-Hcy. Then, this compound is hydrolyzed to Hcy by a specific hydrolase.

Depending on the plasma levels of Me, Hcy metabolism will proceed either to the transsulfuration pathway or the transmethylation pathway. In the former, Hcy leads to cysteine (Cys) through to reactions, with the participation of vitamin B_6, and the enzymes cystathionine-beta-synthase (CbS, responsible of the condensation of Hcy with serine), and cystathionine-gamma-lyase (CgL, driving to the release of Cys and alpha-ketobutyrate) (Blanco-Mudd, 1995). Through two re-methylation pathways, Hcy can form Me, with either the participation of the enzyme Me-synthase (cosubstrate, 5-Me-tetrahydrofolate; methylcobalamine as coenzyme), or the enzyme Betain: Hcy-methyltransferase, which uses betain as the source of methyl-groups.

Genetics of Hyperhomocysteinemia

Cystathionine Beta-Synthase Deficiency

The cystathionine beta-synthase (CBS) gene has been is mapped to the subtelomeric region, 21q22 [16]. Seventeen CBS mutations have been described so far. Homozygous mutations are most frequent cause of homocystinuria, inherited as an autosomic recessive pattern. Heterozygosity results in hyperhomocysteinemia carriers.

Methylene Tetrahydrofolate Reductase (MTHFR) Deficiency

This polymorphism, in its homozygotic form is responsible of mild hyperhomocysteinemia, which occurs only in association with low folate levels. The gene is located on 1p36.3. Mutations leading to the substitution C → T at nucleotide 677 (C677G) of the coding region, leading to the change of valine for alanine at the position 226 of the aminoacid sequence, is linked to hyperhomocysteinemia in homozygotic subjects [17–20].

Other Causes of Hyperhomocysteinemia

Many non-genetic factors influence plasma Hcy levels. *Age* is responsible of increasing fasting plasma levels.

Estrogen affects the activity of enzymes involved in Hcy metabolism. Plasma Hcy levels raise before and after Me load in postmenopausal women. Hormone replacement therapy (HRT) exerts beneficial effects on cardiovascular risk, and significantly decreased plasma Hcy [21], like tamoxifen [22]. Elevated Hcy levels have been reported in cases of *hypothyroidism* [23].

Increased plasma levels of Hcy have been depicted in *variable stages of renal insufficiency*, which has been attributed to the impairment of Hcy renal metabolism [24-27].

Reduction of plasma folate is associated to increased plasma Hcy [28]. Dietary supplementation of folate reduces plasma Hcy levels [29]. Randomized clinical trials with addition of folate (0.5-5.0 mg) and vitamin B_{12} (0.5 mg) have been effective, decreasing plasma Hcy levels [30].

Pyridoxine is an important cofactor of CBS. Vitamin B_6 deficiency may be suspected in subjects showing increased plasma Hcy after a methionine load (frequently associated with premature cardiovascular disease).

Hyperhomocysteinemia as a Cardiovascular Risk Factor

Many clinical investigation protocols have shown evidence, supporting the hypothesis that hyperhomocysteinemia is an independent cardiovascular risk factor. Children affected of homozygous homocysteinemia usually die at young age.

Strong relationship between plasma Hcy levels and overall mortality in individuals with established coronary artery disease has been observed [31]; plasma Hcy performed in the regression analysis like a continuous variable, without a critical threshold. Relative increase of plasma Hcy levels depicted in Irish people in comparison to French ones may explained the higher prevalence and mortality in Ireland in subjects that suffered an episode of myocardial infarction (MI) [32]. Not all studies have pointed out hyperhomocysteinemia as an independent risk factor; for example, homocysteine was not found to be a risk factor for coronary disease at the Multiple Risk Factor Intervention Trials (MRFIT) [33].

Plasma Hcy has been found elevated in patients with peripheral vascular disease (Endo Rev, 136). Several studies have suggested a strong association between hyperhomocysteinemia and cerebrovascular disease. In the Framingham Heart Study, the incidence of carotid disease was about twice in patients with the highest percentiles of plasma levels of Hcy, in comparison with the lowest [34]. Similar results were derived from the Atherosclerosis Risk in Community Study [35]. It has been estimated that 42% of patients with cerebrovascular disease, 28% of patients with peripheral vascular disease, and 30% of patients with coronary artery disease depict hyperhomocysteinemia [36].

A meta-analysis has shown that hyperhomocysteinemia is responsible for as much as 10% of the risk of coronary disease in the general population [37]. Furthermore, increased plasma levels of Hcy over 22 mcmol per liter have been reported to increase the odds ratio for deep venous thrombosis to 4.0 [38].

Experimental data suggest that hyperhomocysteinemia induces endothelial activation, platelet accumulation and increased thrombus formation. Auto-oxidation of Hcy produces cytotoxic reactive oxygen radicals [39 – 40], initiating lipid peroxidation, activating the oxidation of LDL particles, at least in vitro [41 – 42]. Hcy in excess enhances the effects of various coagulation factors, facilitating the formation of thrombin through various mechanisms, including the inhibited expression of thrombomodulin [43]. Chronic exposure to hyperhomocysteinemia damages the endothelium, impairing the synthesis of nitric oxide [44], and the substance leads to vascular smooth-muscle proliferation in vitro [45 – 46].

The Consequences of Hyperhomocysteinemia in Diabetes Mellitus

Type 1 Diabetes

Type 1 diabetic subjects have depicted increased basal and postload plasma homocysteine levels, when compared to controls. Those diabetic patients showing increased plasma Hcy over the normal range, displayed also higher plasma thrombomodulin concentration, higher albumin excretion rate, and higher rate of diabetic complications (retinopathy, nephropathy, neuropathy, atherosclerotic disease), regarding Type 1 diabetic subjects with normal plasma Hcy [47]. Experimental evidence, in vitro, with human umbilical vein cells demonstrated increased release of thrombomodulin in the supernatant when endothelial cells were preincubated with advanced glycation end products (AGEs), before the addiction of Hcy. This observation leads to the suggestion that AGE proteins and Hcy may act synergistically in the development of endothelium dysfunction and vascular damage.

Type 2 Diabetes

Our group have measured fasting plasma Hcy concentration in control, type 1 and type 2 diabetic populations [9]. Patients with type 2 diabetes depicted higher Hcy levels than control subjects. Univariate correlations and multiple regression analysis showed albumin excretion rate to be the parameter with the strongest independent association with plasma Hcy. Higher plasma Hcy levels were present in both type 1 and type 2 diabetic groups, associated to the existence of diabetic nephropathy. Also, increases in plasma Hcy were related to the severity of the nephropathy.

Values of 12 mcmol/liter or higher were considered to define fasting hyperhomocysteinemia, demonstrated in as much as 18 % of all type 2 diabetic subjects. Albumin excretion rate (AER) and age were independently related with plasma Hcy. Individuals with type 1 diabetes without nephropathy, did not differ significantly, with respect to plasma Hcy levels in relation to the control group. Patients with both type 1 and type 2 diabetes, presenting with hyperhomocysteinemia, showed, in general higher levels of serum creatinine than normohomocysteinemic type 2 diabetes patients.

In the group of investigated patients with diabetes, no significant correlations were found between circulating levels of folate, vitamin B_{12} or plasma piridoxal 5ṕhosphate, and plasma Hcy levels. This lack of correlation contrasts with other studies in which levels of folate and vitamin B_{12} showed a non-linear inverse correlation with plasma Hcy levels. Nevertheless, most of these studies have been conducted in populations from central/northern Europe and north America; therefore, considerable ethnic and dietary differences may justify this discrepancy. Detrimental effects of low serum folate and vitamin B_{12} on plasma Hcy levels occurred only below cut-off levels around 10 nm/l of folate and 375 pmol/l of vitamin B_{12} [48 – 49]. In our study, mean folate and vitamin B_{12} levels were, in diabetic patients, higher than these threshold values.

Patients were classified according to the existence of renal failure as group 1, renal failure; group 2, overt nephropathy; group 3, incipient nephropathy; group 4, without nephropathy. In the diabetic patients as a whole and, preferentially in type 2 diabetic patients, there was a significant increase in plasma Hcy in relation with the presence and severity of the nephropathy. Although without reaching statistical significance, a similar trend was observed in the group of type 1 diabetic individuals. In general, diabetic patients with associated hyperhomocysteinemia presented higher values of creatinine, albumin excretion rate and creatinine clearance. No differences with respect to the plasma levels of folate, vitamin B_{12} and piridoxal 5'-phosphate were found. In the study, all type 1 patients with hypertension had diabetic nephropathy.

Type 2 diabetic patients with hypertension depicted higher plasma Hcy concentrations than Type 2 diabetic patients without hypertension. Also, Type 2 diabetic patients with hypertension had, in general, more severe biochemical signs of nephropathy than type 2 diabetic patients without hypertension. Those patients with type 2 diabetes, nephropathy and hypertension showed a tendency to display higher plasma Hcy than type 2 diabetic patients with nephropathy without hypertension, although Type 2 diabetic patients with hypertension had, in general, more severe biochemical signs of nephropathy than type 2 diabetic patients without hypertension. Finally, patients with type 2 diabetes without nephropathy, but with hypertension, had Hcy levels not statistically different from those type 2 diabetic patients without nephropathy and without hypertension.

In general, diabetic patients with nephropathy who had hyperhomocysteinemia were older and showed more advanced nephropathy than those without hyperhomocysteinemia. The prevalence of macroangiopathy was 25 % in the group of Type 1 diabetes with hyperhomocysteinemia; on the contrary, only 4.2 % of type 1 diabetic subjects with normal homocysteinemia had macroangiopathy. No significant difference was observed between type 2 diabetic patients with and without macroangiopathy.

Treatment of Hyperhomocysteinemia

The therapeutic approach of hyperhomocysteinemia includes the administration of folate, piridoxine and vitamin B_{12}. There is not a general agreement about the doses, and the effects of lowering plasma homocysteine on cardiovascular disease have not been well-defined. For the majority of patients, the treatment with 1 – 5 mg of folic acid is followed by an effective reduction of Hcy concentration, which becomes normalized after 4 – 6 weeks of therapy [50 – 52]. The exception is the case of renal insufficiency, associated to only moderate reduction of plasma Hcy levels.

If the treatment cannot achieve the target, the combined administration of folate with piridoxine (100 – 300 mg/day), or folate with betaine (6 g/day). In general, it is recommended to administer folic acid in association to vitamin B_{12} (0.4 mg/day), to avoid the progression of neuropathy. If the patient display chronic renal failure or marked elevation of plasma Hcy (>30 nmol/ml), higher initial doses of folic acid (5 mg/day) are recommended.

References

1. Schimke RN, McKusick VA, Huang T, Pollack AD. Homocystinuria.Studies of 20 families with 38 affected members. JAMA 1965;193:711–719.
2. McCully KS. Vascular pathology of homocysteinemia. Implications for the pathogenesis of arteriosclerosis. Am J Pathol 1969;56:111–128
3. Boers GH, Smals AG, Trijbels FJ, Fowler B, Bakkeren JA, Schoonderwaldt HC, Kleijer WJ, Kloppenborg PW. Heterozygosity for homocystinuria in premature peripheral and cerebral occlusive arterial disease. N England J Med 1985;313:709–715.
4. Legnani C, Palaretti G, Grauso F, Sassi S, Grossi G, Piazzi S, Bernardi F, Marchetti G, Ferraresi P, Coccheri S. Hyperhomocysteinemia and commom methyleneetetrahydrofolate reductase mutation (Ala-223ValMTHFR) in patients with inherited thrombophilic coagulation defects. Thromb Vasc Biol 1997;17:2924–2929.
5. Ma J, Stampfer MJ, Hennekens CH, Frosst P, Selhub J, Horsford J, Malinow R, Willett WC, Rozen R. Methylene tetrahydrofolate reductase polymorphism, plasma folate, homocysteine, and risk of myocardial infarction in US physicians. Circulation 1996;94:2410–2416.
6. Kang SS, Wong PWK. Genetic and non-genetic factors for moderate hyperhomocysteinemia. Arterioscler Thromb 1993;13:2253.
7. Carson NAJ, Dent CE, Field CMB, Gaull GE. Homocystinuria. Clinical and pathological review of ten cases. J Pediatr 1965;66:565–583.
8. Hoogeveen EK, Kostense PJ, Beks PJ, MacKaay AJC, Jakobs C, Bouter LM, Heine RJ, Stehower CD. Hyperhomocysteinemia is associated with and increased risk of cardiovascular disease,specially in non-insulin-dependent diabetes mellitus: a population-based study. Arterioscler Thromb Vasc Biol 1998;18:133–138.
9. Chico A, Pérez A, Córdoba A, Arcelus R, Carreras G, de Leiva A, González-Sastre F, Blanco-Vaca F. Plasma homocysteine is related to albumin excretion rate in patients with diabetes mellitus : a new link between diabetic nephropathy and cardiovascular disease?. Diabetologia 1998;41:684–693.
10. Lanfredini M, Fiorina P, Peca MG, Veronelli A, Mello A, AstorriE, Dall?Aglio P, Craveri A. Fasting and post-methionine load homocysteine values are correlated with microalbuminuria and could conbtribute to worsening vascular damage in non-insulin-dependent diabetes mellitus patients. Metabolism 1998;47:915–921.
11. Hoogeveen EK, Kostense PJ, Jager A, Heine RH, Jakobs C, Bouter LM, Donker AJ, Stehower CD. Serum homocysteine level and protein intake are related to risk of albuminuria : the Hoorn Study. Kidney Int 1999;54:203–209
12. Fiorina P, LanfredininM, Montanari A, Peca MG, Veronelli A, Mello A, Astorri E, Caraveri A. Plasma homocysteine and folate are related to arterial blood pressure in type 2 diabetes mellitus. Am J Hypert 1998;11:1100–1117.
13. Stehouwer CD, Gall MA, Hougaard P, Jakobs C, Parving HH. Plasma homocysteine concentration predicts mortality in non-insulin-dependent diabetic patients with and without albuminuria. Kidney Int 1999;55:308–314.
14. Bostom AG, Lathrop L. Hyperhomocysteinemia in end-stage renal disease: prevalence, etiology and potential relationshipto arteriosclerotic outcomes Kidney Int 1997; 52:10–20.
15. Pyörälä K, Laakso M, Uusitapa M. Diabetes and atherosclerosis : an epidemiologic view. Diab Metab Rev. 1987;3:463–524.
16. Giusti R, Comeglio P, Attanasio M, Gori AM, Brunelli T, Prisco D, Pepe G, Gensini GF, Abbate R. Different distribution of the doble mutant "T833 C/68 bp Insertion", in cysthatione-beta-synthasa gene in Northern and Southern Italian populations. Letter to the Editor, Thromb Haemost 1997;78:1293–1303
17. Engerbsen AMT, Franken DG, Boers GHJ, Stevens EMB, Trijbels FJM, Blom HJ. Thermolabile 5,10-methylenetetrahydrofolate reductase as a cause of mild hyperhomocysteinemia. Am J Hum Genet 1995;56:142–150.

18. Harmon DL, Woodside JV, Yarnell JWG, McMaster D, Young IS, McCrun EE, GeyKF, Whitehead AS, Evans AE. The common "thermolabile" variant of methylenetetrahydrofolatereductase is a major determinant of mild hyperhomocysteinemia. QJMed 1996;89:571–577.
19. D'Angelo A, Selhub J. Homocysteine and thrombotic disease. Blood 1997;90:1–11.
20. Friedman G, Goldschmidt N, Friedlander Y, Ben-Yehuda A, Selhub J, Babaey S, Mendel M, Kidron M, Bar-On H. A common mutation A1298 C in human methylenetetrahydrofolate reductase gen : association with plasma total homocysteine and folate concentration. J Nutr 1999;129:1656–1661.
21. van der Mooren MJ, Wouters MG, Bom HJ, Schellekens LA, Eskes TJ, Rolland R. Hormone replacement therapy may reduce serum homocysteine in postmenopausal women. Eur J Clin Invest 1994;24:733–736.
22. Anker G, Lonning PE, Ueland PM, Refsum H, Lien EA. Plasma levels of athergenic amino acid homocysteine in postmenopausal women with breast cancer treated with tamoxifen. Int J Cancer 1995;60:365–368.
23. Nedrebo BG, Ericsson UB, Nygard O, Refsum H, Ueland PM, Aakvaag A, Aanderund S, Lien EA. Plasma total homocysteine levels in hyperthyroid and hypothyroid patients. Metabolism 1998;47:89–93.
24. Bostom AG, Brosnan JT, Hall B, Nadeau MR, Selhub J. Net uptake of plasma homocysteine by the rat kidney in vivo. Atherosclerosis 1995;116:59–62.
25. Bostom AG, Shemin D Lapane KL, Hume AL, Yoburn D, Nadeau MR, Bendich A, Selhub J, Rosenberg IH. High dose B-vitamin treatment of hyperhomocysteinemia in dialysis patients. Kidney Int 1996;49:147–152.
26. Massy ZA, Chadefaxu-Vekemans B, Chevalier A, Bader CA, Drueke TB, Legendre C, Lacour B, Kamoun P, Kreis H. Hyperhomocysteinemia : a significant risk factor for cardiovascular disease in renal transplant recipients. Nephrol Dial Transplant 1994;9:1103–1108.
27. Arnadottir M, Hultberg B, Vladov V, Nilsson-Ehle P, Thysell H. Hyperhomocysteine in cyclosporine-treated renal transplant recipients. Transplantation 1996;61:509–512.
28. Selhub J, Jacques PF, Wilson PW, Rush D, Rosenberg IH. Vitamin status and intake as primary determinant of homocysteinemia in an elderly population. JAMA 1993;270:2693–2698.
29. Garg UC, Zheng ZJ, Folsom AR, Moyer YS, Tsai MY, McGovern P, Eckfeldt JH. Short-term and long-term variability of plasma homocysteine measurement. Cin Chem 1997;43:141–145.
30. Homocysteine Lowering Trialists' Collaboration. Lowering blood homocysteine with folic acid based supplements : meta-anlysis of randomised trials. Br Med J 1998;316:894–898.
31. Nygard O, Nordrehaug JE, Refsum H, Ueland PM, Farstad M, Vollset SE. Plasma homocysteine levels and mortality in patients with coronary artery disease. N Engl J Med 1997;337:230–236.
32. Malinow MR, Ducimetiere P, Luc G, Evans AE, Arveiler D, Cambien F, Upson BM. Plasma homocysteine levels and graded risk for myocardial infarction : findings in two populations at contrasting risk for coronary herat disease. Atherosclerosis 1996;126:27–34.
33. Evans RW, Shaten BJ,, Hempel JD, Cutler JA, Kuller LH. Homocysteine and risk of cardiovascular disease in the Multiple Risk Factor Intervention Trial. Arterioscler Thromb Vasc Biol 1997;17:1947–1953.
34. Aronow WS, Ahn C, Schoenfeld MR. Association between plasma homocysteine and extracranial carotid arterial disease in older persons. Am J Cardiol 1997;79:1432–1433.
35. Malinow MR, Nieto FJ, Szklo M, Chambless LE, Bond G. Carotid artery intimal-medial wall thickening and plasma homocysteine in asymptomatic adults. The Atherosclerotic Risk in Communities Study. Circulation 1993;87:1107–1113.
36. Clarke R, Daly L, Robinson K. Hyperhomocysteinemia : and independent risk for cardiovascular disease N Engl J Med 1991;324:1149–1155.
37. Boushey CJ, Beresford SA, OmennGS, Motulsky AG. A quantitative assessment of plasma homocysteine as a risk factor for cardiovascular disease : probable benefits of increasing folic acid intakes. JAMA 1995;274 : 1049–1057.
38. den Heijer M, Kostor T, Blom HJ. Hyperhomocysteinemia as a risk factor for deep-vein thrombosis. N Engl J Med 1996;334 : 759–762.
39. Misra HP. Generation of superoxide free radical during the autooxidations of thiols. J Biol Chem 1974;249:2151–2155.
40. Rowley DA, Halliwell B. Superoxide-dependent formation of hydroxyl radicals in the presence of thiol compounds. FEBS Lett 1982;138:33–36.

41. Heinecke JW, Kawamura M, Suzuki L, Chait A. Oxidation of low density lipoprotein by thiols: superoxide-dependent and -independent mechanisms. J Lip Res 1993;34:2051-2061.
42. Parthasarathy S. Oxidation of low density lipoprotein by thiol compounds leads to its recognition by the acetyl LDL receptor. Biochim Biophys Acta 1987;917:337-340.
43. Lentz SR, Dadler JL. Inhibition of thrombomodulin surface expression and proteinC activation by the thrombogenic agent homocysteine. J Clin Invest 1991;88:1906-1914.
44. Loscalzo J. The oxidant stress of hyperhomocysteinemia. J Clin Invest 1996;98:5-7.
45. Tsai JC, Perrella MA, Yoshimuzi M. Promotion of vascular smooth muscle cell growth by homocysteine : a link to atherosclerosis. Proc Natl Acad Sci USA 1994;91:6369-1373.
46. Tsai JC, Wang H, Perrella MA. Induction of cyclen A gene expression by homocysteine in vascular smooth muscle cells. J Clin Invest 1996;97:146-153.
47. Hofmann MA, Kohl B, Zumbach MS. Hyperhomocysteinemia and endothelial dysfunction in IDDM. Diabetes Care 1997;20:1880-1886.
48. Selhub J, Jacques PF, Bostom AG. Relationship between plasma homocysteine, vitamin status and extracranial carotid-artery stenosis in the Framingham study. J Nutr 1996;126:1258S-1265 S.
49. Pancharutini N, Lewis CA, Sauberlich HE. Plasma homocysteine, folate, and vitamin B12 concentrations and risk for early-onset coronary artery disease. Am J Clin Nutr 1994;59:940-948.
50. Glueck CJ, Shaw P, Lang JE. Evidence that homocysteine is an independent risk factor for atherosclerosis in hyperlipemic patients. Am J Cardiol 1995;75:132-136.
51. Franken DG, Boers GHJ, Blom HJ. Treatment of mild hyperhomocysteinemia in vascular disease patients. Arterioscler Thromb 1994;14:465-471.
52. Brattstrom L, Israelsson B, Norrving B. Impaired homocysteine metabolism in early onset cerebral and peripheral vascular disease: Effects of pyridoxine and folic acid treatment. Atherosclerosis 1990;81:51-55.

CHAPTER 16

Cardiac Autonomic Neuropathy: Is it a Cardiovascular Risk Factor in Type 2 Diabetes?

P. Kempler

Abstract. The autonomic nervous system, through the sympathetic and parasympathetic pathways, supplies and influences every organ in the body. It closely integrates vital processes such as heart rate, blood pressure, myocardial contractility and as a consequence plays a pivotal role in the regulation of the cardiovascular system.

Cardiac autonomic neuropathy represents a serious complication as it carries an approximately fivefold risk of mortality in patients with diabetes just as in those with chronic liver diseases. The high mortality rate may be related to silent myocardial infarction, cardiac arrhythmia, cardiovascular and cardiorespiratory instability and to other causes not explained yet. Resting tachycardia due to parasympathetic damage may represent one of the earliest signs. Typical findings refering to autonomic dysfunction may include exercise intolerance, orthostatic hypotension and cardiac dysfunction to rest or exercise. Severe autonomic neuropathy may be responsible for spontaneous respiratory arrest and unexplained sudden deaths, which are not rare among diabetic patients. A relationship between the presence and/or severity of CAN and corrected QT interval prolongation is well documented.

Our better understanding on clinical and prognostic importance of autonomic neuropathy was closely related to the widespread use of simple non-invasive cardiovascular reflex tests. The most commonly used battery of non-invasive tests for assessment of cardiovascular reflexes includes heart rate variation in response to deep breathing, standing and Valsalva maneouvre as well as blood pressure responses to standing and sustained handgrip.

Near normoglycaemia is now generally accepted as the primary approach to the prevention of diabetic neuropathy, but is not achievable in a considerable number of patients. The antioxidant alpha-lipoic acid can be recommended as first choice drug for the treatment of cardiac autonomic neuropathy.

Introduction

Langley coined the term "autonomic nervous system" in 1898. Eichorst suggested in 1892 that persistent tachycardia in diabetic patients might be due to damage to the vagus nerve [9]. However, for many years autonomic nerve dysfunction was considered an interesting but rare complication. A remark by the obstetrician Timothy Wheeler to the diabetologist Peter J Watkins in 1972 that loss of heart rate variation in the foetus in utero might be due to hypoxia of autonomic centres, sparked the thought of using a foetal heart rate monitor to assess whether beat to beat variability in heart rate was altered in diabetic patients with neuropathy [56]. Subsequently, a significant decrease in beat to beat heart rate variability was documented in two important studies [54, 11]. Our better understanding on clinical and prognostic importance of autonomic neuropathy was closely related to the widespread use of simple non-invasive cardiovascular reflex tests.

Just at the centennial of the use of the term autonomic nervous system, we should ask whether autonomic disorders are being sufficiently considered, suitably investigated and appropriately managed in clinical practice.

Pathogenesis

Metabolic just as vascular factors have been invoked in the pathogenesis of diabetic neuropathy, but their interrelationships are poorly understood [17]. Vascular factors become more important with age [52]. Considerable evidence implicates nerve ischaemia in the pathogenesis of diabetic nerve conduction slowing. Reduced endoneural blood flow and oxygen tension accompanied by increased vascular resistance has been demonstrated in experimental studies early after the induction of diabetes. Impaired blood flow and artery-venous shunting has been shown by nerve photography and fluorescent angiography in human diabetic neuropathy [47].

Metabolic changes include polyol pathway hyperactivity, oxidative stress, increased advanced glycation and impaired essential fatty acid metabolism [17, 52, 15, 8]. These effects are exacerbated by weakened trophic support. Hyperglycaemia have been reported to increase diacylglycerol concentration and protein kinase C activity in the peripheral nerve.

Nitric oxide may be the link between the metabolic and vascular hypotheses of diabetic neuropathy [17]. Early metabolic effect may lead to a decrease in synthesis of nitric oxide in either the vascular endothelium or in the sympathetic ganglia leading to decreased nerve blood flow. Nitric oxide may also be involved in more distal defects of somatic nerve metabolism that impairs the activity of the nerve Na^+, K^+-ATP-ase by a mechanism involving phosphoinositide signalling and diacylglycerol. This may impair nerve conduction velocity independently of ischemia. It should be noted that neuropathies accompanying Type 1 and Type 2 diabetes are different. Etiological factors other than hyperglycaemia seems to be more important in patients with Type 2 diabetes [43].

Prevalence and Risk Factors

Due to different definitions of neuropathy and to variable diagnostic procedures extreme wide ranges of prevalence rates (between 5 and 100 %) have been published. The frequency of neuropathy in most relevant studies among patients with Type 1 and Type 2 diabetes was between 13 – 54 % (median: 32 %) and 17 – 45 % (median: 32 %), respectively [30]. The prevalence of autonomic neuropathy in the EURODIAB IDDM Complications Study was 36 % [29]. Significant correlation was observed between the presence of autonomic neuropathy with age, duration of diabetes, HbA1c, the presence of retinopathy and microalbuminuria, severe hypoglycaemia and ketoacidosis, cigarette smoking, lower HDL cholesterol, total cholesterol / HDL cholesterol ratio, diastolic blood pressure and fasting triglyceride [29]. Data of the study suggest that autonomic neuropathy is associated with an increased cardiovascular risk and at the first time a highly significant correlation between autonomic nerve dysfunction and cardiovascular disease has also been observed [29].

Autonomic neuropathy in Type 2 diabetes is associated with an unfavourable metabolic risk profile including hyperinsulinemia and hypertriglyceridemia [16]. Parasympathetic neuropathy in patients with Type 2 diabetes has been reported to be associated with obesity, microalbuminuria, hyperinsulinemia and increased plasminogen activator inhibitor 1 activity [46]. It has been suggested that cardiac parasympathetic damage should be considered as a new component of the insulin resistance syndrome [50].

Clinical Presentation

The autonomic nervous system, through the sympathetic and parasympathetic pathways, supplies and influences every organ in the body. It closely integrates vital processes such as heart rate, blood pressure, myocardial contractility and body temperature and as a consequence plays a pivotal role in the regulation of the cardiovascular system. Cardiac autonomic neuropathy (CAN) represents a serious complication. Survival patterns of patients with CAN compared to those without CAN are similar in diabetes mellitus and in chronic liver diseases. Metaanalysis of 9 studies showed that mortality after 5,8 years in diabetic patients with CAN was 29%, while it was 6% in those without CAN [58]. Corresponding data of the only 4-year-long follow-up study performed in patients with chronic liver diseases were 30% and 6%, respectively [18]. Factors leading to increased mortality of AN have not been definitely identified till now.

Resting tachycardia due to parasympathetic damage may represent one of the earliest signs of CAN. Experiences from large epidemiological studies indicate that tachycardia of any origin is a major risk factor for cardiovascular and noncardiovascular death [41]. The heart rate–mortality association is present at any age. The hemodynamic effects of faster ejection are independently conducive to vascular damage and to the development of atherosclerosis. A practical implication is that tachycardia cannot be considered as an indicator of an essentially benign condition, merely reflecting a temporary state of anxiety [41].

Dizziness, faintness, blackouts or visual impairment on standing are clinical presentations of postural hypertension. Sometimes these symptoms may mistakenly thought to represent hypoglycaemia.

CAN is associated with a high risk of unexpected and sudden death, possibly related to silent myocardial ischaemia/infarction, cardiac arrhythmia and hypoxia [58]. Cardiorespiratory arrests during or right after anaesthesia has been described. Any diabetic with CAN is at a considerable anaesthetic risk. The mechanisms by which CAN has been most frequently postulated to increase mortality include increased susceptibility to fatal ventricular arrhythmia and increased propensity to cardiovascular events [3]. A relationship between the presence and/or severity of CAN and corrected QT (QTc) interval prolongation is well demonstrated in patients with diabetes mellitus and chronic liver diseases [58, 21, 26, 24] indicating that changes in QT interval appear to be due to autonomic impairment, rather than diabetes per se. QT interval prolongation predisposes the subject to cardiac arrhythmia and the risk of sudden death. It has been shown that QTc prolongation correlated significantly with both parasympathetic and sympathetic test results, indicating that besides the established role of sympathetic dysfunction, even parasympathetic damage may contribute to the development of QTc prolongation [26]. Autonomic neuropathy should be taken into consideration when the aetiology of QT interval lengthening is not clear. Both CAN and QTc prolongation may be present in patients with newly diagnosed type 1 diabetes [28]. Studies must establish whether prolonged QTc interval among these patients is reversible [28].

Cardiac dysfunction at rest or exercise may be associated with CAN even in the absence of ischemic heart disease. Impaired diastolic relaxation precedes the development of decreased ejection fraction due to systolic dysfunction.

Autonomic neuropathy has been shown to be associated with hypertension [33, 44, 37]. Recently, we assessed cardiovascular autonomic function and 24-hour-long blood pressure profiles in patients with type 1 diabetes [27]. The decrease of parasympathetic parameters (30/15 ratio and Valsalva ratio) correlated significantly with systolic and diastolic hypertensive time indices as well as with systolic and diastolic hyperbaric impact (mm Hgxh) values. These data may suggest that a relative sympathetic hyperactivity due to predominant parasympathetic neuropathy might be responsible for hypertension [27]. A similar mechanism is supposed to have primary importance in the pathogenesis of essential hypertension.

The degree of loss of day-night rhythm of blood pressure is associated with the proportional nocturnal sympathetic predominance. Decreased blood pressure fall combined with relative sympathetic predominance during the night might represent a risk factor for cardiovascular accidents and could modify the circadian pattern of cardiovascular event in the diabetic population. As a consequence, even nornotensive diabetic patients are characterised by an increased left ventricular mass [13], which is an independent cardiovascular risk factor. The "non-dipper" phenomenon could be identified in both normotensive and hypertensive diabetic patients with asymptomatic autonomic neuropathy [22]. A reduction in the circadian heart rate variability due to more frequent sleeping heart rates was found in diabetic patients with CAN [20]. Diminished circadian heart rate variability as well as blunted or absent day-night blood pressure variation should be considered as potential mechanisms leading to acute ischaemic heart disease with specific diurnal pattern in patients with CAN [20]. Recent data suggest that diminished systolic and diastolic diurnal indices are associated with impaired blood pressure response to standing in patients with type 1 diabetes [27].

Vascular instability, exercise intolerance, poor heat adaptation due to defective sympathetic thermoregulation, denervation hypersensitivity and abnormal hormonal regulation may be present in subjects with CAN [51].

Autonomic Neuropathy and Coronary Artery Disease – Risk Stratification After Myocardial Infarction

There is a general agreement that the prevalence of both symptomatic and asymptomatic coronary artery disease is increased in diabetic patients [58]. It is also generally assumed that CAN is responsible for an altered perception of myocardial ischaemia, painless myocardial ischaemia and silent acute myocardial infarction [58]. However, the major drawback of most studies dealing with this topic is the lack of data on coronary morphology. In a recently published study CAN was independently associated with asymptomatic coronary artery disease in patients with type 2 diabetes [4]. In this study planar scintigraphy and SPECT has been performed as well. The authors suggest that patients with CAN should routinely screened for the presence of coronary artery disease, regardless of the presence of symptoms. Silent myocardial infarction should always be suspected in a diabetic patient with acute left ventricular failure (especially pulmonary oedema), collapse, vomiting and ketoacidosis.

On the other hand, the heart rate variability (HRV) decreases and its components alter their relative contribution in patients with coronary heart disease, acute myocardial infarction, chronic heart failure and hypertension. A large longitudinal observational study provided the first clinical evidence that decreased HRV was a powerful predictor of cardiac mortality after myocardial infarction [31]. The analysis of HRV in the frequency domain has also provided data of prognostic value; power spectral band calculated over 24 hour, particularly frequencies below 0.04 Hz were strongly related to all cause mortality and arrhythmic death independently of left ventricular ejection fraction [5]. These studies showed that HRV was an independent predictor of death additive to other post-infarction risk variables, such as left ventricular ejection fraction and heart rate.

In the last few years, more and more clinical attention was drawn to the key role played by the vagus nerve in the mediation of HRV. The arrhythmogenic role of sympathetic hyperactivity is firmly established and can be antagonised by vagal activation and the ability to augment vagal activity can be quantified by the baroreflex sensitivity. The ATRAMI Study (Autonomic Tone and Reflexes After Myocardial Infarction) provided clinical evidence that after myocardial infarction the analysis of baroreflex sensitivity has significant prognostic value independently of left ventricular ejection fraction and ventricular arrhythmia and that it significantly adds to the prognostic value of HRV [34]. It has been shown more recently analysing HRV and

Table 16.1. Possible factors associated with high mortality and sudden death due to autonomic neuropathy

---

Silent myocardial ischaemia/infarction
Cardiorespiratory arrest/increased perioperative and peri-intubation risk
Resting tachycardia
Ventricular arrhythmias/prolongation of the QT-interval
Hypertension
Orthostatic hypotension
Flattening of the nocturnal reduction of blood pressure and heart rate ("non-dipper" phenomenon)
Exaggerated blood pressure responses with supine position and exercise
Abnormal diastolic/systolic left ventricular function
Poor exercise tolerance
Impaired cardiovascular responsiveness
Heat intolerance due to defective sympathetic thermoregulation
Susceptibility to foot ulcers and amputations due to arteriovenous shunting and sudomotor dysfunction
Hypoglycaemia unawareness (?)
Increased risk of severe hypoglycaemia
Obstructive sleep apnoea syndrome

baroreflex sensitivity that cardiovascular adaptation mechanisms in type 1 diabetic patients with long-term diabetes are severely impaired [36].

As an important new finding, a highly significant correlation between CAN and cardiovascular disease has been shown by the EURODIAB IDDM Complications Study [29]. Data indicate that silent myocardial ischaemia in diabetic patients may result either from CAN or from autonomic dysfunction due to coronary artery disease or both.

To sum up, in a more direct or indirect way, many factors may contribute to the poor prognosis of CAN in diabetic patients. Putative mechanisms are summarised in Table 16.1. Nevertheless, other causes and mechanisms not explained yet might be of importance as well. Going back to the question in the title of this chapter – *cardiac autonomic neuropathy represent a cardiovascular risk factor in type 2 diabetes.*

Diagnosis

Symptoms possibly reflecting autonomic neuropathy should not, by themselves be considered markers for its presence. Symptoms are important in the individual patients, however, they are difficult to evaluate and quantitative as they are often nonspecific [27]. Our better understanding on clinical and prognostic importance of CAN was closely related to the widespread use of simple non-invasive cardiovascular reflex tests. The most commonly used battery of non-invasive tests for assessment of cardiovascular reflexes was proposed by Ewing and Clarke [10] which includes heart rate variation in response to deep breathing, standing and Valsalva manoeuvre as well as blood pressure responses to standing and sustained handgrip. These five tests are validated, are reliable and reproducible, correlate with each other and with tests of peripheral somatic nerve function and are of prognostic value [2, 49]. These tests still form the core of diagnosis of CAN. Normal, borderline and abnormal values [10, 40] of the five standard cardiovascular reflex tests are summarised in Table 16.2. Heart

Table 16.2. Normal, borderline and abnormal values in tests of cardiovascular autonomic function

	Normal	Borderline	Abnormal
Tests reflecting mainly parasympathetic function			
Heart rate response to Valsalva Manoeuvre (Valsalva ratio)	>1.21	1.11–1.20	<1.10
Heart rate (R-R interval) variation during deep breathing (maximum–minimum heart rate)	>15 beats/min	11–14 beats/min	<10 beats/min
Immediate heart rate response to standing (30:15 ratio)	>1.04	1.01–1.03	<1.00
Tests reflecting mainly sympathetic function			
Blood pressure response to standing (fall in systolic blood pressure)	<10 mm Hg	11–29 mm Hg	>30 mm Hg
Blood pressure response to sustained handgrip (increase in diastolic blood pressure)	>16 mm Hg	11–15 mm Hg	<10 mm Hg

rate tests evaluating mainly parasympathetic function appear to be abnormal more frequently and earlier in cardiac autonomic involvement, whereas sympathetic damage assessed by blood pressure tests usually occur later and are more often associated with clinical symptoms.

Data of the EURODIAB IDDM Complications Study confirmed that cardiovascular reflex tests rather than a questionnaire should be used for the diagnosis of autonomic neuropathy [29] and indicate that the frequency of orthostatic hypotension is closely related to diagnostic criteria [55]. According to different diagnostic criteria of abnormal blood pressure response to standing (>30 mmHg, >20 mmHg, and >10 mmHg fall in systolic blood pressure), the frequency of abnormal results were 5,9%, 18% and 32%, respectively. The frequency of feeling faint on standing in the same study was 18%, thus, it was identical with the prevalence of abnormal blood pressure response to standing when >20 mmHg fall in systolic blood pressure was considered as abnormal [1]. These results may indicate that a fall >20 mmHg in systolic blood pressure after standing up seems to be the most reliable criterion for the assessment of orthostatic hypotension in the diagnosis of CAN.

Measurement of heart rate response to deep breathing may allow evaluating autonomic function in simple, quick and non-invasive ways in general practice.

According data of a recent meta-analysis, corrected QT – interval prolongation is a specific albeit insensitive indicator of autonomic failure [55]. Although QTc – prolongation is relatively accurate for men, accuracy may be even greater for young men at low QTc threshold [55]. QTc interval alone should not be used for the diagnosis of the severity of AN [26]. However, evaluation of QTc interval may provide a simple additional diagnostic aid to identify individuals with an increased cardiovascular risk [26]. Myocardial infarction is the prime cause of death among type 2 diabetic patients. The prognostic importance of QTc interval at discharge after myocardial infarction has been proved [1]. It should be noted that QT interval is influenced by many other factors including electrolyte abnormalities, myocardial ischemia and alcohol toxicity. QT interval measurement could be used as a screening test as well to select diabetic patients for more extensive cardiac investigation [39]. In the case of prolonged QTc interval, beside more extensive cardiac investigations even standard autonomic reflex tests are suggested being performed [28]. Assessment of QT dispersion just as circadian oscillations of QT interval represents a more comprehensive diagnostic approach [39, 35].

Assessments of HRV represent a more sophisticated method in the diagnosis of CAN. HRV is usually characterised in the time domain by simple statistical methods and in the frequency domain by spectral analysis [36, 35, 38]. Evaluation of baroreflex sensitivity provides a more focused measure of autonomic control [34, 36]. Scintigraphic assessment using ^{123}I-metaiodobenzylguanidine (^{123}I-MIBG) and single photon – emission computed tomography are more sensitive in detecting cardiovascular autonomic neuropathy than conventional autonomic function tests [38, 42]. Using ^{123}I-metaiodobenzylguanidine (^{123}I-MIBG) Schnell et al. has reported on evidence of cardiac sympathetic dysinnervation in newly diagnosed IDDM patients [42]. It should be noted, however, that autonomic nerve dysfunction could be shown by standard cardiovascular reflex tests among patients with newly diagnosed type 1 and type 2 diabetes just as in those with gestation diabetes [25].

It worth to mention another aspect as well: it seems to be controversial that according to the San Antonio Consensus Statement [2] autonomic neuropathy can be diagnosed if at least two of the five standard tests are abnormal. Thus, on the one hand abnormality of one standard test in a diabetic patient is judged to be normal, while on the other hand reduced ^{123}I-MIBG-uptake or decreased HRV in a patient with five normal tests should be considered as a sign of autonomic dysinnervation.

Autonomic Neuropathy and Glycaemic Control

The natural history of neuropathy is governed by the degree of glycaemic control. The unfavourable impact of long-term poor glycemic control on the development and progression of CAN is now generally accepted. In the light of evidence from prospective large-scale cohort studies including the DCCT and UKPDS, tight glycaemic control is clearly a priority in primary and secondary prevention of neuropathy. A close relationship between CAN and glycaemic control has been documented in the EURO-DIAB IDDM Complications Study as well [29]. Data suggest that intensive diabetes therapy resulting in long term HbA1c levels of approximately 7% prevents the onset and slows the progression of neuropathy in both Type 1 and Type 2 diabetic patients. Intensive insulin therapy reduced the risk for the development of clinical neuropathy by 64% within 5 years in Type 1 diabetics during the DCCT and it could be documented that intensive diabetes therapy was able to slow the progression and development of abnormal autonomic function tests as well [48]. Recently, the beneficial effect of tight glycaemic control on myocardial sympathetic innervation assessed by [^{123}I] metaiodobenzylguanidine scintigraphy was shown in a 4-year prospective study in patients with type 1 diabetes [61]. Unfortunately, near normoglycaemia is not achievable in a considerable number of patients.

Therapy of Cardiac Autonomic Neuropathy

Autonomic and sensory nerve dysfunction represent progressive forms of neuropathies and are therefore of utmost clinical and prognostic importance [53, 23]. With that in mind even a retarding effect on autonomic function may have particular importance. Is there a need for specific treatment for CAN? The answer is undoubtedly yes. On the one hand, CAN is associated with poor prognosis and carries a fivefold risk for mortality. On the other hand CAN evolve early in the course of diabetes even in the absence of other microvascular complications. Moreover, it is well known that the onset of Type 2 diabetes occurs at least 4–7 years before clinical diagnosis. As a consequence, neuropathy is a common complication even in patients with newly diagnosed Type 2 diabetes [58, 25]. Thus, its prevention in these patients is not more available.

Preferably, pathogenetically based therapeutical strategies are recommended. It should be noted that peripheral neural damage was the target of most studies on the field of neuropathy in diabetic patients. Experiences with aldose-reductase inhibitors in human individuals in general are disappointing [58], favourable effects has been observed using tolrestat [14]. Supplementation of the diet of diabetic subjects with gamma-linolenic acid failed to improve autonomic function [57].

Inhibition of advanced glycation endproducts formations proved to be more effective by thiamine pyrophosphate and pirydoxamin compared to aminoguanidin [7].

The lipidsolubile derivate benfotiamine is characterised by five times higher bioavailability compared to water-soluble compound [6] and was shown to be effective in the treatment of diabetic polyneuropathy [45]. Experiences from cardiology indicate the long-term increase in heart rate variability and reduction in sudden cardiac death has only been clearly shown with lipophilic agents that readily penetrate the blood nerve/blood brain barrier [3]. In accordance with these observations experimental data indicate a preventive effect of benfotiamine on the development of CAN [32].

Alpha-lipoic acid (thioctic acid), a powerful free radical scavenger improves nerve blood flow, reduces endoneurial hypoxia, lipid peroxidation and oxidative stress [40]. Improvement of insulin-stimulated glucose disposal was documented in patients with type 2 diabetes after administration of thioctic acid [19]. During treatment with alpha-lipoic acid beneficial effect on symptomatic peripheral neuropathy was observed [59] in the ALADIN Study (Alpha-Lipoic Acid in Diabetic Neuropathy), while improvement of cardiac autonomic function assessed by heart rate variability has been documented [60, 62] in the DEKAN (Deutsche Kardiale Autonome Neuropathie) Study. Results of the DEKAN Study can be assigned as one of the most important findings on the field of therapy of CAN. The anti-oxidant alpha-lipoic acid can be recommended by now as first choice drug for the treatment of cardiac autonomic neuropathy.

References

1. Ahnve S, Gilpin E, Madsen EB, Froelicher V, Henning H, Ross J (1984) Prognostic importance of QT_c interval at discharge after acute myocardial infarction: a multicenter study of 865 patients. Am Heart J 108: 395-400.
2. American Diabetes Association, American Academy of Neurology (1988) Consensusstatement. Report and recommendations of the San Antonio conference on diabetic neuropathy. Diabetes Care 11: 592-596.
3. Aronson D (1997) Pharmacologic modulation of autonomic tone: implications for the diabetic patient. Diabetologia 40: 476-481.
4. Beck MO, Silveiro SP, Friedman R, Clausell N, Gross JL (1999) Asymptomatic coronary artery disease is associated with cardiac autonomic neuropathy and diabetic nephropathy in type 2 diabetic patients. Diabetes Care, 22: 1745-1747.
5. Bigger JT, Fleiss JL, Rolnitzky LM, Steinman RC (1993) Frequency domain measures of heart period variability to assess risk late after myocardial infarction. JACC 21: 729-36.
6. Bitsch R, Wolf M, Möller J, Heuzeroth L, Grüneklee D (1991) Bioavailability assessment of the lipophilic benfotiamine as compared to a water-solubile thiamin derivate. Ann Nutr Metab 35: 292-296.
7. Booth AA, Khalifah RG, Hudson BG (1996) Thiamine pyrophosphate and pyridoxamine inhibit the formation of antigenic advanced glycation end-products: comparison with aminoguanidine. Biochem Biophys Res Commun 220: 113-119.
8. Boulton AJM (1997) ed. Diabetic neuropathy. Marius Press, Carnforth, UK, pp 41-61.
9. Eichorst H (1892) Beiträge zur Pathologie der Nerven und Muskeln. Archiv Pathol Anat Physiol Klin Med 127: 1-17
10. Ewing DJ, Clarke BF (1982) Diagnosis and management of diabetic autonomic neuropathy. BMJ 285: 916-8.
11. Ewing DJ, Campbell IW, Burt AA, Clarke BF (1973) Vascular reflexes in diabetic autonomic neuropathy. Lancet II: 1354-1356.
12. Ewing DJ, Marty CN, Young RJ, Clarke BF (1985) The value of cardiovascular autonomic function tests: 10 years experiences in diabetes. Diabetes Care 8: 491-498.
13. Gambardella S, Frontoni S, Spallone V, Maiello MR, Civetta E, Lanza G, Menzinger G (1993)

Increased left ventricular mass in normotensive diabetic patients with autonomic neuropathy. Am J Hypertens 6: 97–102.
14. Giugliano D, Marfella R Quatraro A, De Rosa N, Salvatore T, Cozzolino D, Ceriello A, Torella R (1993) Tolrestat for mild diabetic neuropathy. A 52-week, randomized, placebo-controlled trial. Ann Intern Med 118: 7–11.
15. Giugliano D, Ceriello A, Paolisso G (1996) Oxidative stress and diabetic vascular complications. Diabetes Care 19: 257–267.
16. Gottsäter A, Ahmed M, Fernlund P, Sundkvist G (1999) Autonomic neuropathy in Type 2 diabetic patients is associated with hyperinsulinaemia and hypertriglyceridaemia. Diabet Med 16: 49–54.
17. Greene DA, Stevens MJ (1995) Interaction of metabolic and vascular factors in the pathogenesis of diabetic neuropathy. In: Hotta N, Greene DA, Ward DJ, Sima AAF, Boulton AJM, eds. Diabetic neuropathy: New concepts and insights, Elsevier Science B.V. pp 37–41.
18. Hendrickse MT, Thuluvath PJ, Triger DR (1992) The natural history of autonomic neuropathy in chronic liver disease. Lancet 339: 1462–1464.
19. Jacob S, Henriksen EJ, Tritschler HJ, Augustin HJ, Dietze GJ (1996) Improvement of insulin-stimulated glucuse disposal in type 2 diabetes after repeated parenteral administration of thioctic acid. Exp Clin Endocrinol Diabetes 104: 284–288.
20. Jermendy Gy (1995) Sympathovagal balance and cardiovascular diseases in diabetic patients with autonomic neuropathy. Diab Nutr Metab 8: 123–124.
21. Jermendy Gy, Tóth L, Vörös P, Koltay MZ, Pogátsa G (1990) QT-interval in diabetic autonomic neuropathy. Diabet Med 7: 750.
22. Jermendy Gy, Ferenczy J, Hernandez E, Farkas K, Nádas J (1996) Day-night blood pressure variation in normotensive and hypertensive NIDDM patients with asymptomatic autonomic neuropathy. Diabetes Res Clin Pract 34: 107–114.
23. Kempler P (1997) ed. Neuropathies. Nerve dysfunction of diabetic and other origin. Springer Verlag, Budapest, Hungary
24. Kempler P, Váradi A, Szalay F (1992) Autonomic neuropathy and prolongation of QT-interval in liver disease. Lancet 340: 318.
25. Kempler P, Váradi A, Tamás Gy (1993) Autonomic neuropathy in newly diagnosed diabetes mellitus. Diabetes Care 16: 848–849.
26. Kempler P, Váradi A, Szalay F, Tamás Gy (1994) Autonomic neuropathy and corrected QT interval prolongation: there is a relationship. Diabetes Care 17: 454–456.
27. Kempler P, Hermányi Zs, Keresztes K, Marton A (1998) Klinische und prognostische Bedeutung der kardialen autonomen Neuropathie.In: Gries FA, Federlin K, eds. Benfotiamin in der Therapie von Polyneuropathien. Thieme Verlag, Stuttgart-New York, 39–44.
28. Kempler P, Keresztes K, Hermányi Zs, Marton A (1998) Studies must establish whether prolonged QTc interval in newly diagnosed type 1 diabetes is reversible. Br Med J 317: 678–679.
29. Kempler P, Tesfaye S, Chaturvedi N, Stevens LK, Ward JD, Fuller JH and the EURODIAB IDDM Study Group. (1998) Autonomic neuropathy and the cardiovascular risk: the EURODIAB IDDM Complications Study. Diabetologia 41 (Suppl 1): A51 (Abstract).
30. Kempler P, Tesfaye S, Stevens LK, Kerényi Zs, Tamás Gy, Ward JD, Fuller JH and the EURODIAB IDDM Study Group (1999) Blood pressure response to standing in the diagnosis of autonomic neuropathy: the EURODIAB IDDM Complications Study. Diabetologia 42 (Suppl 1): A297 (Abstract).
31. Kleiger RE, Miller JP, Bigger JT, Moss AJ and the Multicenter Post-Infarction Research Group (1987) Decreased heart rate variability and its association with increased mortality after acute myocardial infarction Am J Cardiol 59: 256–262.
32. Koltai MZ, Pósa I, Winkler G, Kocsis E, Pogátsa G (1997) The preventive effect of benfotiamine on the development of cardiac autonomic neuropathy in diabetic dogs. Hung Arch Int Med 50: 443–448.
33. Krahulec B, Strobová L, Balaľovjech I (1996) Hypertension is a prominent feature of diabetic autonomic neuropathy. a 10-year follow-up study. Diabetologia 39 (Suppl 1): 36 A (Abstract)
34. La Rovere MT, Bigger JT, Marcus FI, Mortara A, Schwartz PJ, for the ATRAMI Investigators (1998) Baroreflex sensitivity and heart-rate variability in prediction of total cardiac nortality after myocardial infarction. Lancet 351: 478–484.
35. Lengyel Cs, Thury A, Várkonyi T, Ungi I, Boda K, Fazekas T, Csanády M (1997) Disturbances

of heart rate variability and spatial and circadian QT intervals in diabetic patients with cardiac autonomic neuropathy. Hung Arch Int Med 50: 431–438.
36. Lengyel Cs, Török T, Várkonyi T, Kempler P, Rudas L (1998) Baroreflex sensitivity and heartrate variability in insulin-dependent diabetics with polyneuropathy. Lancet 351: 1436–1437.
37. Maser RE, Pfeifer MA, Dorman JS, Kuller RH, Becker DJ, Orchard TJ (1990) Diabetic autonomic neuropathy and cardiovascular risk. Arch Intern Med 150: 1218–1222.
38. Murata K, Sumida Y, Murashima S et al (1996) A novel method for the assessment of autonomic neuropathy in Type 2 diabetic patients: a comparative evaluation of ^{123}I-MIBG myocardial scintigraphy and power spectral analysis of heart rate variability. Diabetic Med 13: 266–272.
39. Naas AAO, Davidson NC, Thompson C, Cummings F, Ogston SA, Jung RT et al (1998) QT and QTc dispersion are accurate predictors of cardiac death in newly diagnosed non-insulin dependent: cohort study. BMJ 316: 745–746.
40. Nagamatsu M, Mickander KK, Schmelzer JD, Raya A, Wittrock DA, Tritschler H, Low PA (1995) Lipoc acid improves nerve blood flow, reduces oxidative stress, and improves distal nerve conduction in experimental diabetic neuropathy. Diabetes Care 18: 1160–1167.
41. Palatini P, Julius S (1997) Heart rate and the cardiovascular risk. J Hypertens 15: 13–17.
42. Schnell O, Muhr D, Dresel S, Tatsch K, Ziegler AG, Haslbeck M, Standl E (1996) Autoantibodies against sympathetic ganglia and evidence of cardiac sympathetic dysinnervation in newly diagnosed and long-term IDDM patients. Diabetologia 39: 970–975
43. Sima AAF, Sugimoto K (1999) Experimental diabetic neuropathy: an update. Diabetologia 42: 773-788.
44. Spallone V, Maiello MR, Cicconetti E, Menzinger G (1997) Autonomic neuropathy and cardiovascular risk factors in insulin-dependent and non-insulin-dependent diabetes. Diab Res Clin Pract 34: 169–179.
45. Stracke H, Lindemann A, Federlin K (1996) A benfotiamine-vitamin B combination in treatment of diabetic polyneuropathy. Exp Clin Endocrinol Diabetes 104: 311–316.
46. Szelag B, Wroblewski M, Castenfors J, Henricsson M, Berntorp K, Fernlund P, Sundkvist G (1999) Obesity, microalbuminuria, hyperinsulinemia and increased plasminogen activator inhibitor 1 activity associated with parasympathetic neuropathy in Type 2 diabetes Diabetes Care 22: 1907–1908.
47. Tesfaye S, Harris N, Jakubowski JJ, Mody C, Wilson RM, Rennie IG, Ward JD (1993) Impaired blood flow and arterio-venous shunting in human diabetic neuropathy: a novel technique of nerve photography and fluorescein angiography. Diabetologia 36: 1266–1274.
48. The Diabetes Control and Complications Trial Research Group (1998) The effect of intensive diabetes therapy on measures of autonomic nervous system function in the Diabetes Control and Complications Trial. Diabetologia 41: 416–423.
49. Valensi P, Attali JR, Gagant S and the French Group for Research and Study of Diabetes Neuropathy (1993) Reproducibility of parameters for assessment of diabetic neuropathy. Diabet Med 10: 933–939.
50. Valensi P, Paries J, Lormeau B, Assad N, Attali JR (1999) Cardiac parasympathetic changes: a new component of the insulin resistance syndrome. Diabetes 48: (Suppl 1) A149 (Abstract).
51. Vinik AI, Zola BE (1995) The effects of diabetic autonomic neuropathy on the cardiovascular system. In: Schwartz CJ, Born GVR, eds. New horizons in diabetes mellitus and cardiovascular disease. Current Science Ltd, London, UK, 159–171.
52. Ward JD. Diabetic neuropathy (1992) In: International textbook of Diabetes Mellitus. Eds: KGMM Alberti, RA DeFronzo, H Keen, P Zimmet. John Wiley and Sons Ltd. Chichester. 59: 1385–1414.
53. Watkins PJ (1992) Clinical observations and experiments in diabetic neuropathy. Diabetologia 35: 2–11.
54. Wheeler T, Watkins PJ (1973) Cardiac denervation in diabetes. Br Med J IV: 584–586.
55. Whitsel EA, Boyko EJ, Siscovick DS (2000) Reassessing the role of QTc in the dignosis of autonomic failure among patients with diabetes. Diabetes Care 23: 241–247.
56. Wieling W, Smit AAJ, Karemaker JM (1997) Diabetic autonomic neuropathy: conventional cardiovascular laboratory testing and new developments. Neuroscience Research Communications 21: 67–74.
57. Ziegler D, Mühlen H, Rathmann W, Gries FA (1993) Effects of one year's treatment with gamma-linolenic acid (EF4) on diabetic neuropathy. Diabetes 42 (Suppl 1): 99 A. (Abstract).

58. Ziegler D (1994) Diabetic cardiovascular autonomic neuropathy: Prognosis, diagnosis and treatment. Diabetes Metab Rev 10: 339–383.
59. Ziegler D, Hanefeld M, Ruhnau KJ, Meissner HP, Lobisch M, Schütte K, Gries FA. The ALADIN Study Group (1995) Treatment of symptomatic diabetic peripheral neuropathy with the antioxidant alpha-lipoic acid. A 3 week multicenter randomized controlled trial (ALADIN Study), Diabetologia 38: 1425–1433.
60. Ziegler D, Schatz H, Conrad F, Ulrich H, the DEKAN Study Group, Reichel G, Gries FA (1997) Effects of treatment with the antioxidant alpha-lipoic acid on cardiac autonomic neuropathy in NIDDM patients. Diabetes Care 20: 369–373.
61. Ziegler D, Weise F, Langen KJ, Piolot R, Boy C, Hübinger A, Müller-Gärtner HW, Gries FA (1998) Effect of glycaemic control on myocardial sympathetic innervation assessed by [^{123}I] metaiodobenzylguanidine scintigraphy: a 4-year prospective study in IDDM patients. Diabetologia 41: 443–451.
62. Ziegler D, Reljanovic M, Mehnert H, Gries FA (1999) Alpha-lipoc acid in the treatment of diabetic polyneuropathy in Germany: current evidence from clinical trials. Exp Clin Endocrinol Diabetes 107: 421–430.

CHAPTER 17

Thiazolidinediones in Cardiovascular Risk in Type 2 Diabetes Mellitus

M. Khamaisi, L. Symmer, I. Raz

Abstract. Type 2 diabetes mellitus is a growing problem across the world. There is now strong evidence that intensive controls of blood glucose can significantly reduce and retard the microvascular complications. Ultimately however, up to 80% of type 2 diabetics die from macrovascular cardiovascular disease. Insulin resistance, a major pathophysiologic abnormality in type 2 diabetes, is involved in the development of not only hyperglycemia, but also dyslipidemia, hypertension, hypercoagulation, vasculopathy, and ultimately atherosclerotic cardiovascular disease. Thiazolidinediones (Glitazones) are a new family of oral drugs that activate selectively peroxisome proliferator activated receptor γ and increased transcription of genes involved in lipid and glucose metabolism. These compounds, because of their insulin sensitizing action, are already used therapeutically in type 2 diabetes. Recent works suggested that Thiazolidinediones have potentially favorable effects on the diabetes associated proatherogenic metabolic abnormalities including decrease in blood pressure, correction of diabetic dyslipidemia, improvement of fibrinolysis, and decrease in carotid artery intima-media thickness.

In this chapter we summarize the current knowledge about Thiazolidinediones, the intracellular mechanism of action and discuss their potential role in the treatment of diabetes associated micro and macrovascular diseases.

Introduction and Mechanism of Action

Type 2 diabetes mellitus is a chronic disease characterized by hyperglycemia and numerous other metabolic abnormalities and late complications. Of all the long-term complications, cardiovascular disease has been found one of the most serious outcomes in terms of morbidity and mortality.

There are three major pathophysiologic abnormalities associated with type 2 diabetes: impaired insulin secretion, excessive hepatic glucose output, and insulin resistance in skeletal muscle, liver, and adipose tissue. The oral pharmacologic agents available for the treatment of type 2 diabetes act primarily by increasing insulin availability (Sulfonylureas and Meglitinides); delaying gastrointestinal glucose absorption (α-glucosidase inhibitors); suppressing excessive hepatic glucose output (Metformin); and reducing insulin resistance at target tissues, mainly skeletal muscle, adipose tissue, and liver (Thiazolidinediones).

The Thiazolidinediones (also known as glitazones) are a new class of compounds that are chemically and functionally unrelated to the other classes of oral antidiabetic agents. These agents have a thiazolidine-2–4 dione structure (Fig. 17.1), but they differ in their side chains, which alter their pharmacologic and side-effect profile. The efficacy of these drugs in decreasing plasma glucose levels through direct insulin sen-

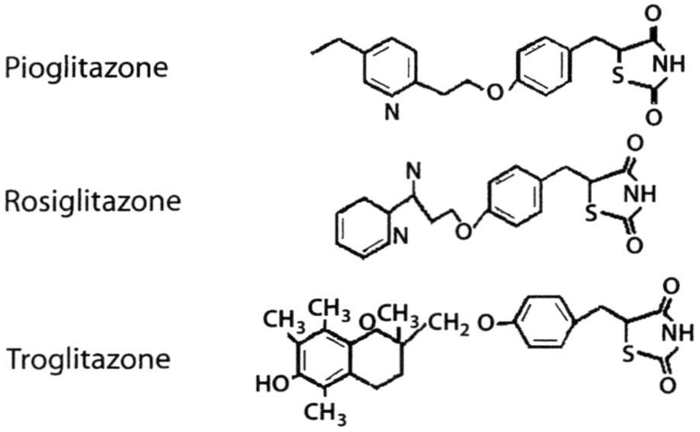

Pioglitazone

Rosiglitazone

Troglitazone

Fig. 17.1. The structure of thiazolidinedione agents. (Reprinted from Mudaliar 2001)

sitizing actions is well established (Parulkar et al. 2001). Troglitazone (Rezulin), the first drug of this new class became available for clinical use in 1997. In March 2000 Troglitazone was withdrawn when the Food and Drug Administration received reports of 61 deaths from hepatic failure and seven liver transplants associated with the drug. In contrast, the more novel thiazolidinediones, Rosiglitazone (Avandia) and Pioglitazone (Actos), became available in 1999 and are approved as monotherapy and in combination with other hypoglycemic agents; Pioglitazone is also approved in combination with insulin. Despite the extensive use of these drugs during the last years, some evidence of hepatic impairment was described.

The mechanism of action of the Thiazolidinediones at the cellular level has not been fully elucidated. However, a variety of experimental data suggested that the Thiazolidinediones stimulate transcriptional events by activating a specific nuclear receptor, the peroxisome proliferator-activated receptor gamma (PPARγ), which has a regulatory role in differentiation of cells, particularly adipocytes (Campbell 2000). Peroxisome proliferator activated receptors (PPARs) are ligand-dependent transcription factors of the nuclear hormone receptor superfamily, that are activated by fatty acids and their eicosanoid metabolites. The three known PPAR subtypes, -α, -β and -γ, show distinct tissue distributions and can be activated by selective ligands (Mudaliar and Henry 2001; Campbell 2000). PPARα is highly expressed in liver, kidney, heart and muscle, and regulates the production of enzymes involved in the β-oxidation of fatty acids and lipoprotein metabolism. PPARγ receptors are found in key target tissues for insulin action, such as adipose tissue, skeletal muscle, and liver, and evidence indicates that these receptors are important regulators of adipocyte differentiation, lipid homeostasis and insulin action. Fibrates, weak agonists of PPARγ, are used to treat hypertriglyceridemia, and thiazolidinediones (TZDs), which are potent and selective synthetic PPARγ agonists, are used to treat type 2 diabetes. There is a close relationship between the potency of various Thiazolidinediones to stimulate PPARγ and their antidiabetic action. PPARβ is ubiquitously expressed and its biological roles are less established than PPARα and -γ but recent studies suggest roles in the development of colon cancer ligands (Mudaliar and Henry 2001; Parulkar et al. 2001).

The lipophilic Thiazolidinediones readily enter the cells and bind to PPARγ, which results in activation of regulatory sequences of DNA that control the expression of

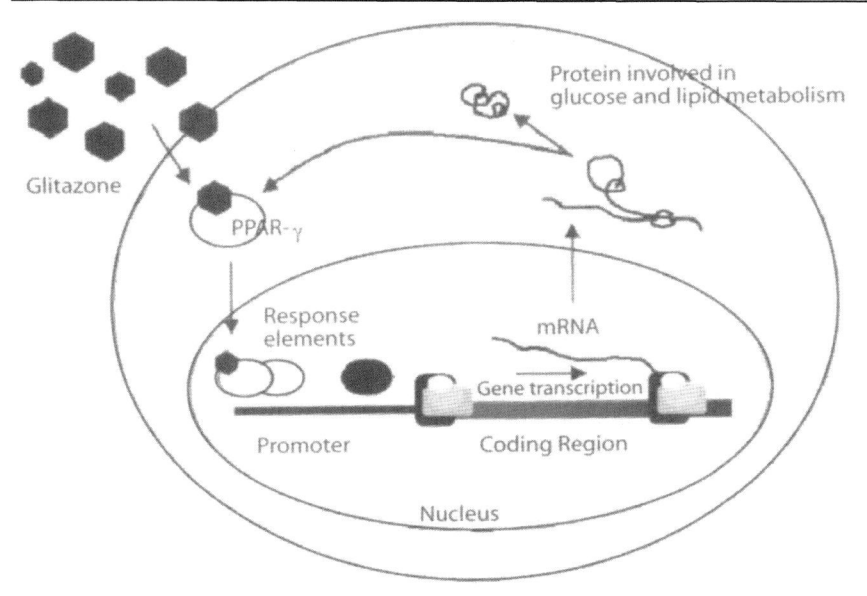

Fig. 17.2. Glitazone activation of the nuclear receptor PPARγ. (Reprinted from Mudaliar 2001)

specific genes, some of which are also controlled by insulin (Fig. 17.2) (Mudaliar and Henry 2001). In freshly isolated human adipocytes, Rosiglitazone increased p85-phosphatidylinositol 3-kinase (p85-a PI3K) and decreased leptin expression. P85-a PI3K is a major component of insulin action and the induction of its expression might explain, at least in part, the insulin-sensitizing effect of the Thiazolidinediones. In animal studies, glitazones have been shown to stimulate GLUT 1 and GLUT 4 (glucose transporters) gene expression and hepatic glucokinase expression through activation of PPARγ.

The Effect of Thiazolidinediones on Cardiovascular Complications and Cardiac Function

Before the introduction of Troglitazone in 1997, Metformin was the only drug able to sensitize target tissues to insulin. In the United Kingdom Prospective Diabetes Study (UKPDS), treatment with Metformin was shown to produce greater reduction in cardiovascular disease events and mortality compared to Sulphonylureas and Insulin treatment (UKPDS 34). Moreover, intensive treatment of type 2 diabetes with Sulphonylureas or Insulin significantly reduced microvascular complications, but did not have a significant effect on macrovascular complications after 10 years (UKPDS 33). The influence of treatments on macrovascular disease is particularly important: although 9% of patients with type 2 disease develop a microvascular complication within 9 years of diagnosis, 20% have a macrovascular complication. Furthermore, macrovascular disease is 70-fold more likely to result in death, than a microvascular complication in these patients.

The effect of Thiazolidinediones on cardiac function was evaluated in animals and human studies. In vivo, Shimoyama et al. investigated the direct cardiac hemodynamic effects of Troglitazone in isolated perfused rat hearts. Troglitazone administration (0.2, 0.5, and 1.0 micromol) has direct positive inotropic, positive lusitropic, negative chronotropic, and coronary artery dilating effects. The inotropic and chronotropic actions of Troglitazone were not mediated via adrenergic receptors or calcium channels (Shimoyama et al. 1999). In Streptozotocin (STZ)-induced diabetic rats and age-matched controls animals, Troglitazone treatment (0.2% food admixture for 6 weeks) partially restored the basal heart rate and cardiac work of diabetic rats to nearly control values. In addition, Troglitazone improved the postischemic functional deficits of diabetic rats: heart rate, left ventricular (LV) developed pressure, and cardiac work. Diabetic animals showed ultrastructural damage including disarray of sarcomere, disorganization of mitochondrial matrix, cytoplasmic vacuolization, and invagination of nuclear membrane; these were partially protected by Troglitazone treatment (Shimabukuro et al. 1996). Similarly, Rosiglitazone treatment protects against cardiac tissue following ischemic events or ischemia/reperfusion-induced cardiac damage through reduction in the accumulation of neutrophils and macrophages in cardiac tissue and inhibition of JNK/AP-1 pathway (Yue et al. 2001; Khandoudi et al. 2001).

A clinical study by Ghazzi and his colleagues demonstrated that treatment with 800 mg/day Troglitazone for 48 weeks changed significantly left ventricular mass index (Ghazzi et al. 1997). There was a substantial increase in stroke volume index and cardiac index and a statistically significant decrease in diastolic pressure and estimated peripheral resistance in Troglitazone-treated patients. Similarly no adverse effect on cardiac mass or function was observed in the Rosiglitazone and Pioglitazone treated patients. Nevertheless, Thiazolidinediones are currently not recommended in patients with advanced heart failure because of their tendency to significantly expand the plasma volume.

The Effect of Thiazolidinediones on Cardiovascular Risk Factors

Improvement in lipid profile appears to be a class effect of Thiazolidinediones, however, there are some subtle differences in the effects on individual lipid parameters. Studies using high dosages of Troglitazone demonstrated significant reduction in serum triglyceride and non-esterified fatty acid levels (Day 1999). Marked reductions in serum triglyceride levels have been observed with all dosages of Pioglitazone (15–45 mg/day), whereas changes in serum triglyceride levels during Rosiglitazone therapy were variable and not significantly different from placebo. Dose-dependent reductions in free fatty acid levels have been observed with Rosiglitazone treatment (Goldstein and Salzman 1999). Serum HDL cholesterol levels are significantly increased with Pioglitazone within the first 24 weeks of treatment, but are only slightly increased during Rosiglitazone therapy. Pioglitazone shows no significant changes in serum LDL cholesterol and total cholesterol levels over placebo, whereas Rosiglitazone is associated with significant increase in serum LDL cholesterol and total cholesterol levels compared with placebo (Campbell 2000).

Insulin resistance is associated with a predominance of small, atherogenic LDL particles (sLDL-C). SLDL-C increases the risk of coronary artery disease 3.6-fold and is present in 50% of males with coronary artery disease. Diabetic patients that received 4 mg Rosiglitazone or 15 mg Pioglitazone daily for 10 weeks show a significant reduction in sLDL-C accompanied by increased levels of the less atherogenic intermediate and large LDL-C. There is also a significant increase in the atheroprotective large HDL-C subfraction (Thomas and Taylor 2001).

Oxidation of the LDL cholesterol particles confers their atherogenic properties, and individuals with insulin resistance and/or type 2 diabetes are more likely to have small, dense, triglyceride-rich LDL cholesterol particles, than nondiabetic persons. These characteristics may make LDL cholesterol susceptible to oxidation (Suter et al. 1992; Brown 1996). In a randomized double-blined study, Tack shows that Troglitazone treatment (400 mg/day) for 8 weeks decreases the proportion of small to dense LDL and increases the resistance of LDL to oxidation in obese subjects (Tack et al. 1998). This should be explained by the fact that oxidized LDL cholesterol regulates macrophage and foam-cell gene expression through activation of PPARγ (Yamasaki et al. 1997; Nagy et al. 1998; Tontonoz et al. 1998). Atherosclerosis is a macrovascular pathology hallmarked by cholesterol accumulation in macrophages, resulting in their transformation into foam cells. Recent data provide conclusive evidence that Troglitazone does not promote foam-cell formation, but stimulates pathways of cholesterol efflux (Staels 2001).

The overall effect of long term treatment with Thiazolidinediones on lipid metabolism and its impact on the related cardiovascular risk needs to be further investigated.

The Effect of Thiazolidinediones on Vascular and Endothelial Function

In healthy individuals, Insulin has a dilatory effect on the arterioles that supply skeletal muscle (Steinberg et al. 1994). In obese individuals with insulin resistance and patients with type 2 diabetes, this vasodilatory action of insulin may be decreased and it is possible that by enhancing insulin action, the Thiazolidinediones may enhance the tonic vasodilator response to insulin and thereby reduce peripheral vascular resistance (Steinberg et al. 1996). This defect is important in the pathogenesis of cardiovascular disease in type 2 diabetics.

An in vitro study in cultured endothelial cells treated daily with 10^{-8} M Troglitazone or Pioglitazone for 5 days showed a significant elevation in the secretion of C-type natriuretic peptide, a novel endothelium-derived relaxing peptide, and suppressed the secretion of endothelin, a powerful vasoconstrictor peptide (Fukunaga et al. 2001).

Vascular reactivity or flow-mediated dilatation in response to stimuli, including ischemia, was assessed by a noninvasive brachial artery vasoactivity method (Lehmann et al. 1997). Since endothelial injury is an early event in atherogenesis, it has been suggested that abnormal flow-mediated dilatation precedes development of structural changes in the vessel wall. Diabetes mellitus, smoking, hypercholesterolemia and other factors, predisposing atherosclerosis, were associated with impaired flow-mediated dilatation in young adults. Avena and his colleagues demonstrated that treatment with Troglitazone (400 mg/day) for 2 or 4 months normalize the impaired brachial artery vasoactivity in persons with peripheral vascular disease

(Avena et al. 1998). In contrast, Troglitazone administration to obese persons with insulin resistance had no effect on endothelin-dependent or endothelin independent vascular response, despite improved insulin sensitivity (Tack et al. 1998). Endothelium-dependent response to acetylcholine in the coronary arteries has been studied in a small number of diabetic patients with vasospastic angina. The vasodilatory response improved substantially and anginal episodes decreased after therapy with Troglitazone (Murakami et al. 1999).

The Effect of Thiazolidinediones on the Vascular Wall

The expression of PPARγ is well established in human endothelial cells (EC) (Marx et al. 1999), vascular smooth muscle cells (VSMC) (Marx et al. 1998), monocytes and macrophages (Marx et al. 1998), and human arterial lesions (Ricote et al. 1998), all of which play important pathogenic roles in atherosclerosis. Proliferation and migration of VSMC in response to arterial injury are important in atheromatous plaque formation and restenosis after PTCA. In vitro studies have demonstrated that Troglitazone, Rosiglitazone, Pioglitazone, and prostaglandin J2 (the endogenous ligand of PPARγ) inhibit vascular smooth-muscle cell proliferation and migration, and thus can limit restenosis and atherosclerosis(Marx et al. 1998; Law et al. 2000; Law et al. 1996). Also, both Troglitazone and Pioglitazone inhibit vasopressin and platelet-derived growth factor (PDGF) induced Ca^{+2} entry and proliferation in rat VSMC (Law et al. 2000; Law et al. 1996). In vivo, Law and his colleagues demonstrated that Troglitazone treatment attenuates neointimal thickening after balloon injury to the aorta (Law et al. 2000). In type 2 patients, using intravascular ultrasound Takagi showed that Troglitazone treatment significantly reduced intimal hyperplasia in patients who underwent coronary stenting (Takagi et al. 2000).

The finding that increased intima-media complex thickness of carotid artery correlates with a higher rate of cardiovascular events was used as a surrogate marker of atherosclerosis (Lehmann et al. 1997; O'Leary et al. 1999). Significant decrease in the intima-media complex thickness was demonstrated after as early as 3 months of Troglitazone treatment and was maintained over 6 months (O'Leary et al. 1999). There was no correlation between the thickness of intima-media complex and glycosylated hemoglobin or postprandial triglycerides, suggesting that this effect of Thiazolidinediones may be due to direct cellular effect on the atherosclerosis and probably is not linked to the insulin resistance.

The current concept of acute coronary events includes disruption of the fibrous cap or plaque rupture, that exposes the highly thrombogenic lipid core present in most arterial atherosclerotic lesions, to the coagulation factors present in the circulation, thereby precipitating most acute myocardial events (Lee and Libby 1997; Jiang et al. 1998). Monocyte-derived macrophages and VSMC are sources of highly regulated matrix metalloproteinases that can degrade collagen and other matrix proteins and so contribute to this process. Troglitazone was shown to inhibit the expression and activity of matrix metalloproteinase-9 in human monocyte derived macrophages and human VSMC (Marx et al. 1998).

Thiazolidinedione Effects on Peripheral Vascular Resistance and Blood Pressure

Patients with type 2 diabetes are about twice as likely to have hypertension than non diabetics (Rosenstock and Raskin 1988; Simonson 1988). As mentioned above, insulin resistance is etiologically related to hypertension, so Thiazolidinediones, through their capability to decrease insulin resistance, may also decrease blood pressure. This theoretical suggestion was observed in patients with type 2 diabetes and hypertension (Sung et al. 1999) and in obese non diabetics (Ogihara et al. 1995; Nolan et al. 1994). Sung et al described that Troglitazone treatment for 6 months, attenuates the stress induced increase in blood pressure and decreases significantly peripheral vascular resistance (Sung et al. 1999). A significant correlation was found between decrease mean blood pressure and reduction in plasma insulin level (Ogihara et al. 1995). Additionally, by reducing hyperinsulinemia and plasma insulin levels, these agents may reduce the potential blood pressure raising actions of insulin, such as renal sodium retention and increased symphatetic activity. These findings are consistent with the hypothesis that Troglitazone decreases blood pressure by improving insulin resistance. Other potential mechanisms for the hypotensive effects of these drugs include improved endothelium dependent vasodilatation, decrease in calcium influx and calcium sensitivity of the contractile apparatus, and inhibition of the expression and secretion of endothelin-1, a potent vasoconstrictor, in bovine vascular endothelial cells through activation of PPARγ. Limited data suggest that the Glitazones may have a beneficial effect on blood pressure. Early studies show that Troglitazone treatment (800 mg/day) over 48 weeks significantly reduced diastolic blood pressure by 6.5 mm Hg (8%). Rosiglitazone treatment (4 mg twice a day) over 52 weeks has also been associated with a significant decrease in systolic blood pressure (3.5 mm Hg) and diastolic blood pressure (2.7 mm Hg) (Bakris et al. 2000).

Thiazolidinedione Effect on the Thrombotic/Fibrinolytic Systems

Plasminogen activator inhibitor type 1 (PAI-1) is an endogenous inhibitor of fibrinolysis. An elevated plasma level of PAI-1 associated with cardiovascular disease (Davidson 1995), and usually elevated in diabetics and obese non diabetics with insulin resistance. Impaired fibrinolytic function is a risk factor for myocardial infarction in both diabetics and nondiabetics patients (Jokl and Colwell 1997) and it correlate with the severity of vascular disease in diabetic patients. An increased PAI-1 level is now recognized as an integral part of the insulin resistance syndrome and correlates significantly with plasma insulin and triglyceride levels. Insulin infusion during and after infarction, which is known to improve outcomes, has been shown to decrease plasma PAI-1 levels (Melidonis et al. 2000). Randomized clinical studies show that Troglitazone treatment (400 mg/day) for 12 or 26 weeks decreased significantly plasma level of PAI-1 in individuals with various insulin resistance conditions (including even the polycystic ovary syndrome), probably directly through decreasing synthesis in the vessel wall (Fonseca et al. 1998; Ehrmann et al. 1997). Rosiglitazone has a similar effect on PAI-1, and therefore PAI-1 reduction may be a class effect of insulin sensitizers.

Platelet aggregation is also increased in diabetic subjects. Troglitazone treatment (0.1-1 µmol/l for 6 min) has been shown to have potent inhibitory effects on human platelet aggregation via suppression of thrombin-induced activation of phosphoinositide signaling in platelets (Ishizuka et al. 1998). Clinical trials that are now in progress will hopefully address the question, whether these changes in the thrombotic /anti thrombotic systems will have clinical benefits in preventing cardiovascular events.

Roles of PPARγ in the Development of Inflammation and Atherosclerosis: Antiatherogenic Effect of Thiazolidinediones

Although most studies on PPARγ have focused on the understanding of how PPARγ regulates glucose and lipid metabolism, research reports over the past few years suggest that this receptor might play several additional roles in inflammation and atherosclerosis. PPARγ have been found to be expressed in cells of the arterial wall, with PPARγ being highly expressed in macrophages foam cells within atherosclerotic lesions. PPARγ modifies transcription factors, such as nuclear factor κB, and inhibits activation of many proinflammatory genes such as tumor necrosis factor α, interleukin 1β, and interleukin 6 that are responsible for plaque development and maturation (Jiang et al. 1998). These observations have led to investigations into the effects of synthetic agonists in these cells. Thiazolidinediones have been shown to inhibit the expression of tumor necrosis factor α (TNF-α), gelatinase B, scavenger receptor A (SR-A) and inflammatory mediators, suggesting that they might inhibit inflammatory component of atherosclerosis. In addition, PPARγ agonists inhibit expression of the chemokine monocyte chemoattractant protein 1 and inflammatory enzymes such as inducible nitric oxide synthase (Ricote et al. 1998; Murao et al. 1999), and reduce the production of metalloproteinases by activated plaque macrophages, thus promoting plaque stability (Marx et al. 1998). Crucially, PPARγ agonists (100 µmol/l Troglitazone) also reduce expression of vascular cell adhesion molecules (VCAM-1), and intracellular adhesion molecule (ICAM-1) in cultured endothelial cells, thereby reducing macrophage homing to plaques in vivo (Pasceri et al. 2000).

Direct evidence for an antiatherogenic role of PPARγ was recently provided by a series of recent articles using two different animal models of atherogenesis. Li et al. demonstrated that synthetic PPARγ ligand Rosiglitazone exert potent antiatherogenic effects in LDL-receptor deficient (LDLR-/-) male mice fed a high fat and high cholesterol diet (Li et al. 2000). This effect was striking and revealed a reduction in both number and size of lesions. More recently, Collins has shown in the same model that Troglitazone treatment (4 g/kg for 12 weeks) inhibited lesion formation and decreased the accumulation of macrophages in intimal xanthomas (Collins et al. 2001). Furthermore, these results have been confirmed using apolipoprotein E knockout mice as a model of atherosclerosis (Chen et al. 2001). A 7-day Troglitazone treatment (400 mg/kg) significantly reduced monocyte/macrophage homing to atherosclerosis plaques in apoE-deficient mice (Pasceri et al. 2000).

Conclusions

The Thiazolidinediones are a unique new class of oral antidiabetic agents that exert direct effects on the mechanisms of insulin resistance, which is a major pathophysiologic abnormality in type 2 diabetes. In human subjects with diabetes, who have a high risk for coronary disease, Thiazolidinediones improve insulin resistance and other various components of the insulin resistance syndrome, and therapy with these drugs may therefore reduce the risk for cardiovascular disease. The potential beneficial non hypoglycemic effects of the Thiazolidinediones include decrease in plasma insulin and triglyceride levels, an increase in HDL cholesterol level, decreased lipid oxidation, favorable redistribution of body fat, a decrease in vascular resistance, and improvement in endothelial function. However, these drugs increase low-density lipoprotein cholesterol levels, tend to cause weight gain, decrease hematocrit, cause edema, and rarely liver failure.

Long-term clinical studies are needed to determine whether these drugs can prevent or delay cardiovascular disease, morbidity, and mortality in type 2 diabetic patients.

References

Avena R, Mitchell ME, Nylen ES, Curry KM, Sidawy AN (1998) Insulin action enhancement normalises brachial artery vasoactivity in patients with peripheral vascular disease and occult diabetes. J Vasc Surg 28:1024–1031
Bakris GL, Dole JF, Porter LE (2000) Rosiglitazone improves blood pressure in patients with type 2 diabetes. Diabetes 4: Abstract 388-P
Brown V (1996) Detection and management of lipid disorders in diabetes. Diabetes Care (Suppl 1): S96-S102
Campbell IW (2000) Antidiabetic drugs present and future: will improving insulin resistance benefit cardiovascular risk in type 2 diabetes mellitus? Drugs 60:1017–1028
Chen Z, Ishibashi S, Perrey S, Osuga Ji, Gotoda T, Kitamine T, Tamura Y, Okazaki H, Yahagi N, Iizuka Y, Shionoiri F, Ohashi K, Harada K, Shimano H, Nagai R, Yamada N (2001) Troglitazone inhibits atherosclerosis in apolipoprotein E-knockout mice: pleiotropic effects on CD36 expression and HDL. Arterioscler Thromb Vasc Biol 21:372–377
Collins AR, Meehan WP, Kintscher U, Jackson S, Wakino S, Noh G, Palinski W, Hsueh WA, Law RE (2001) Troglitazone inhibits formation of early atherosclerotic lesions in diabetic and nondiabetic low density lipoprotein receptor-deficient mice. Arterioscler Thromb Vasc Biol 21:365–371
Davidson MB (1995) Clinical implications of insulin resistance syndromes. Am J Med 99:420–426
Day C (1999) Thiazolidinediones: a new class of antidiabetic drugs. Diabet Med 16: 1–14
Ehrmann DA, Schneider DJ, Sobel BE, Cavaghan MK, Imperial J, Rosenfield RL, Polonsky KS (1997) Troglitazone improves defects in insulin action, insulin secretion, ovarian steroidogenesis, and fibrinolysis in women with polycystic ovary syndrome. J Clin Endocrinol Metab 82:2108–2116
Fonseca VA, Reynolds T, Hemphill D, Randolph C, Wall J, Valiquet TR, Graveline J, Fink LM (1998) Effect of Troglitazone on fibrinolysis and activated coagulation in patients with non-insulin-dependent diabetes mellitus. J Diabetes Complications 12:181–186
Fukunaga Y, Itoh H, Doi K, Tanaka T, Yamashita J, Chun TH, Inoue M, Masatsugu K, Sawada N, Saito T, Hosoda K, Kook H, Ueda M, Nakao K (2001) Thiazolidinediones, peroxisome proliferator-activated receptor gamma agonists, regulate endothelial cell growth and secretion of vasoactive peptides. Atherosclerosis 158:113–119
Ghazzi MN, Perez JE, Antonucci TK, Driscoll JH, Huang SM, Faja BW, Whitcomb RW (1997) Car-

diac and glycemic benefits of Troglitazone treatment in NIDDM. The Troglitazone Study Group. Diabetes 46: 433–439

Goldstein B, Salzman A (1999) Rosiglitazone is effective in poorly controlled type 2 diabetes patients. Diabetologia 42:229

Ishizuka T, Itaya S, Wada H, Ishizawa M, Kimura M, Kajita K, Kanoh Y, Miura A, Muto N, Yasuda K (1998) Differential effect of the antidiabetic thiazolidinediones troglitazone and pioglitazone on human platelet aggregation mechanism. Diabetes 47:1494–1500

Jiang C, Ting AT, Seed B (1998) PPAR-γ agonists inhibit production of monocyte inflammatory cytokines. Nature 391:82–86

Jokl R, Colwell JA (1997) Arterial thrombosis and atherosxlerosis in diabetes. Diabetes Reviews 5: 316

Khandoudi N, Delerive P, Berrebi-Bertrand I, Buckingham R, Staels B, Bril A (2001) Rosiglitazone protects the diabetic heart from ischmia-reperfusion injury by inhibiting the JNK/AP-1 pathway. Diabetes 50: Abstract 478-P

Law RE, Goetze S, Xi XP, Jackson R, Kawano Y, Demer L, Fishbein MC, Meehan WP, Hsueh WA (2000) Expression and function of PPARγ in rat and human vascular smooth muscle cells. Circulation 101:1311–1318

Law RE, Meehan WP, Xi XP, Graf K, Wuthrich DA, Coats W, Faxon D, Hsueh WA (1996) Troglitazone inhibits vascular smooth muscle cell growth and intimal hyperplasia. J Clin Invest 98:1897–1905

Lee RT, Libby P (1997) The unstable atheroma. Arterioscler Thromb Vasc Biol 17:1859–1867

Lehmann ED, Riley WA, Clarkson P, Gosling RG (1997) Non-invasive assessment of cardiovascular disease in diabetes mellitus. Lancet 350: SI14–119

Li AC, Brown KK, Silvestre MJ, Willson TM, Palinski W, Glass CK (2000) Peroxisome proliferator-activated receptor gamma ligands inhibit development of atherosclerosis in LDL receptor-deficient mice. J Clin Invest 106:523–531

Marx N, Bourcier T, Libby P, Plutzky J (1999) PPARγ activation in human endothelial cells increases plasminogen activator inhibitor type-1 expression: PPARγ as a potential mediator in vascular disease. Arterioscler Thromb Vasc Biol 19:546–551

Marx N, Schönbeck U, Lazar MA, Libby P, Plutzky J (1998) Peroxisome proliferator- activated receptor γ activators inhibit gene expression and migration in human vascular smooth muscle cells Circ Res 83:1097–1103

Marx N, Sukhova G, Murphy C, Libby P, Plutzky J (1998) Macrophages in human atheroma contain PPAR-γ differentiation dependent peroxisomal proliferator-activated receptor γ expression and reduction of MMP-9 activity through PPAR-γ. activation in mononuclear phagocytes in vitro. Am J Pathol 153: 17–23

Melidonis A, Stefanidis A, Tournis S, Manoussakis S, Handanis S, Zairis M, Dadiotis L, Foussas S (2000) The role of strict metabolic control by insulin infusion on fibrinolytic profile during an acute coronary event in diabetic patients. Clin Cardiol 23:160–164

Mudaliar S, Henry RR (2001) New oral therapies for type 2 diabetes mellitus: The glitazones or insulin sensitizers. Annu Rev Med 52:239–257

Murakami T, Mizuno S, Ohsato K, Moriuchi I, Arai Y, Nio Y, Kaku B, Takahashi Y, Ohnaka M (1999) Effects of troglitazone on frequency of coronary vasospastic-induced angina pectoris in patients with diabetes mellitus. Am J Cardiol 84: 92–94

Murao K, lmachi H, Momoi A, Sayo Y, Hosokawa H, Sato M, Ishida T, Takahara J (1999) Thiazolidinedione inhibits the production of monocyte chemoattractant protein-1 in cytokine treated human vascular endothelial cells. FEBS Lett 454:27–30

Nagy L, Tontonoz P, Alvarez JG, Chen H, Evans RM (1998) Oxidized LDL regulates macrophage gene expression through ligand activation of PPAR-γ. Cell 93:229–240

Nolan JJ, Ludvik B, Beerdsen P, Joyce M, Olefsky JM (1994) Improvement in glucose tolerance and insulin resistance in obese subjects treated with Troglitazone. N Engl J Med 331:1188–1193

Ogihara T, Rakugi H, Ikegami H, Mikami H, Masuo K (1995) Enhancement of insulin sensitivity by Troglitazone lowers blood pressure in diabetic hypertensives. Am J Hypertens 8:316–320

O'Leary DH, Polak JF, Kronmal RA, Manolio TA, Burke GL, Wolfson SK Jr (1999) Carotid-artery intima and media thickness as a risk factor for myocardial infarction and stroke in older adults. Cardiovascular Health Study Collaborative Research Group. N Engl J Med 340:14–22

Parulkar AA, Pendergrass ML, Granda-Ayala R, Lee TR, Fonseca VA (2001) Nonhypoglycemic Effects of Thiazolidinediones. Ann Intern Med 134: 61–71

Pasceri V, Wu H, Willerson JT, Yeh ET (2000) Modulation of vascular inflammation in vitro and in vivo by peroxisome proliferator-activated receptor- γ activators. Circulation 101:235–238

Ricote M, Huang J, Fajas L, Li A, Welch J, Najib J, Witztum JL, Auwerx J, Palinski W, Glass CK (1998) Expression of the peroxisome proliferator-activated receptor g (PPARγ) in human atherosclerosis and regulation in macrophages by colony stimulating factors and oxidized low density lipoprotein. Proc Natl Acad Sci U S A 95:7614–7619

Ricote M, Li AC, Willson TM, Kelly CJ, Glass CK (1998) The peroxisome proliferator-activated receptor-gamma is a negative regulator of macrophage activation. Nature 391:79–82

Rosenstock J, Raskin P (1988) Hypertension in diabetes mellitus. Cardiol Clin 6:547–560

Shimabukuro M, Higa S, Shinzato T, Nagamine F, Komiya I, Takasu N (1996) Cardioprotective effects of troglitazone in streptozotocin-induced diabetic rats. Metabolism 45:1168–1173

Shimoyama M, Ogino K, Tanaka Y, Ikeda T, Hisatome I (1999) Hemodynamic basis for the acute cardiac effects of troglitazone in isolated perfused rat hearts. Diabetes 48:609–615

Simonson DC (1988) Etiology and prevalence of hypertension in diabetic patients. Diabetes Care 11:821–827

Staels B (2001) New roles for PPARs in cholesterol homeostasis. TRENDS in Pharmacological Sciences 22:444

Steinberg HO, Brechtel G, Johnson A, Fineberg N, Baron AD (1994) Insulin mediated skeletal muscle vasodilatation is nitric oxide dependent. A novel action of insulin to increase nitric oxide release. J Clin Invest. 94:1172–1179

Steinberg HO, Chaker H, Leaming R, Johnson A, Brechtel G, Baron AD (1996) Obesity/insulin resistance is associated with endothelial dysfunction. Implications for the syndrome of insulin resistance. J Clin Invest 97:2601–2610

Sung BH, Izzo JL Jr, Dandona P, Wilson MF (1999) Vasodilatory effects of Troglitazone improve blood pressure at rest during mental stress in type 2 diabetes mellitus. Hypertension 34:83–88

Suter SL, Nolan JJ, Wallace P, Gumbiner B, Olefsky JM (1992) Metabolic effects of new oral hypoglycemic agent CS-045 in NIDDM subjects. Diabetes Care 15:193–203

Tack CJ, Demacker PN, Smits P, Stalenhoef AF (1998) Troglitazone decreases the proportion of small, dense LDL and increases the resistance of LDL to oxidation in obese subjects. Diabetes Care 21:796–799

Tack CJ, Ong MK, Lutterman JA, Smits P (1998) Insulin-induced vasodilatation and endothelial function in obesity/insulin resistance. Effects of Troglitazone. Diabetologia 41:569–576

Takagi T, Akasaka T, Yamamuro A, Honda Y, Hozumi T, Morioka S, Yoshida K (2000) Troglitazone reduces neointimal tissue proliferation after coronary stent implantation in patients with non-insulin dependent diabetes mellitus: a serial intravascular ultrasound study. J Am Coll Cardiol 36:1529–1535

Thomas JC, Taylor KB (2001) Effects of Thiazolidinediones on lipoprotein subclasses in patiens who are insulin resistant. Diabetes 50: Abstract 1902-PO

Tontonoz P, Nagy L, Alvarez JG, Thomazy VA, Evans RM (1998) PPAR-γ promotes monocyte/macrophage differentiation and uptake of oxidized LDL. Cell 93:241–252

UK Prospective Diabetes Study Group (1998). Effect of intensive blood-glucose control with metformin on complications in overweight patients with type 2 diabetes (UKPDS 34). Lancet 352:854–865

UK Prospective Diabetes Study Group (1998). Intensive blood-glucose control with sulphonylureas or insulin compared with conventional treatment and risk of complications in patients with type 2 diabetes (UKPDS 33). Lancet 352: 837–853

Yamasaki Y, Kawamori R, Wasada T, Sato A, Omori Y, Eguchi H, Tominaga M, Sasaki H, Ikeda M, Kubota M, Ishida Y, Hozumi T, Baba S, Uehara M, Shichiri M, Kaneko T (1997) Pioglitazone (AD-4833) ameliorates insulin resistance in patients with NIDDM. AD-4833 Glucose Clamp Study Group, Japan. Tohoku J Exp Med 183: 173–183

Yue TL., Chen J, Ohlstein EH (2001) In vivo cardioprotective effects of rosiglitazone in nondiabetic and diabetic rats subjected to myocardial ischemia. Diabetes 50: Abstract 694-P

CHAPTER 18

Hyperglycemia and Cardiovascular Disease in Type 2 Diabetes Mellitus: Evidence-based Approach to Primary and Secondary Prevention

Z. Milicevic, N. Hancu, I. Raz

Abstract. Cardiovascular (CV) disease is recognized as the most common and the most serious complication of Type 2 diabetes. Up to 70% of diabetic patients die from CV causes. Major CV risk factors play a significant role in the progression of diabetic CV disease, and diabetes-specific abnormalities contribute further to the magnitude of the problem. Data from interventional studies are indicating that management of the standard risk factors decreases CV risk. However, it is still unclear whether lower overall glycemic exposure or improved treatment of the post-meal abnormalities, yield improved outcomes. This chapter reviews current studies to address this issue.

Introduction

Cardiovascular (CV) disease is the most serious complication of Type 2 diabetes in terms of morbidity and mortality (Laakso 1999). Although, diabetic CV disease has been the focus of research for decades, data to support an optimal treatment strategy remain incomplete. Some of the most critical questions relate to the problem of the contribution of hyperglycemia to the development of diabetic CV disease, interplay between diabetes-specific risk factors and general CV risk factors, and efficacy of various forms of treatment interventions on the incidence of CV outcomes. In this overview, some aspects of the diabetic CV disease and current known interventional studies are presented and discussed, including possible directions in clinical investigation of the effect of hyperglycemia reduction on CV morbidity and mortality.

Epidemiology of CV Disease in Diabetic Populations

Epidemiological studies indicate that the risk of CV outcomes, including myocardial infarction (MI), stroke, peripheral vascular disease, and CV death, is two to three times higher in patients with diabetes compared to non-diabetic patients with a comparable profile of risk factors (Wingard et al. 1995; Haffner et al. 1998; de Vegt et al. 1999; Kuller et al. 2000; Stamler et al. 2001). Up to 70% of these patients die from CV causes.

Although, atherosclerotic vascular disease is not the only mechanism of heart damage in people with diabetes, it plays a primary role in increasing CV morbidity and mortality in these individuals. Those with diabetes show not only an increased frequency of atherosclerosis, but also a greater severity of its course. This is reflected in more widespread morphological changes in the blood vessels and a higher risk of complications of the disease, namely, increased incidence of MI, stroke, and amputations in patients with Type 2 diabetes and atherosclerosis vs. nondiabetic individuals with similar degree of atherosclerotic vascular changes. A subgroup with the highest risk are diabetic patients with previous MI, who have a several times higher risk of CV death, nonfatal MI, and stroke when compared to matched, non-diabetic individuals (Malmberg et al. 1995; Haffner et al. 1998).

Conventional Risk Factors

All known non-glycemic risk factors for atherosclerotic vascular disease operate in diabetic patients. Among them, cigarette smoking, hypercholestrolemia, hypertriglyceridemia, low HDL-cholesterol and high blood pressure are probably the most important.

Epidemiological data that confirmed relationship between cigarette smoking and increased CV risk have been published in 1960s (U.S. Public Health Service: Smoking and Health 1964). People who quit smoking reduce their excess risk of coronary event by 50% in the first year or two after cessation. This period is followed by more gradual decline (The Health Benefits of Smoking Cessation: A report of the Surgeon General 1990). Compared to the non-diabetic population, diabetic patients show similar or higher prevalence of smoking (up to 33% vs. 27%)(Dierkx RIJ. Et al Nether J Med).

Serum total cholesterol is a powerful predictor of ischemic heart disease (IHD) morbidity and mortality in both middle-aged healthy and diabetic subjects (Pyrola et al. 1997). However, the impact of hypercholesterolemia in diabetics is much greater as they have a two to three times higher risk for IHD than their non-diabetic counterparts for the same level of total serum cholesterol (Vaccaro et al. 1998). Besides total cholesterol, elevated triglycerides, high LDL-cholesterol, and low HDL-cholesterol have also been shown to independently increase cardiovascular mortality in those with diabetes (Lehto et al. 1997).

Most clinical trials of lipid intervention and IHD prevention have been conducted in study population that excluded diabetic individuals. However, some of these trials have conducted post hoc analysis of their diabetic subgroups. In diabetic patients who participated in the Scandinavian Simvastatin Survival Study, lowering cholesterol with simvastatin, a HMG-CoA reductase inhibitor, significantly decreased risk of a major IHD event as well as the risk for any other type of atherosclerotic event (Pyrola et al. 1997). Similarly, subgroup analysis of the Helsinki Heart Study, a 5-year IHD primary prevention trial using gemfibrozil, provided additional evidence for the potential benefit of lipid-lowering agents for both non-diabetics and diabetics (Koskinen et al. 1992). In the Veterans Affairs HDL Intervention Trial (VA-HIT) patients who received 1200 mg of gemfibrozil had a 24 % reduction in the combined outcome of death from coronary heart disease, non-fatal myocardial infarction, and stroke ($p<0.001$)during 5-year follow-up period vs. those patients who received placebo (Bloomfield Rubins et al. 1999 and 2001). A subgroup analysis of this secondary prevention study showed that patients with diabetes also benefited ($p=0.05$).

Several trials that focus primarily on the effect of various lipid agents specifically in diabetic individuals have been reported recently. Some of these studies have been completed, some are still in the recruitment phase. The Diabetes Atherosclerosis Intervention Study (DAIS) was developed and conducted in collaboration with WHO to ask the question whether correction of dyslipoproteinemia seen in Type 2 diabetes would decrease the rate of angiographic progression of coronary artery disease (Diabetes Atherosclerosis Intervention Study Group 2001). A total of 418 patients were randomised to be treated with micronized fenofibrate (200 mg/day) or placebo for at least 3 years. This study showed that treatment with fenofibrate yielded greater reduction in total cholesterol, LDL-cholesterol and triglyceride levels and greater increase in HDL-cholesterol level when compared to placebo. This resulted in significant reduction in progression of atherosclerosic changes in coronary blood vessels. Although, this study was not an endpoint study, it is worth mentioning that in the fenofibrate group a 24% reduction in incidence of clinical endpoints was observed vs. the placebo group. Three additional, primary prevention studies are currently being carried out, and will certainly shed more light on the problem of CV disease prevention in diabetes. These are Fenofibrate Intervention and Event Lowering in Diabetes (FIELD), Collaborative Atorvastatin Diabetes Study (CARDS), and Lipids in Diabetes Study (LDS). In all three, clinical events are primary endpoints.

The role of hypertension as a factor in the increased mortality among type 2 diabetics has been extensively investigated. Not only is the prevalence of hypertension in type 2 diabetes high, but hypertension develops early in the course of the disease. The UKPDS strongly demonstrated the link between hypertension and the high risk for CV complications in type 2 diabetes (Adler et al. 2000). Decreasing blood pressure by use of ?-blocking agents or angiotensin converting enzyme (ACE) inhibitors resulted in a significant reduction in mortality risk and/or acute MI.

Diabetes-specific Risk Factors. Role of Post-meal Hypoinsulinemia and Hyperglycemia

The increased incidence of CV disease in diabetic patients can only be explained by the presence of additional, diabetes-specific risk factors.

In numerous epidemiological reports (Rodriguez et al. 1996; Balkau 1998; Anonymous 1999; Hanefeld and Temelkova-Kurktschiev 2001), postprandial BG levels have shown a positive relationship with risk for various cardiovascular complications. According to the DECODE study, which is the most comprehensive evaluation of the effect of hyperglycemia on mortality, this effect is independent of other risk factors. It seems that hemoglobin A1c level also correlates with the level of risk for macrovascular complications, but to a lesser extent than postprandial glycemia (Laakso and Seppo 1998; Anonymous 1999).

From very early stages in the development of type 2 diabetes, the postprandial state is characterized by two main abnormalities: early phase hypoinsulinemia (lasting 30 to 60 minutes), due to a lack of normal early phase insulin secretion; and consequent prolonged hyperglycemia. As a result of these main abnormalities, additional metabolic changes may occur, including prolonged hyper-free-fatty-acidemia, and exaggerated and prolonged postprandial lipemia. One important possible consequence is the increased risk of progression of atherosclerosis. In addition, postprandial lipemia and large fluctuations in BG concentrations, like those occurring during the postprandial state, may contribute to the pathogenesis of cardiovascular disease; other postprandial events including transient hypertension due to adrenergic stimulation (Marfella et al. 2000), abnormalities of repolarization of the myocardial tissue (Marfella et al. 2000), and a state of hypercoagulation, due to abnormalities in concentration and/or activity of several coagulation factors (Ceriello 1999), may also contribute. Ceriello et al. have extensively studied the effect of hyperglycemia and hypertriglyceridemia on generation of free radicals and formation of nitric oxide, and their effect on endothelial function (Ceriello et al. 2002). The authors have found a clear correlation between postprandial hyperglycemia and postprandial hypertriglyceridemia, and abnormalities of protective mechanisms during oxidative stress, which may have a negative impact on endothelial function, including vasomotor control and intracellular signal transduction. Since early postprandial hypoinsulinemia may be a common pathogenic denominator of all or most of the resultant abnormalities, there is a possibility that by restoring a normal pattern of daily insulin concentrations, it may be possible to correct the above-mentioned abnormalities and prevent complications.

However, a recent American Diabetes Association (ADA) consensus statement (American Diabetes Association 2001) emphasized that until a properly designed interventional trial is conducted, it is impossible to conclude that a specific treatment focused on correcting abnormalities primarily of the postprandial state is justified. Other national or international organizations give more specific recommendations for the treatment of postprandial hyperglycemia. European Diabetes Policy Group (supported by International Diabetes Federation-European Region) and American Association of Clinical Endocrinologists propose blood glucose level of 140 mg/dl (7,5 mmol/L) or higher after meal as a cut-off point for intervention. European Diabetes Policy Group recommended very tight overall blood glucose control in people at risk for CV complications (target HbA1c of 6,5%) (Alberti et al. 1999, AACE Diabetes Guidelines 2002).

Interventional Studies

Data from prospective, randomized trials that address the influence of hyperglycemia on cardiovascular outcomes in patients with type 2 diabetes are very limited. Although various CV endpoints were only one component of the primary endpoint in the UKPDS study, analysis of individual outcomes indicated that more intensive metabolic control reduces risks of complicated IHD (acute MI) (UKPDS 1998). Risk of MI was reduced by 16% in the intensive group of the UKPDS study, with borderline significance, mainly due to lack of power and initial recruitment bias (people with more severe forms of coronary heart disease were mainly excluded from the study). It is also possible that levels of glycemia low enough to reduce CV disease events were not reached, or that reducing total glycemia exposure is not enough to reduce CV risk. The UKPDS researchers have estimated that for a 1% decrease in HbA1c, the risk for MI decreases 14% (Stratton IM et al. BMJ 2000). The Diabetes Control and Complication Trial (DCCT) assessed primarily the effect of blood glucose reduction on microvascular complications, while macrovascular endpoints were only a secondary objective. Despite the fact that the DCCT cohort was comprised of young people with Type 1 diabetes, intensive treatment reduced all major CV and peripheral vascular events by 41%. This difference was not statistically significant due to low number of events as was expected in this cohort. (Anonymous 1993). A similar outcome was reported in the Kumamoto Study which included 110 type 2 diabetic patients in Japan (Schichiri M et al. Diabetes Care 2000). Patients who were treated with an intensive insulin regimen and who had a near-normoglycemic HbA1c target had more than 50% reduction in incidence of major clinical CV endpoints, although, the difference was not statistically significant due to the small number of patients in the study.

Another study that addressed this problem was the Diabetes Mellitus Insulin – Glucose Infusion in Acute Myocardial Infarction (DIGAMI) Study (Malmberg et al. 1995, 1996; Malmberg 1997). The DIGAMI study was a prospective trial of 620 patients with diabetes and acute MI who were randomized either to acute treatment with glucose-insulin infusion followed by multidose subcutaneous insulin for at least 3 months, or to a control group that was treated in most cases with diet and oral hypoglycemic medication, although, some were also treated with insulin. After a follow-up of 12 months, 26.1% of patients in the control group had died, compared to only 18.6% of insulin-treated patients, a relative reduction of mortality of 29%. After a mean follow-up of 3.4 years, 33% of patients in the insulintreated group had died, compared to 44% in the control group. Hemoglobin A1c levels at 3 months were 7.1% in the insulin-treated group, compared to 7.5% in the control group, and at 1 year the levels were at 7.3% and 7.6%, respectively. Fasting BG did not differ between the groups. There are several possible explanations for the results of the DIGAMI study:

1. Increased mortality in the control group relates to the potential negative effect of oral agents (for example, sulfonylureas). The difference in the mortality rate between the groups may be explained by the higher proportion of patients treated with sulfonylurea drugs in the control group (Malmberg et al. 1996). This hypothesis is disputed by the UKPDS results which did not find any evidence to suggest that sulfonylureas may have a pro-atherogenic effect.
2. Acute infusion of insulin and glucose may decrease myocardial tissue damage caused by ischemia, leading to improved survival. It has been suggested that acutely increased levels of free fatty acids may promote cell death and tissue injury, as well as endothelial dysfunction due to an unfavorable interaction with cell defense mechanism (increase oxidative stress, reduced formation of nitric oxide) and interference with the physiologic action of the fibrinolytic system (Sodi-Pallares et al. 1969, Eckel et al. 2002).
3. Since those who benefited the most were patients with the most profound drop in BG levels (the subgroup of patients who were on oral agents before the study and who had low risk for cardiovascular disease), there is a possibility that simple reduction in total glycemic exposure improved survival.
4. Finally, it is possible that postprandial BG was better managed in the intensively treated patients, compared to the conventional group. Fasting BG concentration did not differ between the two groups after 1 year of follow-up, indicating that the significant difference in HbA1c level between groups might have been related to better management of the postprandial phase of the daily glucose profile in the intensively treated patients.

Dysglycemia has been proposed as a continuous CV risk factor (Gerstein HC. et al. 1996, Gerstein HC. et al. 1997). This hypothesis is mainly based on epidemiological evidence, including data on postprandial hyperglycemia, from several studies.

Clearly, more studies are needed to be able to understand the processes that lead to progression of CV disease in diabetic individuals, and propose a more efficacious and safer treatment strategy for patients at risk of developing severe complications of atherosclerotic vascular disease.

There are 3 studies currently underway addressing glycemic control and cardiovascular outcomes in people with type 2 diabetes. The Veterans Affairs Diabetes Trial [VADT] - Glycemic Control and Complications in Type 2 diabetes - plans to determine the effect of intensive therapy versus standard glycemic control on reduction of major cardiovascular events in patients with type 2 diabetes (Duckworth WC. et al 2001). The Action to Control CardiOVascular Risk in Diabetes [ACCORD] plans to evaluate the effects of intensive glycemic control on reduction of CV risk. In addition it will also evaluate treatment to increase HDL and lower triglycerides as well as intensive blood pressure control (both in the context of good glycemic control) on reduction of CV risk. The Bypass Angioplasty Revascularization Investigation - Type 2 Diabetes [BARI-2D] plans to compare revascularization plus medical therapy versus medical therapy alone on cardiovascular benefits in patients with type 2 diabetes. In addition it will compare the glycemic and CV benefits of insulin-sparing (thiazolidinediones or metformin) versus insulin-providing (sulphonylureas or insulin) agents. All 3 studies aim to achieve optimal glycemic control and assess whether it will benefit CV outcomes.

Acknowledgment

Authors are members of the Diabetes International Research and Educational Cooperative Team (DIRECT) which has been established by a board of experts in September 2001 in Prague. DIRECT consists of leading diabetologists from Central, Eastern, Southern Europe, and Mediterranean regions. The mission of DIRECT is to improve concepts for the prevention, management and control of diabetes mellitus as well as to enhance the quality of life of diabetic patients.

References

AACE Diabetes Guidelines. American Association of Clinical Endocrinologists. Endocrine Practice 8 (Suppl): 40-2, 2002.

Adler AI, Stratton IM, Neil HA, Yudkin JS, Matthews DR, Cull CA, Wright AD, Turner RC, Holman RR. Association of systolic blood pressure with macrovascular and microvascular complications of type 2 diabetes (UKPDS 36): prospective observational study. BMJ 321: 412-19, 2000.

Alberti G.: A desktop guide to type 2 diabetes mellitus. European Diabetes Policy Group 1998-999. Exp Clin Endocrinol Diabetes 107:390-20, 1999.

DECODE Study Group. Consequences of the new diagnostic criteria for diabetes in older men and women. DECODE Study (Diabetes Epidemiology: Collaborative Analysis of Diagnostic Criteria in Europe). Diabetes Care. 22:1667-1, 1999.

DCCT Reseach Group. The effect of intensive treatment of diabetes on the development and progression of long-term complications in insulin-dependent diabetes mellitus. The Diabetes Control and Complications Trial Research Group. New England Journal of Medicine. 329:977-6, 1993.

American Diabetes Association: Postprandial blood glucose. Diabetes Care 24:775-78, 2001.

Bloomfield Rubens H., Davenport J., Babikian V., Brass LM, Collins D., Wexler L., Wagner S., Papademetriou V., Rutan G., Robins S.J.: Reduction in stroke with gemfibrozil in men with coronary heart disease and low HDL cholesterol: The Veterans Affairs HDL Intervention Trial (VA-HIT), Circulation 103:2828–833, 2001.
Rubins HB, Robins SJ, Collins D et al. Gemfibrozil for the secondary prevention of coronary heart disease in men with low levels of high density lipoprotein cholesterol. N Eng J Med 341:410–18, 1999.
Balkau B., Shipley M., Jarret RJ., Pyrola K., Pyrola M., Forhan A., Eschwege E.: High blood glucose concentration is a risk factor for mortality in middle-aged nondiabetic man. 20-year follow-up in the Whitehall Study, the Paris Prospective Study, and the Helsinki Policeman Study, Diabetes Care 21: 360–67, 1998.
Ceriello A. The emerging role of post-prandial hyperglycaemic spikes in the pathogenesis of diabetic complications, Diab. Med. 15; 188–93; 1998
de Vegt F, Dekker JM, Ruhé, et al.: Hyperglycaemia is associated with all-cause and cardiovascular mortality in the Hoorn population: the Hoorn Study. Diabetologia 42:926–31,1999.
Diabetes Atherosclerosis Intervention Study Group. Effect of fenofibrate on progression of coronary-artery disease in type 2 diabetes: the Diabetes Atherosclerosis Intervention Study, a randomised study. Lancet 357:905–10, 2001.
Dierkx RIJ, van de Hoek W., Hoekstra J.B.L, Erkelens DW.: Smoking and diabetes, Netherlands J Med 48:150–52, 1996.
Duckworth WC., McCarren M., Abraira C.: Glucose control and cardiovascular complications: The VA Diabetes Trial, Diabetes Care 24:942–45, 2001.
Eckel R., Wassef M., Chait a., Sobel B., Barrett E., King G., Lopes-Virella M., Reusch J., Ruderman N., Steiner G., Vlassara H.: Prevention Conference VI: Diabetes and carddiovascular disease: Pathogenesis of Atherosclerosis in Diabetes. Circulation 105:138–43, 2002.
Gerstein HC: Glucose: a continuous risk factor for cardiovascular disease. Diabetic Med 14:S25–1; 1997.
Gerstein HC, Yusof S: Dysglycemia and risk of cardiovascular disease. Lancet 347:949–0, 1996.
Haffner SM, Lehto S, Ronnemaa T, Pyorala K, Laakso M.: Mortality from coronary heart disease in subjects with type 2 diabetes and in nondiabetic subjects with and without prior myocardial infarction. N Engl J Med 339:229–34, 1998.
Hanefeld M., Temelkova-Kurktschiev T., postchallenge plasma glucose and glycemic spikes are more strongly associated with atherosclerosis than fasting glucose or HbA1c level., Diabetes Care 23: 1830–834, 2001.
Health benefits of smoking cessation: A report of the surgeon general. Washington D.C. US department of health and human services, Public health service, Centers for disease control, Office on smoking and health 1990.
Herlitz J, Bang A, Karlson BW. Mortality, place and mode of death and reinfarction during a period of 5 years after acute myocardial infarction in diabetic and non-diabetic patients. Cardiology 87: 423–28, 1996.
Koskinen P, Manttari M, Manninen V, Huttunen JK, Heinonen OP, Frick MH. Coronary heart disease incidence in NIDDM patients in the Helsinki Heart Study. Diabetes Care 15: 820–25, 1992.
Kuller LH, Velentgas P, Barzilay J, et al.: Diabetes mellitus: subclinical cardiovascular disease and risk of incident cardiovascular disease and all-cause mortality. Arterioscler Thromb Vasc Biol 20:823–29, 2000.
Laakso M., Seppo L.: Epidemiology of risk factors for cardiovascular disease in diabetes and impaired glucose tolerance., Atherosclerosis 137: S65-S73, 1998.
Laakso M. Hyperglycemia and cardiovascular disease in type 2 diabetes. Diabetes 48: 937–42, 1999.
Lehto S, Ronnemaa T, Haffner SM, Pyorala K, Kallio V, Laakso M. Dyslipidemia and hyperglycemia predict coronary heart disease events in middle-aged patients with NIDDM. Diabetes 46: 1354–359, 1997.
Malmberg K, Rydén L, Effendic S, Herlitz J, Nicol P, Waldenström A, Wedel H.: Randomised trial of insulin-glucose infusion followed by subcutaneous insulin treatment in diabetic patients with acute myocardial infarction (DIGAMI Study): Effects on mortality at 1 year. J Am Coll Cardiol 26:57–5, 1995.
Malmberg K, for the DIGAMI Study Group: Prospective randomised study of intensive insulin

treatment on long term survival after acute myocardial infarction in patients with diabetes mellitus. Br Med J 314:1512–515, 1997.

Malmberg K, Ryden L. Myocardial infarction in patients with diabetes mellitus. Eur Heart J 9: 259–64, 1998.

Marfella R. et al., The Effect of Acute Hyperglycaemia on QTc Duration in Healthy Men., Diabetologia, 43 , 571–, 2000.

Pyorala K, Pedersen TR, Kjekshus J, Faergeman O, Olsson AG, Thorgeirsson G. Cholesterol lowering with simvastatin improves prognosis of diabetic patients with coronary heart disease. A subgroup analysis of the Scandinavian Simvastatin Survival Study (4S). Diabetes Care 20: 614–20, 1997.

Rodriguez BL. Curb JD. Burchfiel CM. Huang B. Sharp DS. Lu GY. Fujimoto W. Yano K. Impaired glucose tolerance, diabetes, and cardiovascular disease risk factor profiles in the elderly. The Honolulu Heart Program., Diabetes Care. 19:587–0, 1996.

Shichiri M. Kishikawa H. Ohkubo Y. Wake N. Long-term results of the Kumamoto Study on optimal diabetes control in type 2 diabetic patients. Diabetes Care 23 Suppl 2:B21–, 2000

Sodi-Pallares D., Ponce de Leon J., Bisteni A., Medrano GA.: Potassium, glucose, and insulin in myocardial infarction. Lancet 7609:1315–316, 1969.

Stamler J, Vaccaro O, Neaton JD, Wentworth D.: Diabetes, other risk factors and 12-yr cardiovascular mortality for men screened in the Multiple Risk Factor Intervention Trial. Diabetes Care 16:434–44, 2001.

Stratton IM. Adler AI. Neil HA. Matthews DR. Manley SE. Cull CA. Hadden D. Turner RC. Holman RR.: Association of glycaemia with macrovascular and microvascular complications of type 2 diabetes (UKPDS 35): prospective observational study. BMJ. 321:405–2, 2000.

Turner RC, Millns H, Neil HA, Stratton IM, Manley SE, Matthews DR, Holman RR. Risk factors for coronary artery disease in non-insulin dependent diabetes mellitus: United Kingdom Prospective Diabetes Study (UKPDS: 23). BMJ 316: 823–28, 1998.

UK Prospective Diabetes Study Group. Intensive blood-glucose control with sulphonylureas or insulin compared with conventional treatment and risk of complications in patients with type 2 diabetes (UKPDS 33)UK Prospective Diabetes Study (UKPDS) Group. Lancet 352: 837–53, 1998.

Ulvenstam G, Aberg A, Bergstrand R, Johansson S, Pennert K, Vedin A, Wilhelmsen L. Long-term prognosis after myocardial infarction in men with diabetes. Diabetes 34: 787–92, 1985.

U.S.public health service: smoking and health. Report of the advisory committee to the surgeon general of the public health service. Washington DC, Government printing office, PHS publication 1103, 1964.

Vaccaro O, Stamler J, Neaton JD. Sixteen-year coronary mortality in black and white men with diabetes screened for the Multiple Risk Factor Intervention Trial (MRFIT). Int J Epidemiol 27: 636–41, 1998.

Wingard DL, Barrett-Connor E.: Heart disease and diabetes. In: National Diabetes Data Group, Diabetes in America, 2nd edition. National Institute of Health, NIDDK. Bethesda (MD): NIH publication No. 95–468. p 429–48, 1995.

CHAPTER 19

Cardiac Exploration of Diabetic Patients

R. Căpâlneanu

Abstract. Since the cardiac involvement is highly frequent in type 2 diabetes mellitus, mainly by coronary artery disease, diabetic cardiomyopathy and autonomic neuropathy dysfunction and because these patients are often asymptomatic, the cardiac exploration is essential in the clinical assessment. The noninvasive methods (ECG, echo-Doppler, nuclear perfusion, etc.) are usually sufficient in diagnosis and establishing cardiac disease severity evaluation.
The severe symptomatic patients as well as the noninvasive high risk evidence require invasive techniques (cardiac catheterization, coronarography, electrophysiological study, etc.) to make optimal decisions within the interventional therapy (myocardial revascularization, pacemaker implantation, etc.).

Introduction

Complete evaluation of cardiac function in diabetic patient should include the invasive explorations by cardiac catheterization, coronarography and endomyocardial biopsy besides the noninvasive ones, some already frequently used like electrocardiography and sonography (echo-Doppler investigation) or others more complex like radioisotopic techniques (radionuclide ventriculography and myocardial perfusion scintigraphy). The diabetic patient heart evaluation should ideally include data on the angiographic status of the coronary bed, determination of the systolic and diastolic heart function, estimation of the ventricular parietal kinetics and histologic examination [1]. Nevertheless, the invasive explorations are only carried out in the cardiac severe symptomatic diabetic patients (congestive cardiac failure, angor, kidney transplant need, etc.) while the noninvasive methods (myocardial scintigraphy and Doppler-echocardiography) have been successfully used in the correct estimation and follow up of the cardiac function and structural anomalies. Besides the heart function determination by echographic, scintigraphic, hemodynamic, etc. parameters, the heart evaluation of diabetic patient is meant to identify the cardiac damage etiologic entity, basically brought about by coronary atherosclerosis (extramural and/or intramural vessels), autonomic dysfunction or by the so-called disputed entity of diabetic cardiomyopathy [2]. While the diagnosis in the first two variants is less difficult to establish, the identification of the diabetic cardiomyopathy implies a more sophisticated procedure involving the certification of near-normal epicardial coronaries and the presence of some specific histological changes (interstitial fibrosis, modifications of basal membrane, etc.), that obviously requires endomyocardial biopsy.

Some authors call the diabetes mellitus a real "cardiovascular disease" because of high incidence and bad prognosis of cardiac condition, especially in type 2 diabetes mellitus. The high mortality and morbidity of cardiac causes associated with diabetes mellitus strongly advocate for the importance of the cardiac disease identification, the estimation of its severity and finding the optimal therapy solutions in due time, since the asymptomatic patients rate is known to be high among the diabetic patients. Therefore, besides the clinic examination, the diabetic patient exploration by paraclinic cardiovascular specific methods represents an essential clinical stage with important effects on life prognosis and life quality.

Certainly, the way of applying the different cardiac exploration methods is determined by the clinical status of the patient. When the coronary heart disease is clinically manifested, "aggressive" means are necessary to evaluate the severity and risks of the cardiac involvement. This evaluation is highly important in adopting an accurate therapy, either with drugs or interventional procedures, percutaneous techniques or surgical approach. When the patient is asymptomatic, the exploration methods are meant to identify a clinically silent cardiac disease and to establish its severity [3, 4]. When there are no objective features to indicate a subclinical cardiac disease, the diabetic patient is to be re-evaluated after 2 years at most – this recommendation is motivated mostly by clinical common sense than scientifically grounded [5].

The guideline of the Diabetes American Society concerning the use of cardiac diagnosis tests in diabetic patients is presented in the Table 19.1 [6].

The investigations used in the cardiac evaluation of diabetic patients are non-invasive and invasive. The non-invasive methods mainly include the resting electrocardiogram (ECG), exercise ECG, Holter monitor, x-ray examination, systolic time intervals, echocardiography and cardiac Doppler, radioisotopic techniques and computer tomography. The invasive methods most frequently used are cardiac catheterization, selective coronarography, angiocardiography, electrophysiologic endocavitary study and endomyocardial biopsy.

Table 19.1. Indications for cardiac testing in diabetic patients

1. Typical or atypical cardiac symptoms
2. Resting electrocardiograph suggestive of ischemia or infarction
3. Peripheral or carotid occlusive arterial disease
4. Sedentary lifestyle, age = years, and plans to begin a vigorous exercise program
5. Two or more of the risk factors listed below (a–e) in addition to diabetes
   a) Total cholesterol ≥ 240 mg/dl, LDL cholesterol ≥ 160 mg/dl, or HDL cholesterol < 35 mg/dl
   b) Blood pressure > 140/90 mm Hg
   c) Smoking
   d) Family history of premature CAD
   e) Positive micro/macroalbuminuria test

Non-Invasive tests

Resting Electrocardiography

Resting electrocardiography is used to identify certain myocardial infarction sequelae, ischemic modifications, intraventricular or atrioventricular conduction defects, and arrhythmias. It is important to mention that a normal aspect of the resting ECG does not exclude a coronary heart disease and that the ischemic changes cannot be certainly assigned to ischemic cardiopathy since they sometimes reflect a ventricular "strain" due to a frequently associated hypertension disease. Therefore, the presence of ECG left ventricular hypertrophy type modifications has an independent bad prognosis significance. The identification of an electrical necrosis sequelae requires more subsequent investigations by resting nuclear perfusion scintigraphy (to identify the necrotic area) and by physical or pharmacological stress scintigraphy (to identify an additional ischemia). The patient will be further invasive investigated (selective coronarography, ventriculography) depending mainly on the severity and extent of the necrotic and respectively the additional stress ischemic areas.

Exercise Electrocardiography

When the patient attains a cardiac frequency of about 85% of the maximum age and sex corresponding value, without ischemic changes, a favorable cardiac prognosis is to be expected although coronary artery disease cannot be excluded. The severe changes of the ST-T complex (high risk), the exercise hypotension and the overall low work capacity are important indicators for the presence of a coronary heart disease (Figs. 19.1, 19.2).

To confirm myocardial ischemia and quantify its extent, site and severity as well as to establish the need for further invasive procedures, a nuclear stress perfusion test is necessary (mostly pharmacological, since multiple causes prevent the diabetic patient to perform the physical effort required during the testing exercise) or an echocardiography with dobutamine administration. When the resting ECG indicate basic changes that make the exercise test interpretation more difficult (e.g. intraventricular conduction defects, pre-excitation syndrome) a radionuclide myocardial perfusion is necessary from the beginning of the patient's investigation [7].

Both resting ECG, including the Valsalva maneuver and the exercise ECG test are useful in identification and estimation of the degree of the autonomous dysfunction, based on the R-R interval variation analysis (Table 19.2) [8].

Table 19.2. Range of results for R-R variation and Valsalva maneuver

	R-R variation (ms)	Valsalva maneuver
Abnormal	<20	<1,50
Borderline	20-30	
Normal	>30	>1,50

19 Cardiac Exploration of Diabetic Patients

Fig. 19.1. I.C., 57 years old, male, dg. DM type 2, cardiovascular asymptomatic. *Left*, treadmill test with silent severe ischemia (high-risk type) al 75 watts level. *Right*, coronarography: LAD severe stenosis (85%) in proximity of second artery segment with angioplasty solution (PTCA)

Holter ECG Monitor

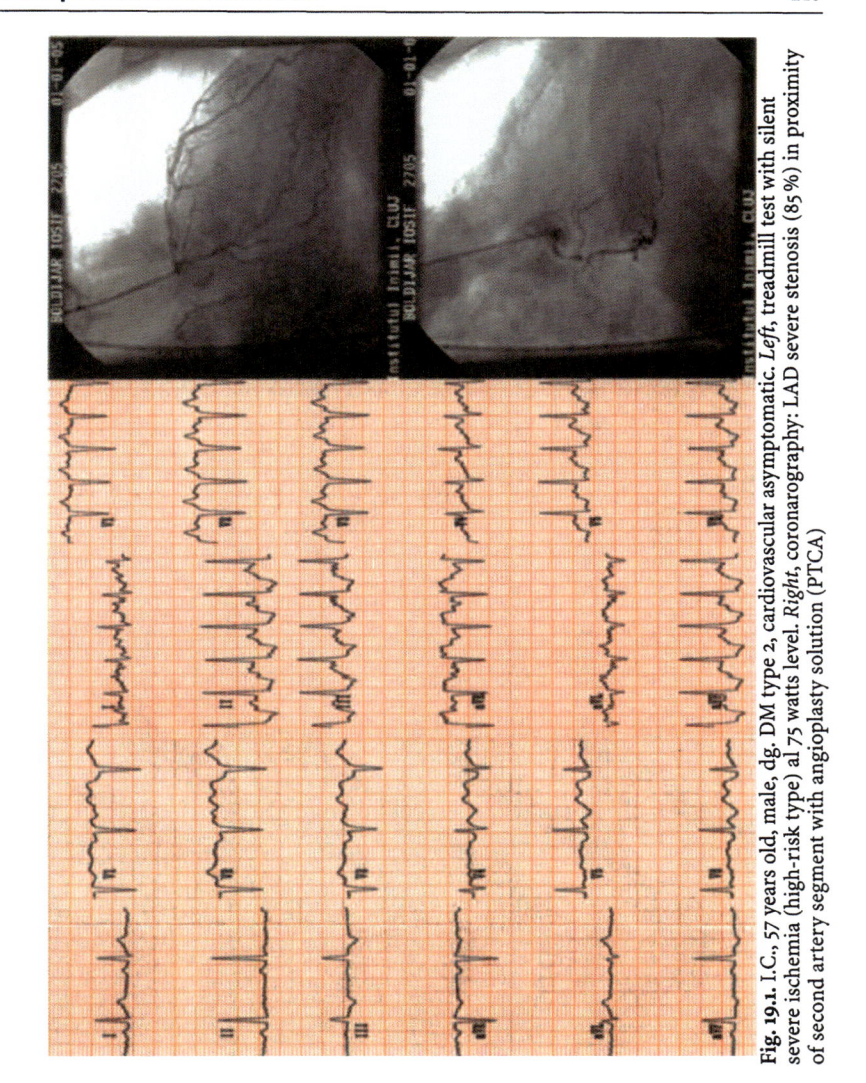

The Holter ECG monitor technique during 24 hours represents a useful method both in establishing the presence and frequency of the silent ischemic episodes, in confirming the rhythm and conduction defects, and in the R-R variations as a marker of latent and intermittent autonomous possible dysfunction. [9, 10] However, this method is not a screening procedure and is rather useful in some patients monitoring as time self-witness comparative criteria for the same person.

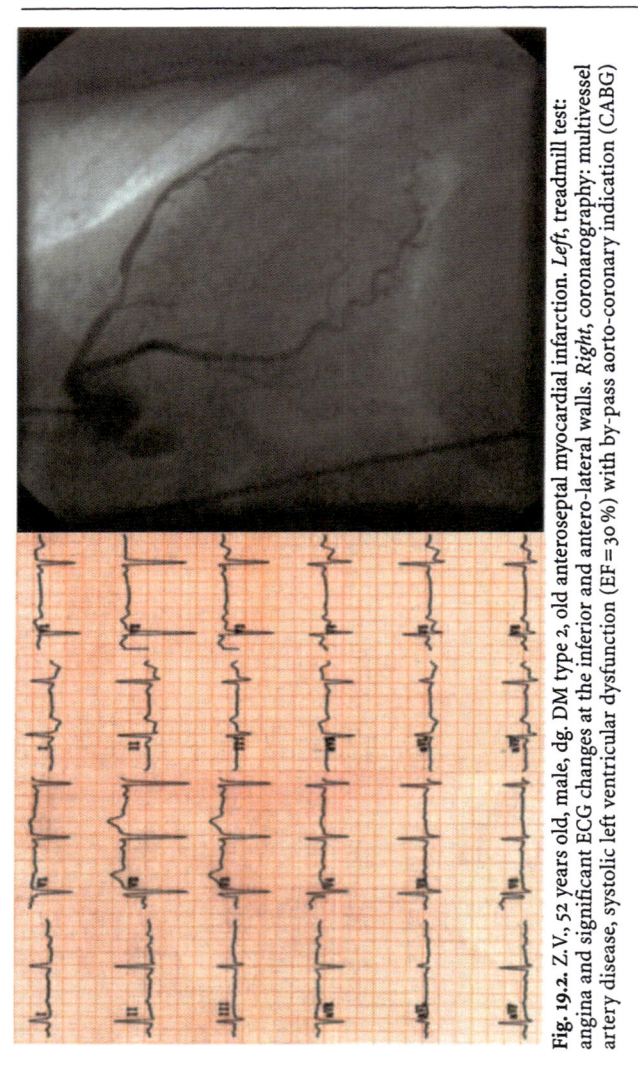

Fig. 19.2. Z.V., 52 years old, male, dg. DM type 2, old anteroseptal myocardial infarction. *Left*, treadmill test: angina and significant ECG changes at the inferior and antero-lateral walls. *Right*, coronarography: multivessel artery disease, systolic left ventricular dysfunction (EF = 30 %) with by-pass aorto-coronary indication (CABG)

Echographic and Doppler Examinations

The echographic and Doppler examination are very useful cardiac evaluations, offering essential data concerning the ventricular mass, left ventricular hypertrophy presence, systolic and diastolic functions, wall kinetic anomalies, coronaries original status, pulmonary hypertension grade, etc. The transthoracic echography (M and B modes) or the transesophageal echography – when the thoracic window is unsatisfactory, allow an accurate evaluation of the chambers size, the parietal hypertrophy identification and the estimation of the main systolic function indices: ejection fraction, shortening fraction by different methods (M mode and B mode by volumes) [11].

19 Cardiac Exploration of Diabetic Patients

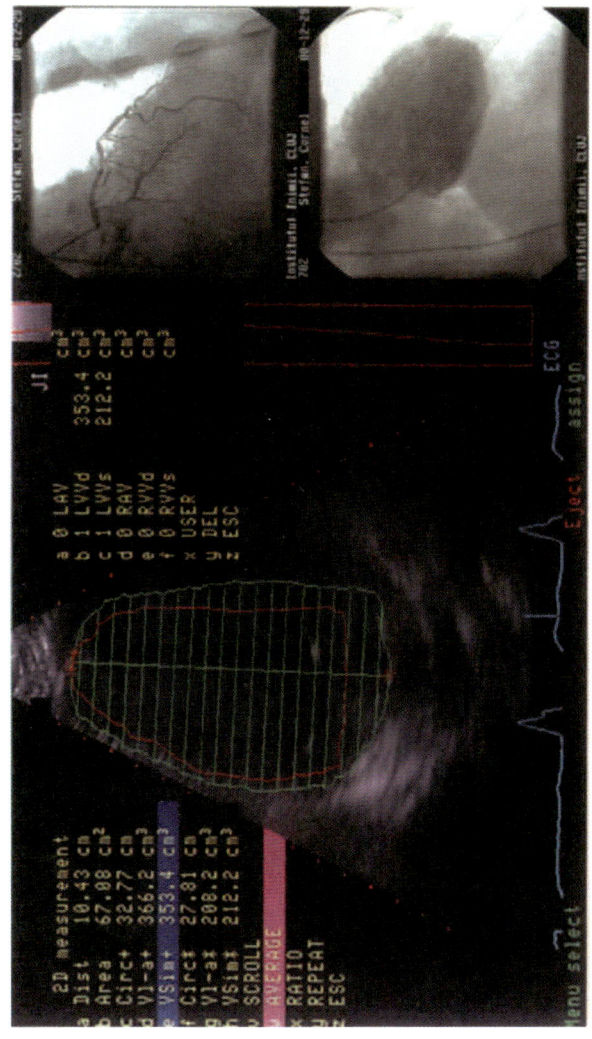

Fig. 19.3. O.T., 59 years old, female, dg. DM type 2, heart failure. *Left*, echo B mode: severe left ventricular systolic dysfunction (EF < 30 %). *Right*, coronarography: multivessel coronary heart disease, global severe left ventricular hypokinesis

These data associated with the Doppler results at the aortic orifice level usually allow to determine the cardiac output and the cardiac index. Minor regurgitation tricuspidian or pulmonary regurgitation at the valvular level – often found in the normal heart – offers the possibility to calculate the systolic and diastolic value in the pulmonary circulation, hemodynamic data especially useful in heart failure. The pulse or continuous Doppler interrogation of the anterograde transmitral flow allows a global evaluation of the ventricular compliance (an expression of the diastolic function or dysfunction), a characteristic physiopathologic element often found in the diabetic cardiopathy (Figs. 19.3, 19.4).

An echo-Doppler examination showing enlarged cavities, systolic and diastolic dysfunctions, absence of some segmentary kinetic abnormalities, aneurysms and

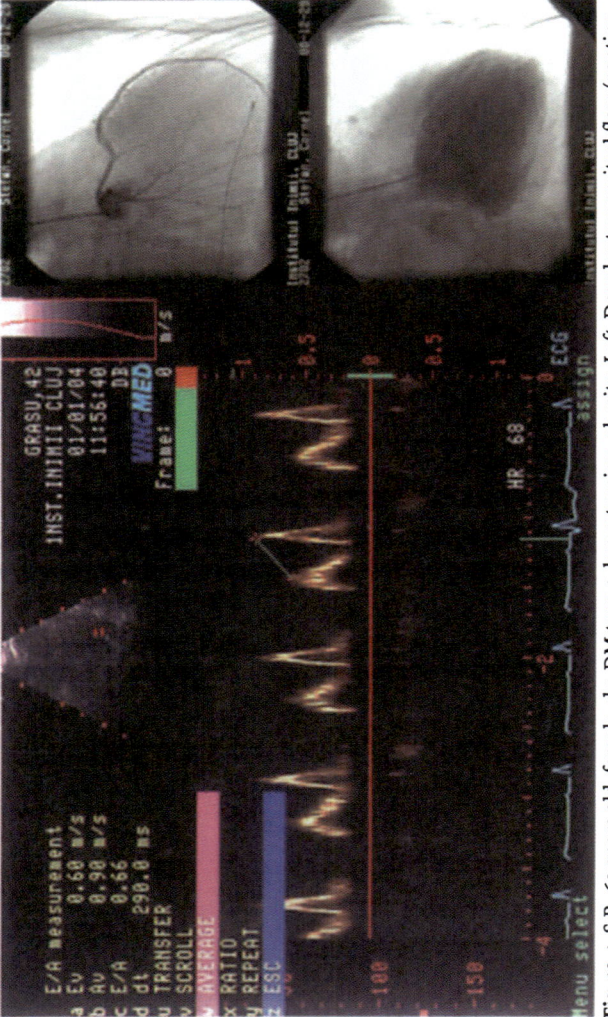

Fig. 19.4. S.P., 60 years old, female, dg. DM type 2, hypertension, obesity. *Left*, Doppler transmitral flow (continuous mode) – diastolic dysfunction with alternate relaxation pattern. *Right*, coronarography: epicardial coronary arteries without significant lesions, dilated left ventricle with severe global hypokinesia

coronary stenosis, no history of coronary heart disease while signs of heart failure are present, is suggestive for a diabetic cardiomyopathy, a pathologic entity still raising controversy.

The Doppler-echocardiography contribution to the diagnosis of ischemic heart disease offers morphological and functional information essential for establishing the diagnosis. Akinetic parietal areas could be identified indicating myocardial necrosis within older myocardial infarctions or hypokinetic zones as an expression of chronic hypoperfusion. The mode B echocardiography can easily reveal the presence of ventricular aneurysms or ostial stenosis in the first sections of the main coronary trunks (right, circumflex and anterior descending arteries). A transesophageal

Doppler evaluation of the coronary flow reserve is an important diagnostic factor, especially in cases with positive stress testing (including perfusion scintigraphy) when the coronary angiography does not indicate significant epicardial vessels stenosis [12].

Associating the echocardiac exploration with stress techniques (physical or pharmacological) can offer additional data on the coronary ischemia or on the identification of hibernating myocardium, susceptible of revascularization.[13] Therefore, the Dobutamine test in low doses is mainly use to identify the hibernating myocardium and in high doses to reveal stress ischemia, exploration method that is considered to have a sensitivity and specificity closed to the nuclear methods [14].

Carotidian Echo-Duplex

The carotidian echo-duplex combines the data offered by the artery echo-biplan mode with the flow information given by Doppler investigation – velocity, gradients, etc. The arterial stenosis can be thus easily determined at the level of common carotid artery, carotid bifurcation and extracranial segment of internal carotid artery level. This procedure allows an accurate estimation of the stenosis severity by flow parameters, mainly by gradient, percent stenosis and morphological aspects of the histogram (Fig. 19.5).

More important than the positive diagnosis and the severity of the carotidian artery stenosis is the possibility of early detection of the atheromatous plaques and, especially to determine their size within a dynamic monitoring follow-up. The carotidian artery echo-Doppler investigation became more important when the mild carotidian artery stenosis has been proved to be a predictive value for the development the coronary events, since the coronary atherosclerosis development has been demonstrated to be "in the mirror" with the carotidian artery one [15]. It is thus known that the patients with carotidian stenosis of 20 % have a 7-fold enhanced risks for coronary heart disease events, among which an important part are present myocardial infarction and/or sudden death as first cardiac manifestation [16]. At present, the most useful and facile non-invasive techniques for the vascular measurements are: carotid artery intima-media thickness (IMT), aortic pulse wave velocity (PWV) and arterial stiffness, and brachial artery flow-mediated dilatation during reactive hyperemia (FMD) [17]. While the last two tests need certain additional procedures – nuclear magnetic resonance, applanation tonometry, etc. – the intima-media thickness is easily determined and monitored only by carotidian echo-duplex.

IMT is the distance between the leading edges of a characteristic double-line pattern seen in longitudinal B-mode ultrasound images of the artery wall [18] or, in Pignoli's opinion (1986), "the distance from the leading edge of the first echogenic line to the leading edge of the second echogenic line". Scanning of the extracranial common carotid artery, the carotid bulb and the internal carotid artery is indicated to be performed from 3 different longitudinal projections as well as the transverse projection [19].

The diabetic patients, mainly of type 2, are known to have a significantly enhanced cardiovascular risk. Therefore, the IMT echo-duplex is an accurate method to evaluate the risk for used in conjunction with other well-known biochemical and constitutional parameters [19]. A direct relation has been demonstrated between the gradual

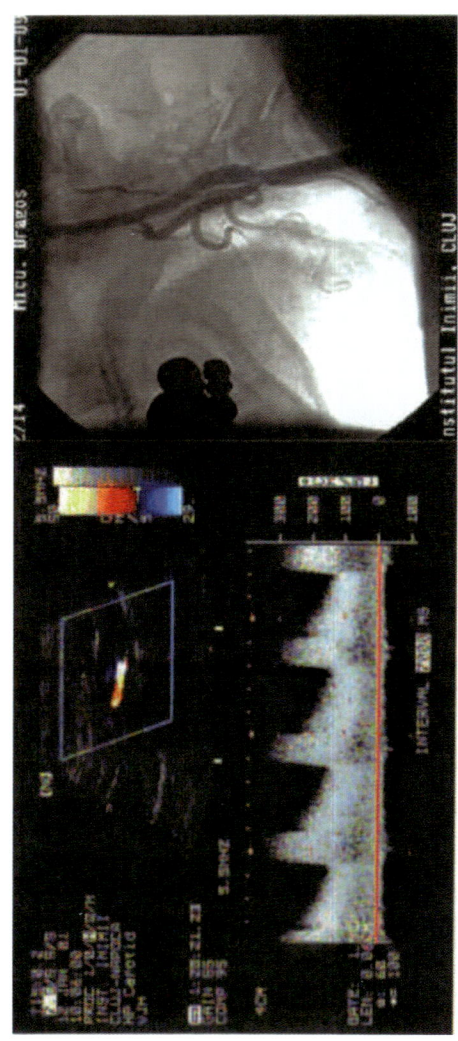

Fig. 19.5. P.V., 52 years old, male, dg. DM type 2, coronary heart disease. Two imaging technique of the same lesion. *Left*, color and spectral Doppler in the origin of the interval carotid artery which indicate a significant stenosis (60 – 70 %). *Right*, angiography with digital substraction which shows a massive plaque burden in the bifurcation of the common carotid artery with tight lesion at the origin of the internal carotid artery

increase of IMT and increasing glycemia [20]. The same relation has been found with the presence of other classical risk factors: LDL cholesterol ↑, HDL cholesterol ↓, hypertension, increased abdominal fat, insulin resistance, smoking, dietary saturated fat, etc. It is also known that the estrogen substitutive therapy, use of aspirin and lipid-lowering agents treatment have a protective effect against the intima-media thickness increase.

19 Cardiac Exploration of Diabetic Patients

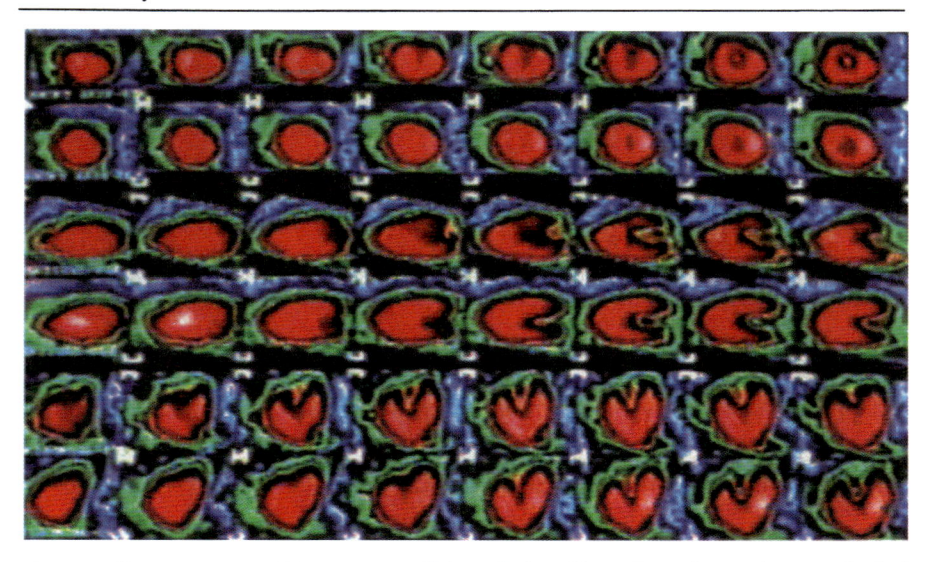

Fig. 19.6. ^{99m}-TcMIBI SPECT rest myocardial perfusion. Normal uptake at pharmacological stress test (Dipiridamol): reversible perfusion abnormality – severe reversible defect (ischemia) on the anterior wall

Myocardial Perfusion Scintigraphy

The myocardial perfusion scintigraphy is a technique using radiotrasors (Thalium, Technicium-labelled MIBI, Tetrofosmin, etc.) which are fixed in myocites depending on the coronary flow degree. The hypofixation present at rest or in stress conditions (physical or pharmacological) allows the retrospective diagnosis of either myocardial necrosis (myocardial infarction) or of reversible ischemia, an expression of hemodynamic significant coronary stenosis (Fig. 19.6).

The 85–93% sensitivity and 90–95% specificity recommend the scintigraphic method for the diagnosis of coronary heart disease and in establishing the algorithm of ischemic severity and risk stratification. [21]. Considering that the ECG exercise test is often non-conclusive in diabetic patients and that frequently they cannot perform maximal or closely maximal test in current clinical practice, certain pharmacological stress testing variants have been taken into consideration: Dipiridamol and Adenosine are mainly used, and Dobutamine for bronchospasm cases [22]. These drugs help to identify the ischemic areas, based on their vasodilator and "arterial steel" effects and are also useful in viable (Nitroglicerin) and hibernating myocardium detection (Dobutamine) (Fig. 19.7).

Such data are essential in the risk stratification and, especially, in selecting optimal therapeutical approach (revascularization).

The stress scintigraphic exercise or pharmacological testing is more frequently used in the following clinical situations:

- Patients unable to perform the exercise ECG test
- Patients with non-conclusive (irrelevant) exercise ECG test

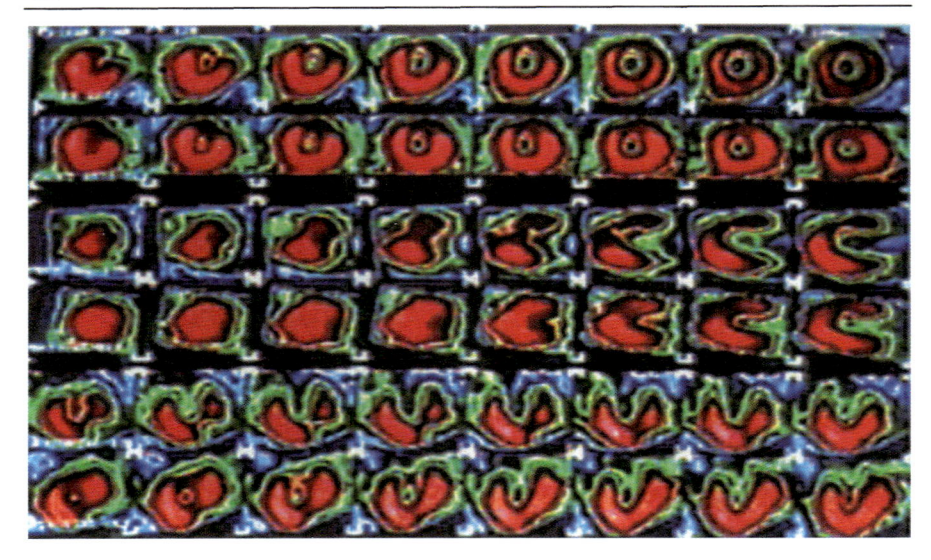

Fig. 19.7. ^{99m}-TcMIBI SPECT rest myocardial perfusion: irreversible defect (necrosis) on the anterior wall (old myocardial infarction). At pharmacological stress test (Dipiridamol): reversible defects (ischemia) on the anterolateral territory

- Patients with negative exercise ECG test but with typical coronary disease symptoms
- Evaluation of ischemic severity in patients with known coronary disease
- Identification of post MI viable and hibernating myocardium in patients with chronic ischemic heart disease for risk stratification and optimal therapeutic approach
- Time monitoring of certain pharmacological (thrombolysis) or interventional (coronary angioplasty, aortocoronary by-pass) therapeutical procedures efficiency over time
- Ischemia risk and prognosis evaluation in diabetic patients before complex general surgery

Invasive Tests

Cardiac Catheterization, Ventriculography and Selective Coronarography

The invasive approach by cardiac catheterization technique is required in a diabetic patient in the following clinical circumstances: (a) asymptomatic patient, with non-invasive tests (exercise ECG, perfusion scintigraphy, etc.) presenting severe silent ischemia (high risk); (b) patient with a history of asymptomatic myocardial infarction (clinically evident or silent) with significant additional ischemia at the physical or pharmaceutical stress testing; (c) progressive symptomatic patient or when the maximal anti-ischemic therapy does not control the clinical status; (d) patients with a need for major vascular surgery, general surgery or kidney transplant.

The cardiac catheterization offers hemodynamic data on the pressure values in the

19 Cardiac Exploration of Diabetic Patients

right or left cardiac chambers and in the pulmonary circulation. The ventriculography with contrast substance offers additional data on the systolic function (by ejection fraction determination), on parietal kinetics, left ventricle and aorta sizes and on the presence of some mechanical complications (mitral insufficiency by rupture or subvalvular apparatus dysfunction, interventricular communication, left ventricular pseudoaneurysm, etc.). Selective contrast substance injection in the right and left coronaries evaluated under several incidences provide the anatomical details necessary to estimated the coronary circulation: presence, number, site and severity of stenosis, vascular occlusions, the extent of collateral circulation development, distal bed sizes, etc., as a result the correct therapeutic option can be selected, either an interventional (PTCA) or surgical (by-pass) revascularization (Fig. 19.8).

In monotroncular or bitroncular coronary heart disease and in the presence of a normal or slightly depreciated left ventricular function, a coronary angioplasty ±

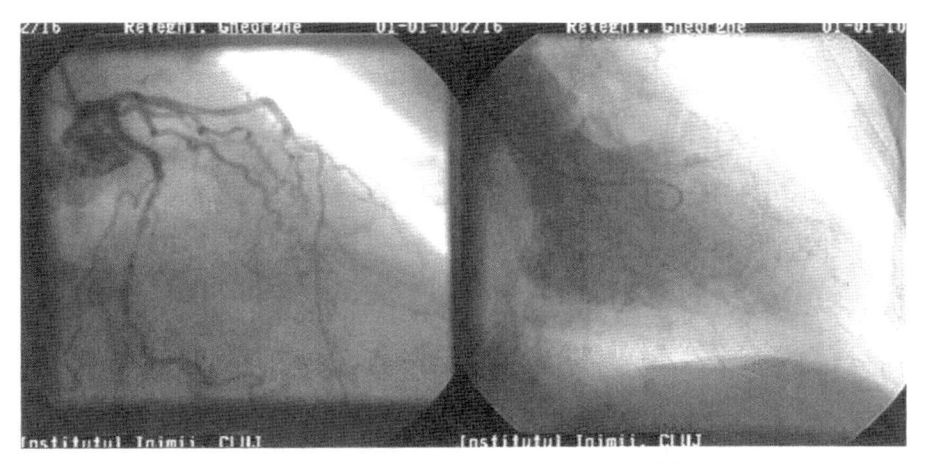

Fig. 19.8. B.B., 51 years old, male, dg. DM type 2, effort angina. *Left*, bitroncular artery disease (LAD and Cx) with severe stenosis – PTCA indication. *Right*, mild depreciate left ventricular systolic function (EF–43%)

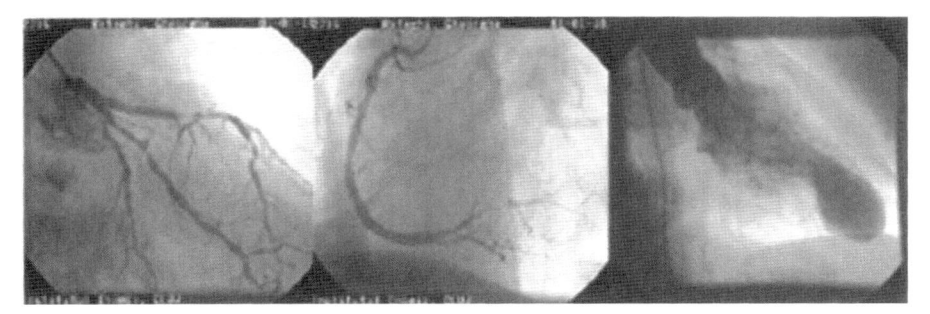

Fig. 19.9. Z.V., 63 years old, female, dg. DM, old anteroseptal myocardial infarction, invalidant angina. *Left*, middle – extensive multivessel coronary artery disease (LAD, Cx, RC). *Right*, left ventricular anteroapical aneurysm; surgical therapeutic option

stent implantation are indicated. In multivessel disease associated with a significant ventricular dysfunction (ejection fraction < 30%) a by-pass surgical revascularization is preferred (in diabetic patient the use of arterial graft is mandatory for the anterior descending artery) [23, 24] (Fig. 19.9).

The invoked risks of the diagnosis invasive methods in diabetic patients are not substantiated if minor precautions are followed: suitable hydration, parsimonious use of contrast substance (possible by substraction technique), adequate hemostasis, etc. Likewise, the invasive therapeutic percutaneous techniques (coronary angioplasty) have prove to be extremely useful and safe, with good results in the diabetic patients, as well [25, 26].

Endocavitary Electrophysiological Investigation

Endocavitary electrophysiological investigation is a diagnosis method required in the presence of certain severe arrhythmias (sustained ventricular tachycardia) or conduction defects (atrio-ventricular, bi- or tri-fascicular blocks), with possible ischemic etiology, due to cardiomyopathy or within the autonomous dysfunction. This procedure allows the reproduction of rhythm or conduction disturbances (inductibility degree) and the evaluation of certain antiarhythmic therapy efficiency. The prognostic value of the test is improved when correlated with the results of late potentials and Q-T interval dispersion, non-invasive parameters usually applied in clinical activity. Finally, the endocavitary electrophysiological study is sometimes indispensable to decide on the implantation of a pacemaker or a cardioverter defibrillator.

Endomyocardial Biopsy

Endomyocardial biopsy is useful in cases of cardiac failure and possible diabetic cardiomyopathy. The bioptic material prelevation is performed by cardiac catheterization technique, more often from the right ventricle [27]. The diagnosis role of the endomyocardial biopsy in diabetes context has mainly the role to exclude some specific cardiomyopathy forms, because the histopathological modifications found in the

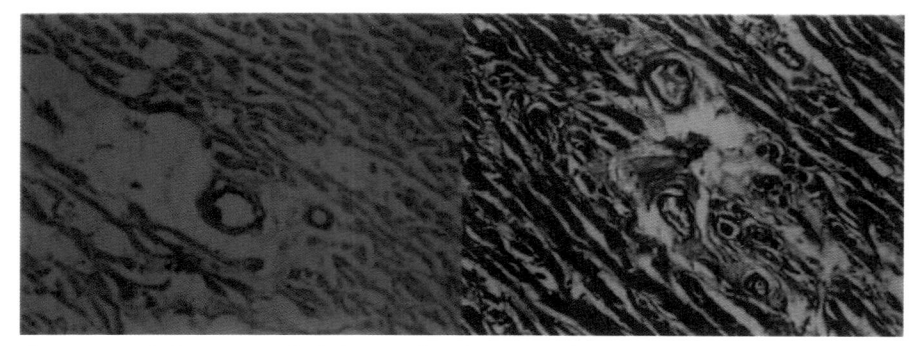

Fig. 19.10. *Left*, intramyocardial, intestinal and perivascular fibrosis. Tricrom Masson stain, ×200. *Right*, focal PAS-positive deposit (*arrow*) within the wall of a small coronary artery. PAS stain, ×200

studies performed on patients with diabetic cardiomyopathies being considered of low specificity (interstitial fibrosis, modifications of basic membrane, etc.) (Fig. 19.10).

In conclusion, the cardiac non-invasive and invasive exploration is useful both in identification and quantification of cardiac disease severity in the patient with type 2 diabetes mellitus as follows:

- For coronary heart disease identification, the resting electrocardiogram, exercise electrocardiogram and especially perfusion scintigraphy with Thalium and Technetium are indicated, associated with pharmacologic stress procedures (dipiridamol, adenozine, dobutamine, etc.).
- For estimation of severity and extension of coronary heart disease and to decide the interventional approach by PTCA or aorto-coronary by-pass, selective coronarography and ventriculography are necessary, associated with perfusion isotopic evaluation and/or stress echocardiography with dobutamine.
- The diabetic cardiomyopathy diagnosis can be considered in asymptomatic patients with diabetes mellitus, but more often when cardiac failure symptoms are present, when the atherosclerotic coronary disease is angiographically excluded, when the coronary flow reserve is not significantly affected and when the microscopic anatomopathological aspects of the endomyocardial biopsy do not show characteristic changes for the specific clinical forms of cardiomyopathies.
- The cardiac autonomic dysfunction can be determined by corroborating the data of a resting electrocardiogram (including Valsalva maneuver), exercise electrocardiogram, and Holter monitor mainly by R-R interval analysis; when the diabetic patient presents syncope or near-syncope symptoms, and/or additional arrhythmias or atrioventricular conduction defects, an endocavitary electrophysiological study is required; these data are necessary to establish the diagnosis, to test possibility of drug control, or to decide on the implant of a pacemaker or cardioverter defibrillator.

References

1. Garber AJ (1998) Non invasive cardiac testing in: "Therapy for Diabetes Mellitus and related disorders, ed Lebobitz HE American Diabetes Ass. Clinical Education Series
2. Bell DSH (1991) Diabetic cardiomiopathy a unique entity or a complication of coronary artery disease? Diabetes Care 18:708–714
3. Nesto RW (1999) Screening for asymptomatic coronary artery disease in diabetes. Diabetes Care 22:1393–1395
4. Janand B et al (1999) Silent myocardial ischemia in patients with diabetes. Diabetes Care 22: 1396–1400
5. Milan Study on Atherosclerosis and Diabetes Group (1997) Prevalence of unrecognized silent myocardial ischemia and its associatiation with atherosclerosis risk factors in non-insulin-dependent diabetes mellitus. Am J Cardiol 79:134–139
6. Consensus Development Conference on the diagnosis of coronary heart disease in people with diabetes (1998) Diabetes Care 21:1551–1559
7. Naka M et al (1992) Silent myocardial ischemia in patients with non-insulin-dependent diabetes mellitus as judged by treadmill exercise testing and coronary angiography. Am Heart J 123:46–53
8. Lebovitz HE (1998) Therapy for diabetes mellitus and related disorders. Third edition, Clinical Education Series, American Diabetes Association

9. Airaksinen KEJ (2001) Early diagnosis of silent coronary artery disease in diabetic subjects. Swiss Med. Wkly 131:425–426
10. Chiariello M et al (2001) Silent myocardial ischemia in diabetic patients. Medicographia (67) 23,2: 119–122
11. Lee M et al (1997) Diabetes mellitus and echocardiographic left ventricular function in freelising elderly men and women. Am Heart J 133:36–43
12. Nahser PJ et al (1995) Maximal coronary flow reserve and metabolic coronary vasodilatation in patients with diabetes mellitus. Circulation 91:635–640
13. Penfornis A et al (2001) Use of dobutamine stress echocardiography in detecting silent myocardial ischaemia in asymptomatic diabetic patients: a comparison with thallium scintigraphy and exercise testing. Diabet Med 18(11): 900–905
14. Kamalesh M et al (2002) Prognostic value of a negative stress echocardiographic study in diabetic patients. Am Heart J 141(10: 163–168
15. Chimowitz MI et al (1994) Cardiac prognosis of patients with carotid prognosis and no history of coronary artery disease: Veterans Affaires Coope, Study Group Stroke 25:759–765
16. Zachny T Bloomgarden (2000) More on cardiovascular disease (American Diabetes Ass. Anmal Meeting, 1999). Diabetes Care, 23:845–852
17. Mudrikova T et al (2000) Carotid intima-media tickness in relation to macrovascular disease in patients with type 2 diabetes mellitus. Wien Klin Wochenschr 27; 112 (20): 887–891
18. Eldon DL et al (1997) Non-invasive assessment of cardiovascular disease in diabetes mellitus. Lancet suppl. 350 (suppl. I): 14–19
19. Yoshimitsu Yamasaki et al (2000) Carotid intima – media thickness in Japanese type 2 diabetic subjects. Diabetes Care 23:1310–1315
20. Foloom AR et al (1994) Relation of carotid artery wall thickness to diabetes mellitus, fasting glucose and physical activity: atherosclerosis risk in communities (ARIC) study investigators. Stroke 25:66–73
21. Shaw GS (2002) Impact of diabetes on the risk stratification using stress single-photon emission computed tomography myocardial perfusion imaging in patients with symptoms suggestive of coronary artery disease. Circulation 1; 105(1): 5–7
22. BARI investigators (1996) Bypass angioplasty revascularisation investigation: comparison of coronary bypass surgery with angioplasty in patients with multivessel disease. N Engl J Med 335:217–225
23. BARI investigators (1997) Influence of diabetes on 5-years mortality and morbidity in a randomized trial comparing CABG and PTCA in patients with multivessel disease. Circulation 96:1761–1769
24. Eichhom EJ et al (1998) Usefulness of dipiridamole-Thallium 201 perfusion scanning for destinguishing ischemic from nonischemic cardiomyopathy. Am J Cardiol 62:945–951
25. Ghali WA et al (2000) Prognostic significance of diabetes as a predictor of survival after cardiac catheterization. Am J Med 109:543–548
26. Van Belle E et al (1997) Restenosis rates in diabetic patients: a comparison of coronary atenting and balloon angioplasty in native coronary vessels. Circulation 96:1454–1460
27. Factor SM (1997) Cardiomyopathy, diabetic in: "Diagnostic criteria for cardiovascular pathology (ed. Bloom S). Lippincot Raven Philadelphia, New York

CHAPTER 20
Assessment of Peripheral Vascular Disease

I.A. Veresiu

Abstract. Although PVD has common patho-physiological and clinical features in patients with DM and in patients without DM, having as underlying process the atherosclerosis, there are some important characteristics of the first group as: younger age of the patients, an almost equal sex distribution and multisegmental and infrapopliteal vessels involvement. The incidence and prevalence of PVD in patients with DM largely depends on the screening and diagnostic method but increases linearly with the age of patients and the diabetes duration. Together with the "classical" ones, some risk factors are considered to have specific influence on producing, progressing and on the clinical picture of PVD in patients with DM. The clinical assessment of PVD in patients with PVD relies on history taking, careful physical examination and instrumental non-invasive and invasive exploration. Due to the topographic characteristics of the arterial obstructions and the association with peripheral neuropathy the intermittent claudication has a low sensitivity. The ischemic rest pain and the diagnosis of chronic critical ischemia require also a careful differential diagnosis. Pulse palpation and bruits presence should be correlated to claudication distance and pain location. The ankle/arm systolic pressure index is a simple, accessible and with good sensitivity and specificity method for routine assessment of PVD in patients with type 2 DM. The toe systolic pressure is a good substitute when ankle pressure is falsely elevated due to medial sclerosis. Other instrumental investigations as pulse volume recordings, transcutaneous oxygen measurement, Doppler ultrasound scanning and magnetic resonance angiographies are used in well-equipped settings. Angiography remains the golden standard when vascular reconstructive surgery is planned. One of the most important characteristic of the patient with PVD and type 2 DM is that their cardiovascular mortality is 4–5 times higher than of those without PVD and therefore annual screening for PVD is mandatory.

Introductory Remarks

The most common form of peripheral vascular involvement in patients with type 2 diabetes mellitus is a progressive impairment of the blood flow in the arteries of the lower limbs produced by an increasing number and/or volume of atherosclerotic plaques. In its natural history the disease has a quite long subclinical stage, then it becomes clinically evident (symptoms and/or signs), initially at effort when an increased blood flow is needed, after that at rest, and finally it can generate tissue necrosis (gangrene) with the need for an amputation. This staged evolution of peripheral vascular disease (PVD) is not the rule, especially in patients with diabetes mellitus (type 1 or type 2) due to specific conditions, and it is not unusual to see patients in which the final stage, foot ulcerations or extensive necrosis, is the first clinical appearance of the disease. It is important to state that progressive evolution is not a fatality. In the well-known Framingham prospective study for general population [18], fewer than 2% of PVD patients required major amputation. Existing data from the general population studies suggest that only 25% of all patients with intermittent claudication will deteriorate progressively [36]. It is also important to mention that for patients with type 2 diabetes, PVD is neither the only nor the most important cause for foot ulcerations and/or amputations. In two recent studies [27, 29], lower limb ischemia was quoted as a component cause in 35% of the studied pathways for ulceration but it was not a sufficient cause for foot ulcers in any patient and, respectively, a component cause in 46% and a sufficient cause in 5% of the patients with amputations.

Even if PVD in patients with diabetes and in patients without diabetes has common patho-physiological and clinical features, there are some important characteristics of the first group [14, 34]. Some of these characteristics are summarized in Table 20.1.

A characteristic of peripheral arterial involvement in patients with diabetes is the high frequency of medial sclerosis (Monckeberg disease), consisting of increased arterial wall stiffness due to calcium deposits in the tunica media. Medial sclerosis leads to non-compressible peripheral vessels and artificially elevated systolic pressure, conditions with a prevalence in the total diabetic population of 5–10% [12] that is increasing with age and diabetes duration. Last but not least, medial sclerosis in patients with diabetes is an important risk indicator of the overall mortality for cardiovascular causes [39]. In one study [15], the mortality rate in patients with medial sclerosis was 3 times higher than in patients without medial sclerosis.

The involvement of microcirculation in lower limb pathology in patients with diabetes has been a matter of intense debate, but a recent international consensus [14] stated: "micro-angiopathy should never be accepted as the primary cause of an ulcer". In spite of the increased thicknes of the basal membrane in the microcirculation, the oxygen diffusion is not impaired and the only determinant of peripheral perfusion is the patency of large and medium arteries.

Table 20.1. Some characteristics of atherosclerotic PVD in patients with type 2 diabetes mellitus compared to those without diabetes

Characteristic	Patients with diabetes mellitus	Patients without diabetes mellitus
Global prevalence (ankle/arm index <0.9)	~21%	~3%
Sex distribution (males/females)	1/1	20/1
Localization	Infrapopliteal Multisegmental Bilateral	Aorto-iliac and femoral segments Unilateral
Collateral circulation impairment	Frequent	Unusual
Risk for amputation	60‰ /yr	28.3‰ /yr

Epidemiological Data Relevant for Clinical Assessment of Peripheral Vascular Disease in Type 2 Diabetes Mellitus

The main criteria used until now in epidemiological studies regarding the incidence and prevalence of PVD in the general population and also in the diabetic population are: the presence or absence of intermittent claudication, the presence or absence of foot arteries pulses and the ankle/arm systolic pressure index. But in patients with type 2 diabetes the usage of these criteria has some important limitation: the late appearance or even the absence of intermittent claudication in spite of severe impairment of blood flow and the relative high frequency of medial sclerosis that can produce false-negative cases when the ankle/arm pressure ratio is used. It is also important to mention that the prevalence of PVD in patients with diabetes increases sharply with the duration of diabetes. In a population-based cohort study in Rochester, the cumulative incidence of PVD was 15% at 10 years after the diagnosis of diabetes and 45% after 20 years, without taking into account the 8% of the patients who already had PVD at the initial diagnosis of diabetes [25].

In a personal evaluation of 350 consecutive patients with type 2 diabetes (unpublished data), the prevalence of PVD (ankle/arm index <0.9) doubled from 10 to 30 years of duration of diabetes, with a significant higher prevalence in males only in the first decade of diabetes evolution (Table 20.2).

All the epidemiological studies, either population-based or hospital settings-based, have demonstrated a higher prevalence of PVD in patients with diabetes than in those without diabetes. In population-based studies, when pulse deficits were used as diagnosis criteria, the prevalence of PVD in patients with diabetes was between 10.5% in the study of Palumbo P.J. et al. [25] and 30.11% in a Finnish study [31]. In this last study, made on randomly selected newly diagnosed male patients with type 2 diabetes, the prevalence of intermittent claudication was 8.8% and an ankle-arm pressure ratio <<0.9 was recorded in 7.3%. In another study conducted in Finland by Laakso M et al [19], the prevalence of intermittent claudication was between 5.4% and 21.6% in men and between 5.8% and 7.7% in women with diabetes and 2.9–5.9% and, respectively, 0.8–1.8% in those without diabetes. The prevalence was greater in the Eastern part of the country than in the Western part.

In the US hospital discharge list, in the period 1989–1991, the codes for peripheral vascular disease was mentioned in 3.3% of the patients with diabetes and in 0.59% in those without diabetes.

Regarding the incidence, in a 5-year prospective study in patients with type 2 diabetes and using the intermittent claudication as diagnostic criteria, the cumulative

Table 20.2. Influence of diabetes duration on prevalence of PVD

Diabetes duration	Prevalence of PVD Females	Males	P value
≤9	20.7	39.1	0.010
10–19	19.4	42.1	0.08
20–29	57.1	75.0	0.95
≥30	21.7	40.0	0.172

incidence was 20.3% in males and 21.8% in females compared to 8% and, respectively, 4.2% in control subjects, meaning a higher incidence in females than in males [38]. These results resemble those of the Framingham study in which after 34 years of follow-up the age-adjusted incidence of intermittent claudication was 2.4 times higher in females and 2 times higher in males with diabetes than in subjects without diabetes [7]. In this study, the adjustments were made also for blood pressure, body mass index, HDL cholesterol and smoking.

The incidence of new episodes of gangrene in patients with diabetes but without PVD is 4.5/1000 patients/year compared to 29.6 ‰ and 37‰ in men and women with PVD [25]. The group of patients with ankle/arm pressure index lower than 0.45 had an adjusted amputation odds ratio of 55.8 compared to those with the index value higher than 0.7 in the Seattle VA study [27].

In comparison with patients with diabetes and without intermittent claudication, the 10 years cardiovascular mortality rate of those with intermittent claudication is 5 times greater [11].

Specific Patterns of Risk for PVD in Patients with Type 2 Diabetes Mellitus

There are by now considerable arguments (experimental, epidemiological and clinical) sustaining that the process of atherogenesis in the lower limbs arteries and its consequences in patients with type 2 diabetes are driven by the same so-called "classical" risk factors (some of them inherited, unmodifiable, others environmental) as in non-diabetic population, but which are acting earlier in life and are more aggressive. Beside this general assumption, there are some specific aspects. The results of the Framingham study have revealed the fact that the incidence of PVD in patients with diabetes compared to the general population was higher than the same comparison for coronary heart disease [17]. It means that the PVD is a more characteristic manifestation of atherosclerosis in the patients with type 2 diabetes than the coronary localization of the disease, at least in terms of epidemiology [39]. The reasons why atherosclerosis preferably affects the legs of patients with diabetes are not fully explained. Some of these will be discussed further on.

Smoking

Confirming a long-standing clinical impression that smoking and hypertension are frequently associated with PVD, Palumbo P J et al. identified that in patients with diabetes, vascular disease, the ankle/arm index, current smoking and the arm systolic blood pressure are independent risk factors for the progression of PVD [25]. Several studies suggested that in the general population the association between smoking and PVD might be even stronger than between smoking and coronary heart disease [36]. A correlation between the severity of PVD and the number of cigarettes has also been demonstrated. An important argument to be used in persuading patients to abandon smoking is that the claudication-free walking distance increases rapidly after smoking cessation. However, in a recent technical review [23] there are several studies mentioned that failed to show an association of cigarette smoking with an increased risk of peripheral vascular disease in patients with diabetes, or the association was present only for proximal localization (pelvic, femuro-popliteal), or even if the association was present, the statistical significance was borderline. However, in the recently published by ADA "Standards of Medical Care for Patients with Diabetes Mellitus" (1), smoking cessation is considered as having A-Level evidence for the prevention and management of diabetes complications.

Insulin Resistance

Being a "common soil" also for type 2 diabetes mellitus and for atherosclerosis [32], the insulin resistance syndrome brings together several aspects as dyslipidemia, hypertension and obesity, that are all accepted as risk factors for PVD [39]. However, until now, there are few and with conflicting results studies regarding the association between insulin resistance / sensitivity and PVD.

Endothelial Dysfunction

Altered endothelial function in patients with type 1 and type 2 diabetes mellitus DM, implying decreased nitric-oxide (NO) synthesis and/or increased NO degradation was demonstrated as an atherogenic mechanism [10, 21]. Several studies revealed that in patients with PVD the level of NO syntethase inhibitors is increased [4], the infusion of arginine (the NO precursor) increased the leg blood flow and increased also the claudication-free walking distance [3, 5].

Neuropathy

The influence of the coexistence of diabetic neuropathy, especially of peripheral diabetic polineuropathy, on the clinical presentation of PVD is a long-standing observation. Several studies during the last years initiated discussion that neuropathy can be also implicated in the pathogenesis of PVD by the loss of the neural control of the smooth muscle cell growth, enhanced synthesis of calcium binding proteins and by the impairment of compensatory enlargement of atherosclerotic vessels (impaired vascular remodeling) and of collateral vessels formation [31].

It is important to recall the well-known effects of autonomic neuropathy on the peripheral microcirculation: increased arterio-venous shunting, redistribution of cutaneous blood flow, loss of postural vasoconstriction and reduced reactive hyperemic response [37].

Other Factors

There are several reviews published concerning other atherogenic risk factors and mechanisms in type 2 diabetes, as the glycation of proteins, inflammation, oxidative stress, haemorheological abnormalities, but without specific references to PVD [19, 30, 31]. Nevertheless, two demographic characteristics, the age and the duration of diabetes, are independent risk factors (as mentioned in epidemiological data) strongly correlated to PVD [21].

Clinical Assessment of PVD

The clinical assessment of PVD in the every day practice must rely initially on the history taking and on careful physical examination. For several reasons mentioned before the clinical presentation of PVD in patients with diabetes can be misleading. Two out of three patients may not be aware of the presence of the disease and may express no complaints [2].

Symptoms

The most common symptom of the chronic and progressive arterial obstruction of the lower limbs, the underlying pathological mechanism of PVD, is the *intermittent claudication*. Rose G A et al. defined it as pain in the calf that develops upon walking and is relieved within 10 minutes of rest [22]. The frequent association of peripheral neuropathy and topographic characteristic of arterial obstruction in patients with diabetes (infrapopliteal localization) are explanations for the fact that intermittent claudication is missing even if the blood perfusion is severely impaired. These are the reasons why the Rose questionnaire has a low sensitivity and a low clinical and epidemiological usefulness in patients with diabetes [14]. In a series of almost 500 volunteers with diabetes the presence of claudication had 22% sensitivity and 96% specificity compared to non-invasive tests [22]. In another study of 687 patients with diabetes [5], using as diagnostic criterion an ankle/arm index < 0.50, the history of claudication sensitivity and specificity was 50%, respectively 87.5%. In the same study, another symptom, the history of cold feet, had 52.6 % sensitivity and 53.8% specificity.

The intermittent claudication can remain relatively stable over years in terms of pain-free walking distance but can also have a progressive trend. The symptomatic stabilization may be due to the development of collaterals, metabolic adaptation of ischemic muscle by an increase in aerobic enzyme content and capillary density, or the patient's self altering of gait in order to favor the nonischemic muscle group [36]. All these adapting mechanisms are less likely to act in patients with diabetes than in non-diabetic subjects.

The *ischemic rest pain* is the result of inadequate blood flow even at rest. This is a persistent or recurrent pain, mostly at night, which is relieved only by lowering the legs and is exacerbated by lifting them, by heat or by the smallest physical exercise. The persistence of rest pain requiring regular analgesia for more than two weeks and/or the presence of ulceration or gangrene, both associated with an ankle systolic pressure of less than 50 mm Hg and/or a toe systolic pressure of less than 30 mm Hg, are the criteria for diagnosing the *chronic critical ischemia* proposed by the European Consensus Document [13]. These criteria are based on the assumption that there are no differences between diabetic and non-diabetic patients concerning critical ischemia. However, studies in diabetic patients suggest that the cut-off pressure levels are inaccurate [13]. Diabetic polineuropathy can mask critical ischemia, meaning that patients with diabetes can tolerate systolic pressure of less than 50 mm Hg without symptoms [34].

The most time-honored classification of PVD is the Fountaine stadialization (1954) that is based on symptoms and includes four stages:

- Stage I: asymptomatic PVD
- Stage II: intermittent claudication (with the subdivision IIa and II b, meaning mild or severe claudication in terms of longer or shorter pain-free walking distance)
- Stage III: ischemic rest pain
- Stage IV: ulceration or gangrene

The usefulness of this classification in patients with diabetes may be limited due to the reasons mentioned before [14].

Finally, it must not be forgotten that lower limb pain is a matter of differential diagnosis and other causes (e.g. venous claudication, peripheral nerve pain, osteoarticular diseases) are to be excluded.

Signs

Inspection of the lower limbs, pulse palpation and auscultation for bruits are the basic methods of clinical examination. Even if the information collected through these methods has a limited sensitivity, specificity and predictive value in patients with type 2 diabetes, simplicity and accessibility are overwhelming advantages.

Muscle atrophy, decreased hair growth, hypertrophied and slow-growing nails, thin and dry skin are signs that can be commonly found, even in patients with mild claudication.

The main task in the physical evaluation of PVD is the palpation of pulses. The common sites where the pulses must be searched are the dorsal part of the foot for dorsalis pedis, the region just behind the internal maleola for the posterior tibial artery, and then the popliteal region and the Scarpa triangle for the popliteal and common femoral arteries. Pulses can be graded as absent, diminished and normal. Room temperature, the training of the examiner, the biological variation and the presence of edema are important determinants of the sensitivity/specificity of the method and explains quite high interobserver variation. The dorsalis pedis artery is congenitally absent in around 12% of children aged from 1 to 10 years (Leng GC, Fowkes FGR, 1992).

The auscultation of bruits together with a diminished/absent pulse to distal arteries is valuable information. If the pulses disappear and the bruits accentuate after a short exercise the information is more worthwhile.

The sensitivity and the specificity of the pulse palpation were 67% and 69% using a standard composed of blood pressure treadmills and Doppler studies [22]. Absent peripheral pulses predicted an ankle/arm index below 0.5, with 65.2% sensitivity and 78.3% specificity in a series of 687 patients with diabetes [6]. In the same study a venous filling time > 20 sec (evaluated with the Ratschow procedure) identified only 4.9% of those with ankle/arm index < 0.5 but excluded 97.4% of those without this value of the index. The sensitivity/specificity of other signs in that group of patients were 47.8%/71% for decreased lower extremity hair, 50%/69.7% for atrophic skin and 65.2% / 47.0% for cool skin.

The recommendation of a consensus committee [36] is that *"pulse palpation should be correlated with claudication distance and location of pain, for they usually indicate location and severity of the responsible arterial lesion(s). Auscultation of bruits may give additional useful information"*. Palpating a normal popliteal but no

Table 20.3. Characteristics of neuro-ischemic and neuropathic foot lesions

Characteristic	Neuroischemic	Neuropathic
Localization	Lateral surfaces of the foot, big toe, heel	Anterior plant (metatarsal heads, high pressure points)
Surrounding skin	Thin, atrophic	Hyperkeratotic
Pulses	Reduced/absent	Evident
Local signs if infection is present	Reduced	Evident
Foot temperature	Decreased	Normal/warm foot
Pain	Present	Absent

pedal pulses associated with moderate claudication indicates infrapopliteal occlusive disease quite common in patients with type 2 diabetes.

As it was mentioned before, it is not unusual for a *foot lesion (ulceration or gangrene)* to be the first clinical sign of PVD in patients with diabetes. So, the correct analysis of the characteristics of the feet lesion is mandatory. The purely ischemic lesion of the foot, with no concomitant neuropathy, is rarely seen in diabetic patients and, for practical purposes, the lesions are classified in neuro-ischemic and neuropathic [12]. The neuroischemic ulcerations are usually smaller, painful (depending on the degree of coexisting neuropathy, with regular edges located on the big toe, lateral surfaces of the foot or on the heel (see Table 20.3). Tissue necrosis is precipitated by a minor trauma and can become quite rapidly extensive.

Last but not least, a careful physical examination must recognize other possible cardiovascular conditions that can affect the peripheral circulation as arrhythmias, valvular heart diseases, anemia or aortic aneurysm.

Noninvasive Assessment of the PVD in Patients with Type 2 Diabetes Mellitus

With a better standardization and an increasing accessibility, the noninvasive exploration of PVD, mainly the ankle/arm systolic pressure index measurement, has become a currently recommended method for screening and diagnosis of PVD in patients with diabetes [24]. There are several reasons for which the instrumental noninvasive methods are useful in patients with diabetes:

- The long subclinical evolution and the atypical clinical presentation of PVD
- The significant cardiovascular morbidity and mortality risk imposed by the discovery of PVD, even in asymptomatic patients:
- PVD is the most important prognostic factor for the outcome of a diabetic foot ulcer [13]
- The invasive exploration – angiography – has a supplemental risk for adverse events in patients with diabetes

Pressure Measurement

The ankle systolic pressure, measured at both foot arteries, anterior and posterior tibial arteries with a hand-held continuous ultrasound Doppler device is now the most widely noninvasive method used for routine assessment of PVD [9, 14, 24, 35, 36]. The cuff used is the same as for brachial pressure (12 cm width) and is placed above the ankle. Then, it is inflated to a pressure sufficient to stop the distal blood flow. The arterial flow sounds heard with a Doppler device on limb arteries with normal hemodynamics are triphasic (or at least biphasic), whereas in the presence of a significant obstruction single phase sounds are heard [9]. The pressure required to stop the flow during inflation of the cuff (closing pressure) is higher than the pressure at which the flow restarts during deflation. The measurement of the systolic pressure is a more sensitive index of the stenotic process than a measurement of blood flow [9].

The ankle/arm systolic pressure index (AAI), named also as Winsor index, is calculated by dividing the ankle pressure by the arm (brachial) pressure. The intra and inter-observer variation can be diminished if the arm and ankle pressure are measured with the same method (hand-held Doppler device) and the arm pressure is measured on both sides and the highest value is used for calculation [34]. Finally, four AA indexes are to be calculated, two for each foot.

In the absence of significant stenosis, as a consequence of the systolic amplification through the vascular tree, the ankle pressure is almost always greater than the arm pressure. The lower normal limit for the AAI has been defined as 0.97 [9]. An AAI below 0.9 has 95% sensitivity and almost 100% specificity in detecting angiogram-positive disease [23]. AAI equal or below 0.6 is a criterion for defining the critical ischemia. Chronic critical ischemia is defined also by the absolute ankle pressure value <50 mm Hg [13].

The ankle pressure measurement in patients with diabetes is complicated by the presence of medial calcinosis which represents the main limitation of this method [9, 23, 35]. Decreased compressibility of the arteries in this situation results in the falsely elevated systolic pressure. An AAI higher than 1.3 is highly specific for the presence of medial sclerosis but medial calcium deposits are present also at normal ranges of AAI and in up to 30% of patients with diabetes with AAI below 1.0 [40]. An AAI >1.15 may be considered unreliable and further evaluations are needed [35].

Ankle pressure measurement before and after treadmill exercise or other means for inducing limb hyperaemia may add valuable information [36].

In a recent consensus conference [24], AAI was recommended to be used together with the claudication history and pulse palpation for screening in patients with type 1 diabetes older than 35 years or with >20 years duration of diabetes and for all patients with type 2 diabetes older than 40 years.

The toe systolic pressure measurement with an adapted (smaller) cuff and using a flow sensor as the photo pletismography may offer a more accurate reflection of blood supply to the foot, being a substitute for ankle pressure measurement when that one is falsely elevated [36]. The toe pressure is normally 10 mm Hg less than the ankle pressure and even in long-standing diabetes the digital arteries are not usually calcified. A toe systolic pressure = 30 mm Hg is also a criterion for chronic critical ischemia [13] and it is in only 45% of the patients with such a toe pressure that a foot ulcer heals [35].

Pulse Volume Recordings and Doppler Velocity Wave Form Analysis

The pulse volume recording (or segmental pletismography) and the Doppler velocity waveform (VWF) analysis are used in some laboratories for noninvasive detection of the site of limb artery occlusion. By detecting volume variation or differences in the magnitude and contour of VWF, at different levels of the legs, these two methods are accurate enough in detecting and localizing arterial occlusion but they cannot further characterize it [36].

Doppler Ultrasound Scanning (Duplex Scanning)

This technique combines echography and Doppler analysis to localize and determine the significance of a stenosis. It offers the opportunity to perform together hemodynamic and morphologic assessment of an arterial segment. The introduction of echo-color Doppler devices aided for earlier and faster vessel exploration. The main limitation of this method is that it offers no information regarding the tissue perfusion. However, arterial reconstructive surgery can be performed on the basis of duplex scanning only in some cases [36].

Magnetic Resonance Angiography

Magnetic resonance angiography (MRA) may be a practical compromise between echo-Doppler scanning and angiography. At present, more studies are required regarding performance, accessibility and cost/effectiveness of this method.

Transcutaneous Oxygen Measurement

Oxygen tension is an accurate parameter of tissue blood perfusion but general factors (respiratory function, cardiac output and hemoglobin level) and local factors (edema, thickness of the tegument) can influence it. The values obtained are directly influenced by the cutaneous blood flow, metabolic activity, hemoglobin dissociation, and oxygen diffusion through the tissues [36]. To exclude the contribution of general factors (see above), a comparison with the value taken in the infraclavicular region is useful. In patients with diabetes, values of transcutaneous oxygen pressure ($TcPO_2$) of 10 mm Hg or less give a minor 20 % probability of healing of a lesion and this probability increases to 80 % at 40 mm Hg or more [14]. Measuring the $TcPO_2$ at rest and during hyperemia (induced by warming of the foot at 44°C) can provide additional information.

Invasive Vascular Diagnostic Procedures

Angiography remains the golden standard for the assessment of PVD including patients with diabetes [14, 23, 36]. The improvements made during the last years (digital subtraction technique, nonionic contrast substances, increased speed in execution) have decreased invasiveness and the complication incidence of this procedure. The objective of angiography is to define whether impaired blood flow in limbs could be approached either by reconstructive surgery (bypass) or by percutaneous angioplasty. The evaluation of the renal function, sufficient hydration of the patient and withholding of biguanides 48 hours before the procedure are mandatory for patients with type 2 diabetes. The specific technique of injecting the contrast media as femoral catheterization and injection of the substance in the infrarenal aorta, the transhumeral catheterization, the anterograde femoral approach and the use of the oblique incidence are chosen by the specialist. It is very important to have the best visualization of the infra polpliteal arteries.

Angiography should be considered in any lesion where there is clinical evidence of significant ischemia [16].

Key Points

- Overwhelming epidemiological data demonstrate that the incidence, prevalence and risk of progression to amputation of PVD are higher in patients with type 2 diabetes than in the general population.
- Together with the loss of protective sensation, bony deformities and a history of ulcer, decreased or absent pedal pulses are conditions associated with an increased risk for amputations.
- The annual screening for PVD through a relatively simple clinical assessment (palpation of foot pulses) can be accomplished in a primary care setting (B-Level of evidence) (1). The annual evaluation of the ankle/arm systolic pressure index is also reccomanded by experts (24).
- Referring the patients with claudication for further vascular assesment has a C-level of evidence.
- The complete cardiovascular workup of patients with diabetes and PVD is mandatory since their cardiovascular mortality is 4 – 5 times higher than of those without PVD.

References

1. American Diabetes Association (2002) Standards of Medical Care for Patients With Diabetes Mellitus.Diabetes Care 25 :S33-S49
2. Banga JD (1994) Lower extremity arterial disease in diabetes mellitus. Diabetes Reviews International 3, 4: 6-11
3. Bode-Boger SM, Boger RH, Alfke H et al (1996) L-arginine induces nitric oxide-dependent vasodilatation in patients with critical ischemia. A randomized, controlled study. Circulation 93: 85-90
4. Boger RH, Bode-Boger SM, Thiele W et al (1997) Biochemical evidence for impaired oxide synthesis in patients with peripheral arterial occlusive disease. Circulation 95: 2068-2074
5. Boger RH, Bode-Boger SM, Thiele W et al (1998) Restoring nitric oxide formation by L-arginine improves the symptoms of intermittent claudication in patients with peripheral arterial occlusive disease. Circulation 32: 1336-1344
6. Boyko EJ, Ahroni JH, Davignon DSV et al (1977) Diagnostic utility of history and physical examination for peripheral vascular disease among patients with diabetes mellitus. J.Clin.Epidemiol.50: 659-668
7. Brand FN, Abbot RD, Kannel WB (1989) Diabetes, intermittent claudication and risk of cardiovascular events. The Framingham study. Diabetes 38: 504-507
8. Carter AS (1985) Role of pressure measurements in vascular disease. Bernstein FE (ed) Noninvasive diagnostic techniques in vascular disease, The CV Mosby Comp. St.Louis, Toronto, Princeton: 513-539
9. Carter SA (1969) Clinical measurement of systolic pressure in limbs with arterial occlusive disease. JAMA 207: 1869-1874
10. Chan NN, Vallence P, Colhoun HM (2000) Nitric oxide and vascular response in type 1 diabetes. Diabetologia 43: 137-147

11. Criqui MH, Langer RD, Froner A (1992) Mortality over a period of 10 years in patients with peripheral arterial disease. N Engl J Med 326: 381-384
12. Edmonds ME, Foster AVM (1994) Classification and management of neuropathic and neuro-ischemic ulcers. In: Boulton AJM, Connor H, Cavanagh PR (eds). The Foot in Diabetes 2nd edition John Wiley & Sons Ltd., Chichester, New York, Brisbane, Toronto, Singapore, pp 109-120
13. European Society of Vascular Surgery: Chronic Critical Leg Ischaemia (1992). Eur J Vasc Surg 6: 6-13
14. International Working Group on the diabetic foot (1999) International consensus on the diabetic foot: 33-41
15. Janka HU, Standl E, Schultz K et al (1980) Mediasclerose bei Diabetikern – eine sonderfarm der macroangipathie. Vasa 9: 281-284
16. Jeffcoate W, MacFarlane R The diabetic foot. An illustrated guide to management. Chapman&Hall Medical London-Glasgow-Weinheim-New York-Tokyo-Melbourne-Madras: 52-68
17. Kannel WB, McGee DL (1979) Diabetes and glucose intolerance as risk factors for cardiovascular disease: the Framingham study. Diabetes Care 2: 120-125
18. Kannel WB, Skinner JJ, Schwartz MJ et al. (1970) Intermittent Claudication: Incidence in the Framingham Study. Circulation 41: 875-883
19. King LG, Wakasaki H (1999) Theoretical mechanisms by which hyperglycemia and insulin resistance could cause cardiovascular disease in diabetes. Diabetes Care 22: C31-C37
20. Laakso M, Rounemmaa T, Pyorala K et al. (1988) Atherosclerotic vascular disease and its risk factors in non-insulin-dependent diabetic and nondiabetic subjects in Finland. Diabetes Care 11, 449-453
21. Makimattila S, Liu ML, Vakkilainen J et al (1999) Impaired endothelium dependent vasodilatation in type 2 diabetes. Relation to LDL size, oxidized LDL and antioxidants. Diabetes Care 22: 973-981
22. Marinelli MR, Beach KW, Glass MJ et al. (1979) Noninvasive testing versus clinical evaluation of arterial disease. J. Ann. Med. Assoc. 241: 2031-2034
23. Mayfield AJ, Reiber EG, Sanders JL et al. (1998) Preventive foot care in people with diabetes. Diabetes Care 21: 2161-2177
24. Orchard TJ, Strandness DEjr (1993) Assessment of peripheral vascular disease in diabetes: report and recommendations of an international workshop sponsored by the American Diabetes Association and the American Heart Association. Circulation 88:818-828
25. Palumbo PJ, Melton LJ (1995) Peripheral Vascular Disease in Diabetes. In: Diabetes care in America 2nd edition National Institute of Health, National Institute of Diabetes and Digestive and Kidney Diseases, NIH Publication 95-1468: 401-408
26. Palumbo PJ, O'Fallon WM, Osmundson PJ et al (1991) Progression of peripheral occlusive arterial disease in diabetes mellitus. Arch Intern Med 151: 717-721
27. Pecoraro RE, Reiber GE, Burgess EM (1990) Pathway to diabetic limb amputations: basis for prevention. Diabetes Care 13: 513-521
28. Reiber GE, Pecoraro RE, Koepsell TD (1992) Risk factors for amputations in patients with diabetes mellitus. A case-control study. Ann Int Med 117: 97-105
29. Reiber GE, Vileikyte L, Boyko JE et al. (1999) Causal pathway for incident lower-extremity ulcers in patients with diabetes from two settings. Diabetes Care 22: 157-162
30. Rivellesse A, Villa V, Sacco M (1999) Macroangiopathy and the diabetic foot. In Faglia E, Giuffrida G, Oriani G (eds)The ischaemic diabetic foot , Editrice Kurtis s.r.l. Milano : 7-15
31. Schaper NC, Nabuurs-Franssen MH, Huijberts MSP (2000) Peripheral vascular disease in type 2 diabetes mellitus. Diabetes Metab Res Rev 16: S11-S15
32. Siitonen O, Uusitupa M, Pyorala K et al. (1986) Peripheral arterial disease and its relationship to cardiovascular risk factors and coronary heart disease in newly diagnosed non-insulin-dependent diabetics. Acta Med Scand 220: 205-212
33. Stern M (1999) Natural history of macrovascular disease in type 2 diabetes. Diabetes Care 22: C2-C5
34. Stiegler H (1977) The burden of peripheral vascular disease in diabetes. Reducing the burden of diabetes: 5-8
35. Takolander R, Rauwerda JA (1996) The use of noninvasive vascular assessment in diabetic patient with foot lesions. Diabetic Med. 13: S39-S42

36. Transatlantic Inter-society Consensus (2000) Management of Peripheral Arterial Disease. European Journal of Vascular and Endovascular Surgery 19, suppl A: S4-S30
37. Uccioli L (1999) The influence of neuropathy on macro- and microcirculation. In Faglia E, Giuffrida G, Oriani G (eds) The ischaemic diabetic foot, Editrice Kurtis s.r.l. Milano : 25-30
38. Uusitupa M, Niskanen LK, Siitonen O (1990) 5 years incidence of atherosclerotic vascular disease in relation to general risk factors, insulin level and abnormalities in lipoprotein composition in non-insulin-dependent diabetic and non diabetic subjects. Circulation 82: 27-30
39. Vaccaro O, Cuomo V (1999) Epidemiology of peripheral vascular disease in diabetes mellitus. In: Faglia E, Giuffrida G, Oriani G (eds). The Ischemic Diabetic Foot. Editrice Kurtis s.r.l., Milano, pp 1-6
40. Young MJ, Adams JE, Boulton AJM, Cavanagh PR (1993) Medial arterial calcification in feet of diabetic patients and matched non-diabetic control subjects. Diabetologia 24: 347-350

CHAPTER 21

Global Approach to Cardiovascular Risk in Type 2 Diabetic Persons

N. Hâncu, A. Cerghizan

Abstract. Type 2 diabetes is associated with a marked increase in both cardiovascular risk and disease. This risk is multifactorial, including from a practical point of view at least five "bad companions": hyperglycemia, hypertension, dyslipidemia, obesity and smoking. The prothrombotic state can also be added.

In clinical setting the global approach to cardiovascular risk is the only recognized way to achieve a control of all these five factors and a subsequent reduction of cardiovascular morbidity and mortality.

The global approach means the following steps: 1) the identification and evaluation of each risk factor, 2) the evaluation of global cardiovascular risk, 3) the intervention for each risk factor.

The implementation of global approach to cardiovascular risk in type 2 diabetes is a huge task for practitioners implying a high effort. But this is worth doing because the significant benefits have been demonstrated.

Overview of Cardiovascular Risk

From the General Population to People with Type 2 Diabetes

Global cardiovascular risk represents the action and consequences of all risk factors which simultaneously or sequentially act on the body, leading to atherogenesis / atherosclerosis with their clinical or subclinical entities: coronary heart disease, cerebrovascular disease, peripheral arteriopathy, aortic aneurism.

As in type 2 diabetes there is a heavy burden of cardiovascular disease (see chapter 1), some authorities have recently considered that *it may be appropriate to say ... diabetes is a cardiovascular disease* [39]. Hence *preventing this complication of diabetes is undoubtedly one of the biggest therapeutic challenges for the new millenium*. In this context the global cardiovascular risk has become one of the most exciting and important problems for people with diabetes mainly type 2.

There is growing evidence that through the control of multiple risk factors these tremendous complications could be reduced. This is *a complex but achievable and affordable task* [90].

It is beyond the scope of this chapter to make an exhaustive analysis of risk factors. We will only comment on the main new concepts in the light of recent guidelines or statements [105, 63, 104, 36, 32, 39, 7, 24, 41], and see how they are reflected in type 2 diabetes. This will be useful for a better understanding of the second part of the chapter where we will focus on the practical approach to the global cardiovascular risk.

Risk Factors and the Concept of the Global Risk

The concept of global risk has emerged from the well-known and already classical investigations: the Framingham Study [66], the Multiple Risk Factors Intervention Trial – MRFIT [91] and the Münster Heart Study – PROCAM [2]. They clearly showed that the development of coronary heart disease is mainly caused by two or more risk factors. Importantly, they have a multiplicative effect. This global risk is *greater than would be expected from a simple addition of each risk* [63].

The importance of the concept of global risk is very high because only through a global approach of risk factors, a real benefit can be attained [76]. In clinical setting the "global risk" is seen as a "multiple risk patient".

It should be mentioned that the true sense of risk factors is mainly referred to coronary heart disease although it has been extrapolated to other atherosclerotic cardiovascular diseases or macrovascular diseases. The facts do not entirely support this extrapolation, but it appears to be useful for practitioners.

Cardiovascular risk factors (or more precisely coronary risk factors) can be characterized as: modifiable or non-modifiable risk factors (Table 21.1); as causal, conditional, predisposing or plaque burden risk factors (Table 21.2); as absolute, relative or attributable risk (Table 21.3). Each of them is important and has to be recognized by practitioners involved in diabetes care and preventive cardiology.

Table 21.1. Lifestyle and characteristics associated with increased risk of future coronary heart disease events (from [105] with kind permission)

Lifestyle	Biochemical or physiological characteristics (modifiable)	Personal characteristics (non-modifiable)
Diet high in saturated fat, cholesterol and calories	Elevated blood pressure	Age
Cigarette smoking	Elevated plasma total cholesterol (LDL-cholesterol)	Sex
Excess alcohol consumption	Low plasma HDL-cholesterol	Family history of CHD or other atherosclerotic vascular disease at early age (in men < 55 years, in women < 65 years)
Physical inactivity	Elevated plasma triglycerides Hyperglycemia/diabetes Obesity Thrombogenic factors	Personal history of CHD or other atherosclerotic vascular disease

Primary and Secondary Prevention

As far as we are aware the concept of risk factors is related to the primary and the secondary prevention of coronary heart disease and other atherosclerotic diseases. In Table 21.4 we have compiled the main data on this subject.

Table 21.2. Categories of risk factors according to mechanism emerge (according to data from [32])

Category	Risk factors
Causal or major	Cigarette smoking High blood pressure Elevated serum cholesterol or LDL cholesterol Low HDL cholesterol High plasma glucose
Conditional	Elevated levels of: Serum triglycerides Lipoprotein (a) Small, dense LDL particles Homocysteine Coagulation factors (fibrinogen, PAI-1)
Predisposing	Obesity Physical inactivity Family history of premature CHD Male sex Possibly behavioral, socio-economic and ethnic factors Insulin resistance
Plaque burden	Age Intimal medial thickness of the carotid arteries (measured by sonography) Coronary calcium scores (measured by electron-beam computerized tomography – EBCT) Subclinical ischemia (during exercise testing)

Table 21.3. Absolute, relative and attributable risk (according to data from [32])

Absolute risk (AR)	Definition	Probability of developing CHD over a finite period
	Stratification of probability	Low risk: low probability of CHD High risk: high probability of CHD
	Stratification according to period of developing CHD	Short-term: ≤ 10 years Long-term: > 10 years or over a lifetime
	Importance	AR should provide a guide to intensify the management in case of: High short-term risk High long-term risk
Relative risk (RR)	Definition	RR is the ratio of two levels of absolute risk (AR): RR = AR of the subject/AR of a baseline population
	Importance	RR has advantage in risk assessment and risk reduction strategy
Attributable risk (ATR)	Definition	ATR is the difference in absolute risk between the considered subject and that of a control group
	Importance	ATR is low in young adulthood and high in older age group

21 Global Approach to Cardiovascular Risk in Type 2 Diabetic Persons

Table 21.4. The concept of primary and secondary prevention (according to data from [36, 105, 63])

Primary prevention (PP)	Definition	All actions to modify risk factors or their development in order to delay or prevent new-onset coronary heart disease
	Importance	PP has to be considered for high risk persons both in short and long term
	Short-term, high risk prevention	The likelihood to develop a major coronary event is similar to that of patients with established coronary heart disease The patients focused are those with coronary heart disease risk equivalents (see below)
	CHD risk equivalents	Are considered for the patients without CHD but having at least one of the follows: 1. Abdominal aortic aneurism 2. Ischemia of the extremities 3. Substantial carotid atherosclerosis documented by clinical cerebral symptoms (transient ischemic attacks or stroke), sonography or angiography 4. Type 2 diabetes mellitus 5. Absolute risk > 20 % in 10 years
	Recommendations	For persons with CHD equivalents the strategy used for secondary prevention is recommended
	Long-term high risk prevention	Focuses the persons either with multiple marginal risk factors or by a single categorical risk factor All persons in this category deserve attention Long-term prevention represents a certain progress in preventive cardiology
Secondary prevention (SP)	Definition	SP means therapy to reduce recurrent CHD events and decrease coronary mortality in patients with established CHD
	Recommendations for:	1. Control of risk factors 2. Direct protection of coronary arteries from plaque eruption

Peculiarity of Cardiovascular Risk in Type 2 Diabetes

Cardiovascular risk in people with type 2 diabetes is similar to that of the general population but also has many and important peculiarities which will be commented later on.

All risk factors are considered potential determinants of macrovascular disease in type 2 diabetes. Their role is important even when atherosclerotic disease had already appeared, because they contribute to disease progression [105, 27, 11, 34].

The causal or major risk factors (Table 21.2) act also as independent determinants of cardiovascular disease. Very often they are clustered as in the metabolic syndrome [31] (Table 21.5) (see also Chapter 10).

The predisposing factors (Table 21.2): obesity, physical inactivity, heredity, sex and advanced age also influence the development of macrovascular disease in type 2 dia-

Table 21.5. The five determinants of the Metabolic Syndrome according to the ATP III [25]. Its diagnosis is made when any three of the five determinants are identified[a]

Determinants	Suggestive values
1. Abdominal obesity: waist circumferences	
Men	>102 cm
Women	>88 cm
2. Plasma triglycerides	≥150 mg/dl [1.7 mmol/l]
3. HDL cholesterol	
Men	<40 mg/dl [1.03 mmol/l]
Women	<50 mg/dl [1.29 mmol/l]
4. Blood pressure	≥130/≥85 mmHg
5. Fasting glucose	≥110 mg/dl [6.1 mmol/l]

[a] According to the WHO Report [99], the definition of the metabolic syndrome is suggested when glucose intolerance (IGT or IFG) or diabetes mellitus and/or insulin resistance is associated with two or more of other components as follows: raised blood pressure, raised plasma triglycerides and/or low HDL cholesterol, central obesity, microalbuminuria.

betes [39]. Nevertheless, their importance has been reconsidered after the results of UKPDS [97]. However, it has to be mentioned that these factors, often clustered as the metabolic syndrome, exacerbate the causal risk factors [31]. Conversely, macrovascular disease and hyperglycemia can be prevented and controlled by controlling some of the predisposing factors [99].

There is much evidence that in diabetics, conventional cardiovascular risk factors have the same impact as in non-diabetic individuals [105, 91, 87].

However, in diabetes, at any given risk factor levels, there is a much higher risk of an atherosclerotic cardiovascular event than in non-diabetic people [105, 91].

Type 2 diabetes is associated with more significant cardiovascular risk factors than type 1 diabetes [105] as shown in Table 21.6.

Premenopausal women with diabetes are not protected from cardiovascular disease: both women and men with diabetes are seen as having similar cardiovascular risks [70].

The cardiovascular risk factors in type 2 diabetes have a distinct spectrum in different manifestations of macrovascular disease as shown in Table 21.7.

Table 21.6. The main cardiovascular risk factors in newly diagnosed type 1 and type 2 diabetes; results from the first 2 years of the EPIDIAB study[a] [51]

Cardiovascular risk factors	Type 1 1,733 subjects	Type 2 26,787 subjects
DLP	2.78%*	50.26%
Obesity	20.80%*	48.50%
Overweight	16.66%*	33.80%
Hypertension	8.80%*	47.61%
Smokers	16.10%*	21.25%

[a] The EPIDIAB is a prospective study concerning the EPIdemia of DIABetes in Romania by focusing on newly diagnosed cases of disease.
* Statistical significant differences ($p < 0.001$).

Table 21.7. The spectrum of risk in macrovascular disease of type 2 diabetes (according to data from [70])

Risk factor	Coronary heart disease	Stroke	Amputation
Hyperglycemia	+	++	+++
Hemoglobin A1c	+	++	+++
Total cholesterol	++	+	+
HDL cholesterol	+++	++	(+)
Total triglycerides	+++	++	(+)
Hypertension	(+)	++	(+)
Duration of diabetes	+	+	+++
Medial arterial calcification	+++	+	+++

Table 21.8. The prevalence of atherosclerotic cardiovascular disease of newly diagnosed type 2 diabetes (data from UKPDS [70] and EPIDIAB study, first 2 years [51])

UKPDS 5,102 subjects	EPIDIAB 26,787 subjects
8%	31.5%

A few cardiovascular risk factors, namely hypertriglyceridemia, low plasma HDL cholesterol, hypertension, abdominal obesity, insulinresistance and hyperinsulinemia are also associated with impaired glucose tolerance which is considered a precursor of type 2 diabetes [70]. This explains why a significant number of people with newly diagnosed type 2 diabetes have already atherosclerotic disease [70] as shown in Table 21.8.

The analysis of baseline risk factors and their predictive power to cardiac end points in UKPDS have shown that [69]:

- Patients without evidence of disease relating to atheroma at diagnosis of type 2 diabetes had a quintet of modifiable risk factors: increased LDL cholesterol, decreased HDL cholesterol, hypertension, hyperglycemia, smoking and age as a non-modifiable risk factor. They have a different position in the model for coronary heart disease, non-fatal or fatal myocardial infarction (Table 21.9).
- Coronary risk factors in the general population change their importance once type 2 diabetes has developed. Abdominal obesity, sedentarism and hyperinsulinism were not found to be major risk factors in type 2 diabetes. Plasma triglycerides level was not found to be an independent risk factor, possibly because of the great variability of this lipid parameter. But postprandial triglycerides values may have an additional atherogenic role to the fasting levels [97].
- The variation of these risk factors and subsequent modification of coronary risk is shown in Table 21.10 according to the UKPDS data [97].

The importance of cardiovascular risk factors in type 2 diabetes has also emerged from impressive interventional trials, where hyperglycemia, hypertension and dyslipidemia have been focused.

Intensive glycemic control as achieved in UKPDS with either sulphonylurea or insulin, reduced significantly only the microvascular but not the macrovascular complications [98, 78, 96]. However in obese people with type 2 diabetes, well controlled

Table 21.9. Risk factors for coronary heart disease in UKPDS: stepwise selection adjusted for age and sex in 2,693 persons with type 2 diabetes with dependant variable as time to first event (according to data from [97])

Position in model	Coronary artery disease	Non-fatal or fatal myocardial infarction	Fatal myocardial infarction
First	LDL cholesterol	LDL cholesterol	Diastolic blood pressure (BP)
Second	HDL cholesterol	Diastolic BP	LDL cholesterol
Third	Hemoglobin A1c	Smoking	Hemoglobin A1c
Fourth	Systolic BP	HDL cholesterol	–
Fifth	Smoking	Hemoglobin A1c	–

Table 21.10. Variation of the main risk factors and modification of coronary risk; compiled from UKPDS data (according to data from [97])

Risk factors	Variation	Coronary risk
LDL cholesterol	↓ 40 mg/dl (1 mmol/l)	36% ↓
HDL cholesterol	↑ 4 mg/dl (0.1 mmol/l)	15% ↓
Hemoglobin A1c	↑ 1%	11% ↑
Systolic blood pressure	↑ 10 mm Hg	15% ↑

with metformin, a significant reduction of macrovascular complication was demonstrated [101].

Another important lesson comes from UKPDS [77,100] where it was concluded that the management of blood pressure should have a high priority in the treatment of type 2 diabetes because the tight control of blood pressure has clearly demonstrated a significant reduction of both microvascular and macrovascular disease. A similar conclusion has been drown from HOPE, microHOPE and HOT studies [59, 61].

The post-hoc analysis of the diabetic subgroups from 4 S and CARE studies has shown that secondary prevention in diabetic patients treated with simvastatin or pravastatin is effective [26, 43, 92, 88]. Moreover, the cardiovascular effect of LDL reduction by statins was greater (4S) or as great (CARE) as in the general population [45]. These results emphasize the role of the control of dyslipidemia in type 2 diabetic persons [20].

In addition, we must mention the beneficial effects of aspirin on macrovascular disease both in primary and secondary prevention [84, 16, 87].

An important fact has risen from studies concerning myocardial infarction and mortality of patients with type 2 diabetes. Haffner [45] based on two prospective studies [58, 80], concluded that patients with type 2 diabetes without preexisting myocardial infarction have a risk of developing myocardial infarction similar to non-diabetic patients with previous myocardial infarction. In addition the prehospital mortality is higher in patients with diabetes than in non-diabetic patients. These patients, who died before any treatment, by definition, could not have benefited from secondary prevention strategies. It means that in people with type 2 diabetes the treatment of cardiovascular risk factors must be as aggressive as in patients with established coronary heart disease [45].

All these facts clearly suggest that:

- The prevention of macrovascular disease in type 2 diabetes could be achieved by controlling the cardiovascular risk [19, 49, 86, 28, 52, 53].
- This can be accomplished only with a multifactorial intervention strategy, which must focus at least five *bad companions* in diabetes: hyperglycemia, hypertension, dyslipidemia, obesity and smoking.
- The interventions should be as aggressive and intensive as for patients with macrovascular disease. This means that in type 2 diabetes the difference between primary and secondary prevention has to be cancelled and all patients must be considered as candidates for secondary prevention irrespective of their cardiovascular status. In this respect it must be noted that in the new AHA guidelines on primary prevention of coronary heart disease, people with type 2 diabetes are included in the group of *coronary heart disease risk equivalents*. For them, secondary prevention is suggested [36, 32].

There is so far no intensive multifactorial intervention in type 2 diabetes to demonstrate the benefits on macrovascular disease endpoints and related mortality [21]. So far this has been shown only for microvascular complications [38]. However, the

Table 21.11. Traditional and so-called novel cardiovascular risk factors for people with diabetes (according to data from [105, 70, 64])

Traditional risk factors	So-called novel risk factors
Poor glycemic control	Increased Lp(a)
Dyslipidemia	Increased IDL
↑ Total cholesterol	Increased small dense LDL
↑ LDL cholesterol	Glycated and oxidized lipoproteins and albumin
↓ HDL cholesterol	Immune response to modified lipoprotein
↑ Triglycerides	Increased cholesterol ester transfer protein
Hypertension	Low level of paraoxonase (PON) and certain PON genotypes
Abdominal obesity	Hyperhomocysteinemia
Insulinresistance/hyperinsulinism	Markers of inflammation:
Physical inactivity	Increased white blood cell count
Hypercaloric/hyperlipidic intake	Increased C-reactive protein
Smoking	Infections with:
Increasing age	*Chlamydia pneumoniae*
Personal and familial history of atherosclerosis	*Helicobacter pylori*
Long duration of diabetes	Periodontal disease
Microalbuminuria	Markers of endothelial dysfunction:
Hemostatic factors	Increased von Willebrand factor
Impaired fibrinolytic activity:	Increased trombomodulin
↑Fibrinogen, ↑PAI-1, ↓tPA activity	Increased adhesion molecules
↑FPA, TAT, f VII	Medial artery calcification
Platelets, leucocytes and erythrocytes abnormalities	Postprandial state
↑Plasma viscosity	Depression
	Erectile dysfunction

PAI-1, plasminogen activator inhibitor 1; tPA, tissue plasminogen activator; FPA, fibrinopeptide A; TAT, thrombin – antithrombin; fVII, coagulation factor VII.

ADDITION study (Anglo-Danish-Dutch Study of Intensive Treatment In People with Screen Detected Diabetes in Primary Care) [73] which began in 2000 proposed this ambitious goal. Concomitantly, the ACCORD study (Action to Control Cardiovascular Risk in Diabetes) [69] will have the same main objectives.

Regarding the concept of risk, this is largely but not totally applied to people with diabetes. In addition there are many other factors both traditional and novel which are not included in Table 21.1. Perhaps the terms *traditional* and *novel* [64] are rather ambiguous or even sophisticated. However, they represent the permanent efforts made in this fascinating field, which remains a dynamic concept. There is an enormous number of risk factors, and only an orientative list is shown in Table 21.11. Not all factors presented here are validated by clinical trials. As a consequence not all of them are mentioned in clinical guidelines. In time, some of them will confirm their usefulness but others will not. Until the large-scale studies define which factors are valid, more important or even specific for diabetes, practitioners should extrapolate the data from the general population to people with diabetes.

From Knowledge to Daily Practice: The Control of Risk in People With Type 2 Diabetes

The golden rule of controlling cardiovascular risk in people with type 2 diabetes is to consider it as:

- A *global approach*, that means
- Global *identification* and *evaluation* of
- *All risk factors* in *every person*
- With an assessment of *global objectives*, and
- The *global achievement* of these objectives through
- *Intensive* and *multifactorial clinical management*
- *Considering all people with type 2 diabetes as candidates for secondary prevention strategy*

The stepwise implementation of all these actions seems to be the only reasonable way to achieve benefits in:

- The *control* of cardiovascular risk,
- The *prevention* of cardiovascular events and
- The *decrease of the burden* of cardiovascular disease in type 2 diabetes

In daily practice the actions shown in Table 21.12 should be considered. These actions are in line with the new proposals from the American Heart Association regarding ... *the pathway from risk assessment to risk reduction* [37] where three steps are involved:

- Measurements of risk factors
- Interpretation of risk – related data with an estimation of risk in both absolute and relative terms
- Intervention to minimize the actual risk or to prevent the development of other risks.

A simple look at these actions is enough to realize that they represent a very difficult task for practitioners [45]. This is due to the complex problems of people we are faced with, including the complexity of actions which they must accomplish. Moreover the

Table 21.12. The stepwise control of cardiovascular risk in persons with type 2 diabetes (see also Figs. 21.5, 21.6)

Actions	Focus on

Step 1: Identification	Cardiovascular risk factors (as much as possible)
	Cardiovascular disease such as:
	  Coronary heart disease (CHD)
	  CHD equivalents: aortic aneurism, ischemia of the extremities, carotid atherosclerosis

Step 2: Interpretation	Global cardiovascular risk: scores and stratification high, medium, low
	Type of prevention:
	  Primary: short-term high risk, long-term high risk
	  Secondary
	Objectives to be achieved for each factor and disease

Step 3: Intervention	For all identified risk factors and disease
	With appropriate clinical management, that is:
	  Lifestyle optimization: diet, physical exercise, alcohol reduction
	  Drugs
	  Therapeutical education
	  Current monitoring
	  Global evaluation

difficulties involved by including the risk control into a busy diabetologist's or family doctor's daily routine should be considered. These problems occur at each step proposed in Table 21.12.

In the light of these considerations we will focus on the practical aspects of identification and evaluation of cardiovascular risk and disease in people with type 2 diabetes, interpreting data in terms of global cardiovascular risk assessment and establishing the objectives and the subsequent intervention with adequate strategies. Many of these risk factors have already been presented in previous chapters and therefore we will only reiterate the principal aspects of the practical problems.

Identification and Evaluation of Cardiovascular Risk and Disease in Type 2 Diabetes

Identification and Evaluation of the Main Risk Factors

Identification and evaluation of the main cardiovascular risk factors in patients with type 2 diabetes is strongly and unanimously recommended in all principal international guidelines [14, 24, 62, 107, 55, 39, 23, 105, 63, 41, 5, 7, 89, 79, 103, 10, 47, 9, 6].

For practical purposes we have to take into account the major risk factors, the predisposing risk factors and if possible, to consider a few of the conditional risk factors (Table 21.13) and other conditions. In clinical setting the depression and erectile dysfunction must also be considered [102, 94, 98].

The identification and evaluation of risk factors in persons with type 2 diabetes should be made according to Grundy's recommendations (1999) [39, 31].

Table 21.13. The priority of identification and evaluation of cardiovascular risk factors (RF) in type 2 diabetes (according to data from [39])

Compulsory assessment Causal or major RF	Predisposing RF	Optional assessment Conditional RF
Cigarette smoking	Body fat: BMI	Lipoprotein (a)
Blood pressure	Fat distribution: waist circumference (insulin-resistance as clinical marker)	Small LDL particles(LDL − B)
Lipids and lipoproteins	Physical activity	Apoprotein B
Albuminuria	Family history	Homocysteine
Glycemic control		Fibrinogen
		Plasminogen activator inhibitor 1

The *major risk factors* to be identified:

- Cigarette smoking: duration, intensity, passive smoke exposure.
- Blood pressure: history, associated factors, physical examination including supine, sitting and standing blood pressure measurements.
- Serum lipids and lipoproteins: history, physical examination for xantomatosis and laboratory: fasting serum cholesterol, triglycerides, HDL cholesterol, calculated LDL cholesterol (if triglycerides < 400 mg/dl). Thyroid, renal and liver function tests are necessary to exclude the secondary forms.
- Macro and microalbuminuria.
- Glycemic status.

The *predisposing risk factors* to be analyzed:

- Body weight, BMI and waist.
- Physical activity: on the job, participation on sport, housework, child care.
- Family history which is positive, i.e., if cardiovascular disease or sudden death occurred in first-degree male relatives before 55 years or in females before 65 years. Investigate the major risk factors in first-degree relatives and if possible also in second-degree relatives.

In Table 21.14, a summary of the levels of main cardiovascular risk factors is presented. Few of them have to be adapted to ADA's recommendations [5].

The identification and evaluation of cardiovascular risk factors as they have been suggested require a few comments:

- The assessment of major (causal) and predisposing risk factors is compulsory, while the evaluation of conditional factors should be optional.
- The glycemic status should be evaluated with HbA1c, fasting and postprandial glycemia [67]. Both will be correlated with the macro- or microvascular risk as it has been recommended by recent guidelines (Table 21.15).
- The assessment of waist circumference will easily offer a clinical marker of insulin resistance. The values have to be interpreted in the light of the *hypertriglyceridemic waist syndrome* (see Chap. 11).

21 Global Approach to Cardiovascular Risk in Type 2 Diabetic Persons

Table 21.14. The levels of main cardiovascular risk factors suggested to be assessed in type 2 diabetes mellitus by the European Arterial Risk Policy Group on behalf of the International Diabetes Federation (adapted from [23, 14], with kind permission)*

Risk factor	Low risk	Moderate risk	High risk
Total serum cholesterol mmol/l	<5.2	5.2–6.5	>6.5
mg/dl	<200	200–250	>250
LDL cholesterol mmol/l	<3.0	3.0–4.0	>4.0
mg/dl	<115	115–154	>154
HDL cholesterol mmol/l	>1.2	1.0–1.2	<1.0
mg/dl	>46	38–46	<38
Serum triglycerides mmol/l	<2.3	2.3–4.0	>4.0
mg/dl	<204	204–354	>354
Blood pressure (mmHg)	<140/90	140/90–160/95	>160/95
Glycated haemoglobin (%Hb)[a]	<6.5	6.5–8.5	>8.5
Body mass index (kg/m^2)	<25.0	25.0–30.0	>30.0
Raised albumin excretion[b]:	–	–	–
Albumin, mg/l	<15	–	>15
Albumin: creatinine ratio mg/mmol	<2.5[c]/3.5[d]	–	>2.5[c]/3.5[d]
Smoking (cigarettes/day)	Not smoking	1–10	>10
Ethnic group	Europid	–	Non Europid
Personal or family history of arterial disease	None	Family history of MI/stroke	Previous MI/stroke /PVD

* According to the newest ADA's recommendations [5], the low-risk category should include: LDL cholesterol <100 mg/dl (<2.6 mmol/l) (B – evidence level); Triglycerides <150 mg/dl (<1.7 mmol/l) (C – evidence level); HDL cholesterol – in men: >45 mg/dl (>1.15 mmol/l) (C – level evidence) – in women: >55 mg/dl (>1.7 mmol/l) (C – level evidence); Blood pressure <130/80 mmHg (A – level evidence); Waist: in men <94 cm; in women <80 cm.
[a] HbA$_{1c}$: assumes a DCCT standardized assay (normal <6.1%).
[b] Early morning urine sample.
[c] Men.
[d] Women.
MI, myocardial infarction; PVD, peripheral vascular disease.

Table 21.15. The blood glucose control assessment (from [24] with kind permission)

	Low risk	Arterial risk	Microvascular risk
HbA1c (DCCT standardized), % Hb	≤6.5	>6.5	>7.5
Venous plasma glucose Fasting/pre-prandial			
mmol/l	≤6.0	>6.0	≥7.0
mg/dl	<110	≥110	>125
Self-monitored blood glucose Fasting/pre-prandial			
mmol/l	≤5.5	>5.5	>6.0
mg/dl	<100	≥100	≥110
Post-prandial (peak)			
mmol/l	<7.5	≥7.5	>9.0
mg/dl	<135	≥135	>160

- The family history of cardiovascular disease or diabetes is very important, because it can confer a genetic basis to the risk. As a consequence, pharmacological control is probably needed [39].
- Regarding the conditional risk factors (Lp(a), LDL type B, apoprotein B, homocysteine, fibrinogen, PAI-1) their role in risk stratification is not yet sufficiently known. In addition, their measurements are not yet widespread recommended in daily practice [36].

Screening and Diagnosis of Macrovascular Disease

Screening and diagnosis of macrovascular disease should be part of the global evaluation of each person with type 2 diabetes.

The objectives of cardiovascular investigations in people with type 2 diabetes are as follows:

- The early detection of clinical and sub-clinical coronary heart disease or cardiomiopathy, cerebrovascular disease and peripheral arteriopathy [54, 18]
- To establish the coronary heart disease risk equivalents (see also Table 21.4): abdominal aortic aneurism, ischemia of the extremities, carotid atherosclerosis [32, 39]
- Their complete diagnosis

This important topic has already been discussed in previous chapters. To complete the global assessment, the evaluation of renal status is also required [39]. Details of this have been provided in Chapter 9.

Assessment of Global Cardiovascular Risk in People with Type 2 Diabetes: Tools and Rules

The multiplicative effects of cardiovascular risk factors has to be known by practitioners. Consequently it should be determined, considering simultaneously all factors. Based on the large prospective studies (Framingham, PROCAM) charts and scores have been developed allowing us to estimate the absolute risk of developing a coronary event in the next 10 years.

Three tools are recommended: the Coronary Chart developed by the Second Joint Task Force of European and other Societies on Coronary Prevention [105] thereafter to be referred to as Euro'98, Risk Stratification Chart for diabetic subjects with or without microalbuminuria [109] (UK'99) and the New Framingham Risk Scores [36, 32, 104, 40].

Coronary Chart "Euro'98"

This chart is based on a risk function derived from the Framingham Study [105]. By knowing five risk factors: total cholesterol level, systolic blood pressure, age, sex and smoking status, the tool is easy to be used. The absolute 10 years risk of developing coronary heart disease (angina, non-fatal myocardial infarction or coronary death) can be estimated in the general population or in people with diabetes (Fig. 21.1).

21 Global Approach to Cardiovascular Risk in Type 2 Diabetic Persons

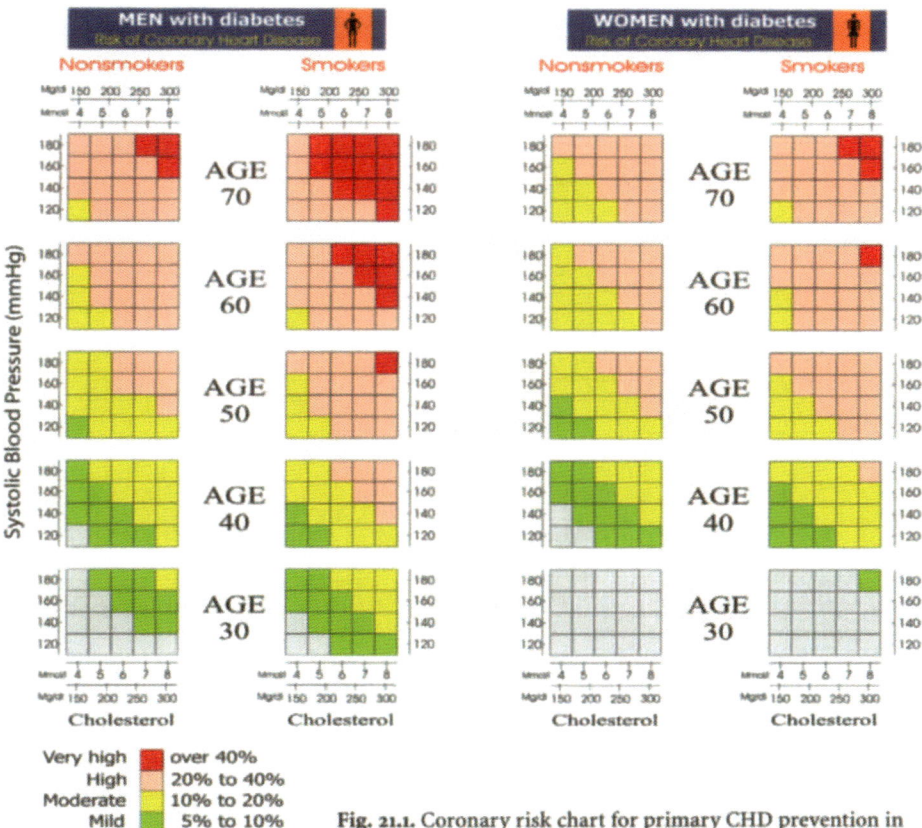

Fig. 21.1. Coronary risk chart for primary CHD prevention in diabetes mellitus. (From [105] with kind permission)

Very high: over 40%
High: 20% to 40%
Moderate: 10% to 20%
Mild: 5% to 10%
Low: under 5%

How to use the Coronary Risk Chart for Primary Prevention

The chart is for estimating coronary heart disease (CHD) risk for individuals who have not developed symptomatic CHD or other atherosclerotic disease. Patients with CHD are already at high risk and require intensive lifestyle intervention and, as necessary, drug therapies to achieve risk factor goals.

- To estimate a person's absolute 10 year risk of a CHD event, find the table for their gender, smoking status and age. Within the table, find the cell nearest to their systolic blood pressure (mmHg) and total cholesterol (mmol/l or mg/dl)
- The effect of lifetime exposure to risk factors can be seen by following the table upwards. This can be used when advising younger people
- High risk individuals are defined as those whose 10 year CHD risk exceeds 20 % or will exceed 20 % if projected to age 60
- CHD risk is higher than indicated in the chart for those with familial hyperlipidemia, those with a family history of premature cardiovascular disease, those with low HDL cholesterol (these tables assume HDL cholesterol to be 1.0 mmol/l or 39 mg/dl in men and 1.1 mmol/l or 43 mg/dl in women), those with raised triglyceride levels > 2.0 mmol/l or 180 mg/dl, as the person approaches the next age category
- To find a person's relative risk, compare their risk category with that for other people of the same age. The absolute risk shown here may not apply to all populations, especially those with a low CHD incidence. Relative risk is likely to apply to most populations
- The effect of changing cholesterol, smoking status or blood pressure can be read from the chart

254   N. Hâncu, A. Cerghizan

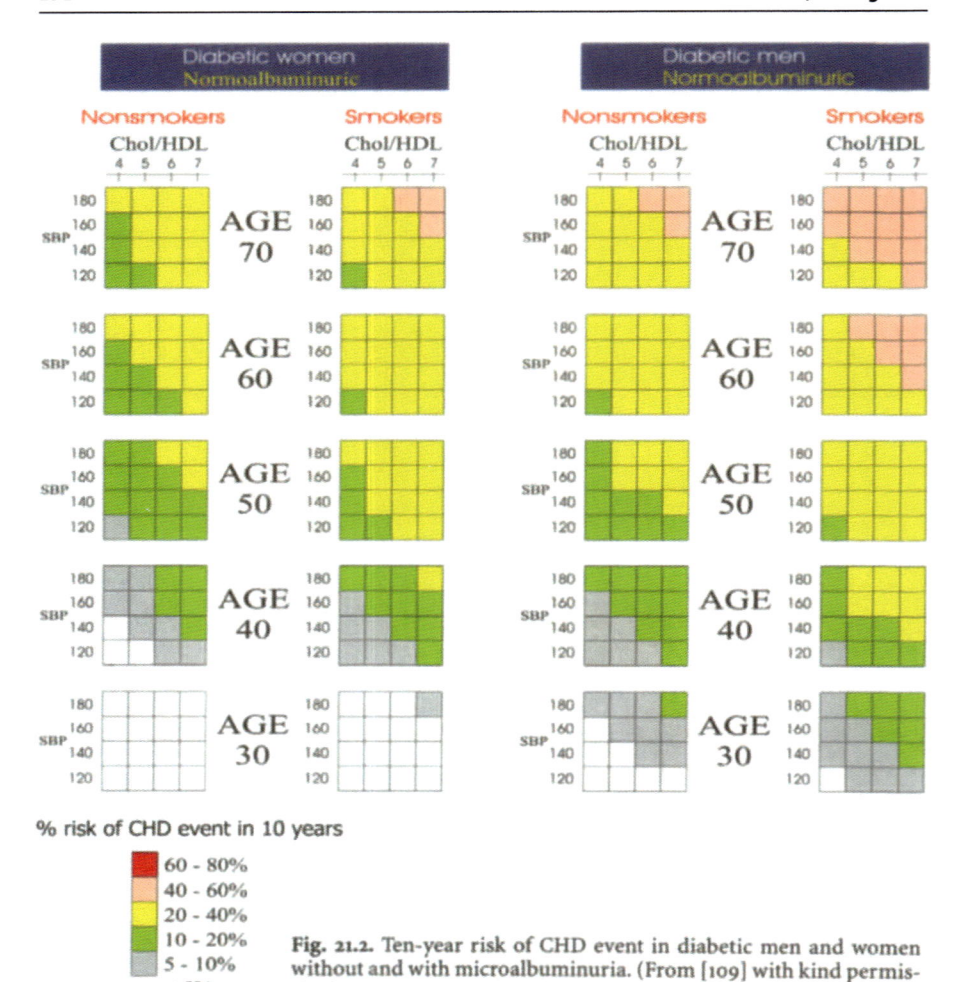

% risk of CHD event in 10 years

- 60 - 80%
- 40 - 60%
- 20 - 40%
- 10 - 20%
- 5 - 10%
- < 5%

Fig. 21.2. Ten-year risk of CHD event in diabetic men and women without and with microalbuminuria. (From [109] with kind permission)

In order to read a person's risk, identify the chart relating to the person's gender, age and smoking status. Within the chart, find the cell nearest to the person's level of total: high density lipoprotein cholesterol ratio and systolic blood pressure. Compare the cell tone with the key and red the risk level. For south Asian subjects, people with symptomatic or asymptomatic cardiovascular disease, a family history of coronary disease at an early age, central obesity, or left ventricular hypertrophy, the risk level will be greater than that indicated in the chart by around one category. The risk will be higher at lower levels, or if concentrations of triglyceride exceed 2.2 mmol/l.
Chol/HDL = total cholesterol: high density lipoprotein cholesterol ratio
SBP = Systolic Blood Pressure in mm Hg

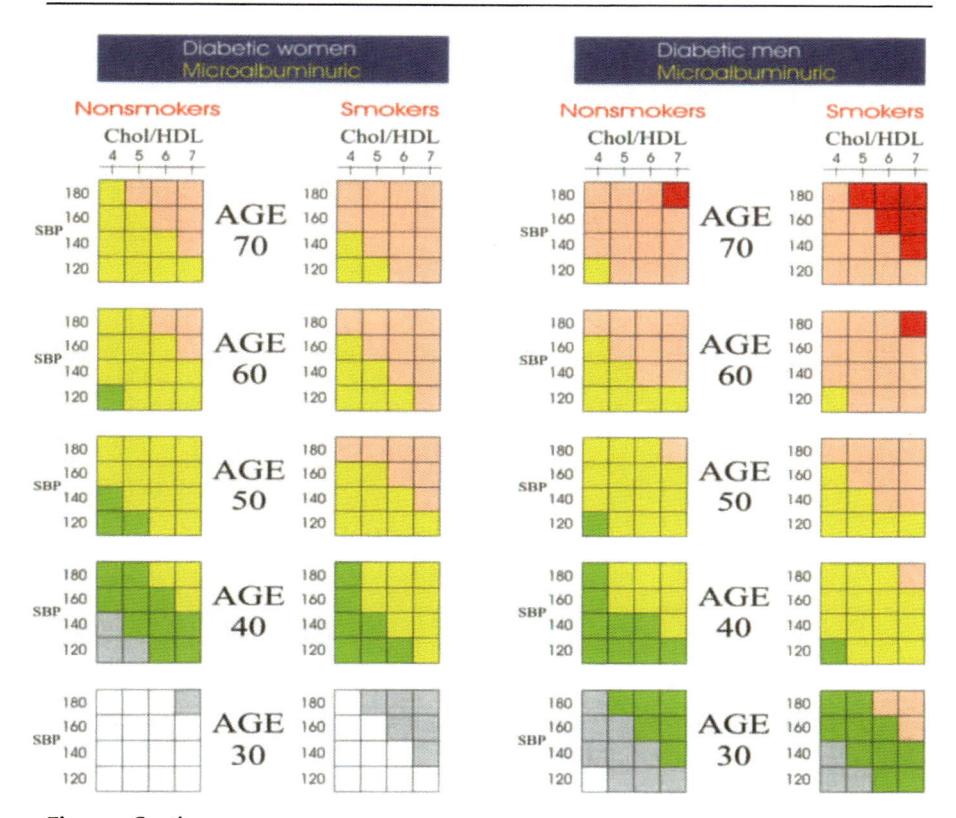

21 Global Approach to Cardiovascular Risk in Type 2 Diabetic Persons   255

Fig. 21.2. Contin.

With Coronary Risk Chart Euro'98, five levels of 10 years risk can be estimated:

- Very high, over 40 %
- High, 20 %–40 %
- Moderate, 10 %–20 %
- Mild, 5 %–10 %
- Low, under 5 %

Risk Stratification Charts "UK'99"

This chart [109] is also based on the Framingham equations. It can estimate the 10 years absolute risk of coronary heart events for non-diabetic and diabetic people, with or without microalbuminuria. The risk has been calculated for men and women according to age (30–70 years), systolic blood pressure, total to high density lipoprotein cholesterol ratio and smoking status. The same levels of risk as those of Euro'98 have been stratified. For microalbuminuric persons with type 2 diabetes 6 levels of risk have been provided: under 5 %, 5 %–10 %, 10 %–20 %, 20 %–40 %, 40 %–60 % and 60 %–80 % [109].

Estimate of 10-Year Risk for Men
Framingham Point Sscores

Age	Points
20-34	-9
35-39	-4
40-44	0
45-49	3
50-54	6
55-59	8
60-64	10
65-69	11
70-74	12
75-79	13

Total cholesterol	Points					
Age	20-39	40-49	50-59	60-69	70-79
< 160	0	0	0	0	0
160-199	4	3	2	1	0
200-239	7	5	3	1	0
240-279	9	6	4	2	1
≥ 280	11	8	5	3	1

	Points					
Age	20-39	40-49	50-59	60-69	70-79
Nonsmoker	0	0	0	0	0
Smoker	8	5	3	1	1

HDL (mg/dl)	Points
≥ 60	-1
50-59	0
40-49	1
< 40	2

Systolic BP (mmHg)	If Untreated	Treated
< 120	0	0
120-129	0	1
130-139	1	2
140-159	1	2
≥ 160	2	3

Point Total	10-Year Risk (%)
< 0	< 1
0	1
1	1
2	1
3	1
4	1
5	2
6	2
7	3
8	4
9	5
10	6
11	8
12	10
13	12
14	16
15	20
16	25
≥ 17	≥ 30

10-Year Risk___%

Estimate of 10-Year Risk for Women
Framingham Point Scores

Age	Points
20-34	-7
35-39	-3
40-44	0
45-49	3
50-54	6
55-59	8
60-64	10
65-69	12
70-74	14
75-79	16

Total cholesterol	Points					
Age	20-39	40-49	50-59	60-69	70-79
< 160	0	0	0	0	0
160-199	4	3	2	1	1
200-239	8	6	4	2	1
240-279	11	8	5	3	2
≥ 280	13	10	7	4	2

	Points					
Age	20-39	40-49	50-59	60-69	70-79
Nonsmoker	0	0	0	0	0
Smoker	9	7	4	2	1

HDL (mg/dl)	Points
≥ 60	-1
50-59	0
40-49	1
< 40	2

Systolic BP (mmHg)	If Untreated	Treated
< 120	0	0
120-129	1	3
130-139	2	4
140-159	3	5
≥ 160	4	6

Point Total	10-Year Risk (%)
< 9	< 1
9	1
10	1
11	1
12	1
13	2
14	2
15	3
16	4
17	5
18	6
19	8
20	11
21	14
22	17
23	22
24	27
≥ 25	≥ 30

10-Year Risk___%

Fig. 21.3. The new Framingham Risk Scores. (From [25] with kind permission)
Risk assessment for determining the 10-year risk for developing CHD is carried out using Framingham risk scoring (for men and for women). The risk factors included in the Framingham calculation of 10-year risk are: age, total cholesterol, HDL cholesterol, systolic blood pressure, treatment for hypertension and cigarette smoking. The first step is to calculate the number of points for each risk factor. For initial assessment, values for total cholesterol and HDL cholesterol are required. Because of a larger data base, Framingham estimates are more robust for total cholesterol than for LDL cholesterol. Note, however, that LDL cholesterol level remains the primary target of therapy. Total cholesterol and HDL cholesterol values should be the average of at least two measurements obtained from lipoprotein analysis. The blood pressure value used is that

The coronary absolute risk predicted refers to angina, myocardial infarction and coronary death [109]. The charts are shown in Fig. 21.2. The number required to treat for 10 years to prevent one coronary heart disease event are also outlined. The calculations reveal that interventions reduce the risk of a coronary risk event by 25% [109].

For a busy practitioner it is wise to count the number of different risk factors. Two additional risk factors in a patient with diabetes aged above 50 years can give a 40% risk of cardiovascular event in 10 years.

The New Framingham Risk Scores

The new Framingham risk scores [36, 32, 104, 40] estimate both absolute risk and relative risk. However, the ATP III [25] do suggest to use in practice the absolute coronary risk, according to the data presented in Fig. 21.3.

The first step is to calculate the points for each major risk factor: age, total and HDL cholesterol, systolic blood pressure, diabetes and smoking status. The score is obtained by adding up the points separately for men and women (Fig. 21.3). This corresponds to the absolute risk for developing, in 10 years, either total coronary heart disease (all forms of clinical coronary heart disease) or hard coronary heart disease (myocardial infarction and coronary death).

Functions, Limits and Interpretation of Results

According to the data in the literature [105, 36, 32, 109, 104, 40, 33] the main functions and the potential uses of these tools are:

- To provide a realistic picture of the global cardiovascular risk in terms of absolute and relative risk
- To help us to tailor a plan for intervention and to predict and evaluate its effect
- To educate and to motivate patients
- To motivate physicians in order to become more involved in cardiovascular risk control

Before using these tools, practitioners should be informed about their limits [105, 36, 32, 109, 104, 40]:

- All these tools can be used only for people without atherosclerotic cardiovascular disease.
- They overestimate the risk in young people and underestimate it in the case of clustering risk factors with people displaying the metabolic syndrome.

---

obtained at the time of assessment, regardless of whether the person is on antihypertensive therapie. However, if the person is on antihypertensive treatment, an extra point is added beyond points for the blood pressure reading because treated hypertension carries residual risk. The average of several blood pressure measurements, as recommended by the Joint National Committee (JNC), is needed for an accurate measure of baseline blood pressure. The designation „smoker" means any cigarette smoking in the past month. The total risk score sums the points for each risk factor. The 10-year risk for myocardial infarction and coronary death (hard CHD) is estimated from total points, and the person is categorized according absolute 10-year risk as indicated

- For certain reasons a few risk factors are not used in the tools: obesity, familial history, physical inactivity, LDL cholesterol, triglycerides, and fibrinogen. Nevertheless they remain an important target for intervention.

To interpret the values provided by this estimation, a few rules have to be taken into consideration:

- People with an absolute risk ≥ 20% have the likelihood of developing a coronary event similar to those with established coronary heart disease. They have to be submitted for short-term high-risk primary prevention [32].
- If the absolute risk is < 20% but the relative risk is moderate or high (Fig. 21.3) a young person should be considered a candidate for long-term high-risk action [40]. These recommendations have to be interpreted in the light of the fact that in time, a moderate or high relative risk will become a high absolute risk [40].
- All those with coronary heart disease equivalents (Table 21.4) must be considered as having a high absolute risk (≥ 20%). Recommendations used for secondary prevention should be applied.
- People with type 2 diabetes represent a coronary heart disease equivalent and must be treated appropriately [32]. However, it is recognized that the absolute risk of these persons is underestimated by Framingham Scores [40]. That is why the risk estimated by means of this tool should be elevated to a higher risk category [40].

These tools with their guidelines are better used in daily practice only when applied with the best clinical judgment which cannot be replaced by any other method.

Targeting Objectives and Planning Interventions

The link between the assessment of cardiovascular risk and intervention should be the interpretations of the results and finally the targeting of objectives and planning of the interventions. The art of clinical judgment has an important role in these actions. After data collection, the following parameters have to be interpreted:

- Levels of individual risk factors and cardiovascular status and how are they modified versus optimal or reasonable standards
- Absolute risk
- Patient education and his or her desire, willingness and possibilities to change

These would allow the picture of a patient's cardiovascular risk status in terms of:

- High risk or multi risk factors patients (≥ 2 risk factors)
- People with ≤ 1 risk factor
- People in danger of being neglected due to the risk factors expressed as *borderline* levels (e.g. blood pressure 130–139/80–89 mmHg, LDL cholesterol 100–139 mg/dl, HDL cholesterol 30–40 mg/dl, triglycerides 150–250 mg/dl, smokers < 10 cigarettes/day, overweight person with waist > 80 cm for women or > 94 cm for men, postprandial glycemia > 180 mg/dl with HbA1c approximate 7.2%–7.5%)
- People with one severe risk factor (heavy smokers > 40 cigarettes/day, familial hypercholesterolemia or combined hyperlipidemia, BMI > 40 kg/m^2, hypertension with high and resistant values)

Table 21.16. Stratification of 26,787 newly type 2 diabetic patients according to the number of risk factors added to diabetes; EPIDIAB Study results (first 2 years) [51]

No risk factors	–
1 risk factor	6.7%
2 risk factors	28.13%
≥ 3 risk factors	65.08%

Table 21.17. The risk stratification (%) estimated with UK'99 charts in 8929 newly diagnosed type 2 diabetic persons; EPIDIAB Study results (first 2 years) [51]. The patients with existing macrovascular disease have not been considered

Risk classes	< 10%	10 – 20%	> 20%
Newly diagnosed type 2 DM (%)	14.9%	32.2%	> 52.8%

It seems that in daily practice the *multiple risk factor patient* is the most frequent *person type* met, as shown in Table 21.16.

The absolute risk estimated with the charts or Framingham Scores also reveal that even in newly diagnosed patients the cardiovascular risk is high (Table 21.17).

This interpretation would further allow establishing:

- The realistic and individualized objectives for each risk factor, which have to be agreed by the persons
- The priorities of the objectives which are to be approached
- The methods of intervention
- The stepwise implementation of these methods

The following actions should therefore be envisaged:

- Good communication with the person and his/her family
- To empower the person and to involve him/her in self control
- To involve the family members in these actions
- To insure an adequate organizational setting for the control in short and long terms

In turn, the intervention should accomplish at least six conditions. These are called by us the "*6S conditions*" for successful control of cardiovascular risk.

Accordingly, each intervention should be:

- Structured on the four components of clinical management, namely: therapy, education, monitoring, and evaluation
- Standardized as minimum, reasonable and optimal qualitative levels
- Stratified according to primary, secondary and tertiary care
- Specified for each individual
- Synchronized – that means synchronization of all factors for a good control
- Strategized in short and long term

Regarding the clinical management it should be emphasized that this is the most important part of the intervention. It is adapted to each focused factor and encompasses four programs:

- Therapeutical program: lifestyle optimization and pharmacotherapy
- Education or more precisely *therapeutical education* as a specific part of a global education program to be applied for people with type 2 diabetes [35]
- Monitoring program that is a regular control of the patient's specific parameters
- Evaluation that is an annual full review of the person

The acronym of these actions is THEME, a suggestive term for practitioners [50].

Some cardiovascular risk factors have been dealt with in previous chapters and we do not wish to repeat what has already been discussed. We will only present in the next pages a synthesis of the recommendations for a global intervention for cardiovascular risk in persons with type 2 diabetes, with or without cardiovascular disease.

Table 21.18. Lifestyle and therapeutic goals for patients with CHD, or other atherosclerotic disease, and for healthy high-risk individuals (from [105] with kind permission)

Patients with CHD or other atherosclerotic disease	Healthy high-risk individuals; absolute CHD risk ≥ 20% over 10 years, or will exceed 20% if projected to age 60
Lifestyle Stop smoking, make healthy food choices, be physically active and achieve ideal weight	
Other risk factors Blood pressure < 140/90 mm Hg, total cholesterol < 5.0 mmol/l (190 mg/dl) LDL cholesterol < 3.0 mmol/l (115 mg/dl) When these risk factor goals are not achieved by lifestyle, blood pressure and cholesterol lowering drug therapies should be used	
Other prophylactic drug therapies Aspirin (at least 75 mg) for all coronary patients, those with cerebral atherosclerosis and peripheral atherosclerotic disease β-blockers in patients following myocardial infarction ACE inhibitors in those with symptoms or signs of heart failure at the time of myocardial infarction, or with chronic LV systolic dysfunction (ejection fraction < 40%) Anticoagulants in selected coronary patients	Aspirin (75 mg) in treated hypertensive patients and in men at particularly high CHD risk
Screen close relatives Screen close relatives of patients with premature (men < 55 yrs, women < 65 yrs) CHD	Screen close relatives if familial hypercholesterolaemia or other inherited dyslipidaemia is suspected

Interventions for the Global Control of Cardiovascular Risk

Secondary Prevention

These recommendations represent the secondary prevention of atherosclerotic cardiovascular disease. In Table 21.18 the strategies proposed by the Second Joint Task Force of European and other Societies on Coronary Prevention [105] for the general population are shown.

For the people with diabetes and cardiovascular disease, American Heart Association has proposed the following prophylactic measures [39]:

- Smoking cessation
- Blood pressure control
- Glucose control
- Regular physical activity
- Weight management
- Antiplatelets agents
- ACE inhibitors in post MI patients
- β Blockers
- Estrogens

Table 21.19. Primary prevention in coronary asymptomatic patients at high short-term risk (CHD risk equivalents) (from [32] with kind permission)

Patient selection (CHD risk equivalents)
Symptomatic peripheral arterial disease
Abdominal aortic aneurysm
Symptomatic carotid artery disease
Type 2 diabetes*
Multiple risk factors (Framingham risk for hard CHD > 20% / 10 years)**
Smoking goal: complete cessation
Blood pressure goal: ≤ 140/90 mm Hg (≤ 130/85 mm Hg in type 2 diabetes)†
Primary lipid goal: LDL cholesterol ≤ 100 mg/dl***
Glucose goal: near normal glucose and near normal hemoglobin A1c (<7%)
Antiplatelet therapy: aspirin 80 mg/day if not contraindicated
Life habits: NCEP/AHA step II diet, weight loss in overweight patients (goal body mass index 21–25 kg/m^2), moderate-intensity exercise (30–60 min) 3 or 4 times weekly

*Includes Americans of white, Hispanic, black, and South Asian origin. May not include Americans of East Asian origin.
†The newest ADA's recommendations: < 130/80 mm Hg.
**Accuracy of absolute risk enhanced by substitution of noninvasive estimates of coronary plaque burden for age as a risk factor.
***Most patients with baseline LDL cholesterol levels > 130 mg/dl will require cholesterol-lowering drugs to achieve the target of therapy. When on-treatment serum LDL cholesterol is in the range of 100 to 129 mg/dl, several therapeutic options are available: to increase the drug dose (or to combine with another cholesterol-lowering drug) to achieve an LDL cholesterol < 100 mg/dl, to add another lipid-lowering drug to improve triglyceride and HDL cholesterol levels, or to aggressively modify other risk factors. Clinical judgment is required whether to start (or to increase the dose of) cholesterol-lowering drugs in patients > 65 years old.

Primary Prevention

According to the concept of primary prevention of coronary heart disease and other atherosclerotic cardiovascular disease [32] the strategies for general population are shown in Tables 21.19 and 21.20.

The greatest part of the measures used for secondary prevention can also be used for primary prevention in people with diabetes [39].

Some Practical Aspects of Clinical Management Related to the Global Cardiovascular Risk in Type 2 Diabetes

The main problems of clinical management related to the cardiovascular risk factors in persons with type 2 diabetes, have been presented in the previous chapters. We only want now to underline some practical aspects: 1) lifestyle optimization, 2) glycemic control, 3) the management of hypertension and microalbuminuria, 4) weight management, 5) lipids control and 6) the anti – aggregant treatment. These will be analyzed in the light of the quality of evidence proposed in the recent ADA's recommendations for clinical practice [5]. Accordingly, three levels of evidence have been distinguished [5]:

A Level of evidence based on large well-designed clinical trials or well done meta-analysis
B Level of evidence that comes from well- conducted cohort studies
C Level of evidence from poorly controlled or uncontrolled studies

Table 21.20. Long-term primary prevention in the clinical setting (from [32] with kind permission)

All categorical risk factors should be treated professionally
Smoking goal: smoking cessation
Blood pressure goal: < 140/90 mm Hg*
Serum cholesterol and lipid goals
Desirable LDL cholesterol: < 130 mg/dl
Very high LDL cholesterol (≥ 190 mg/dl)
Most patients will require cholesterol-lowering drugs
Two or more risk factors** (absolute risk < 20 %/10 years for hard CHD)
LDL cholesterol goal: < 130 mg/dl
Zero to 1 risk factor**:
Acceptable LDL cholesterol: 130 to 159 mg/dl
Elevated triglycerides (> 200 mg/dl) or low HDL cholesterol (< 35 mg/dl)
Emphasize weight reduction and increase physical activity
Consider nicotinic acid or fibric acid only after LDL cholesterol goal of < 130 mg/dl is achieved (limited clinical trial evidence of efficacy)
Life habits: NCEP/AHA step I diet, weight loss in overweight patients (goal: body mass index 21 – 25 kg/m^2), moderate-intensity exercise (30 – 60 min) 3 or 4 time weekly

*The newest ADA's recommendations: < 130/80 mm Hg.
**Includes risk factors other than LDL cholesterol > 160 mg/dl. Ie. cigarette smoking, hypertension, low HDL cholesterol (< 35 mg/dl), family history of premature CHD, age (men ≥ 45 years; women > 55 years or postmenopausal).

A separate category of recommendations is based on expert opinion (E – level) in which there is as yet no evidence from clinical trials, in which clinical trials may be unpractical, or in which there is conflicting evidence [5].

There are many components of clinical decision-making. The evidence is only one of them. The clinical judgment will also help to care the patients not populations. As a consequence all peculiarities and all needs of the individuals ought to be considered in daily practice decisions.

Lifestyle Optimization

Lifestyle optimization is a compulsory objective. According to IDF recommendations [24] a four-point plan should be implemented: 1) a balanced diet, 2) physical exercise, 3) seeking good medical advice and taking control of your life and 4) social events. The first two points are strongly related to cardiovascular risk and ample evidence was provided (A, B and C levels) [5, 6] supporting their importance. The therapeutic education is the best method to accomplish these objectives. More than this, in the curriculum of every educational program the problems of cardiovascular risk factors have to be included.

If a patient is simultaneously confronted with multiple risk factors, he should approach them step-by-step. This would allow a better long-term compliance.

Smoking cessation is extremely important and must be maintained [30]. This can be achieved with intensive therapeutic education [35]. For counseling on smoking cessation and its prevention, health care providers should follow the ADA's recommendations (A and B level of evidence) [5].

Glycemic Control

According to the international guidelines [14] the management of hyperglycemia should be based on four steps [14]: 1) lifestyle optimization, 2) oral monotherapy, 3) oral combined therapy and 4) insulin therapy (Fig. 21.4). Achievement of metabolic control is a step-by-step process. The effectiveness of each therapeutic step should carefully be evaluated. If the glycemic objectives are not achieved, the next step has to be initiated [14].

Regarding insulin therapy in type 2 diabetes mellitus, the following indications are recommended [14]: failure to achieve glycemic control despite maximum doses of combinations of blood glucose lowering agents, decompensation due to intercurrent events, perioperative management, pregnancy and lactation, failure of vital organs,
allergy or other serious reactions to oral drugs, marked hyperglycemia at the time of presentation and acute myocardial infarction. It should be mentioned that in every patient who needs prandial insulin, the use of a rapidly-acting insulin analogue should be prescribed [14], while as basal insulin, glargine would be preferred [56]. Pharmacotherapy used for glycemic control should comply with: 1) minimum cost strategy, 2) minimum weight gain strategy, 3) minimum injections strategy, 4) minimum peripheral insulin strategy, 5) minimum patient's effort strategy [12]. The optimal influences on cardiovascular risk profile should also be taken into consideration [13, 68, 12].

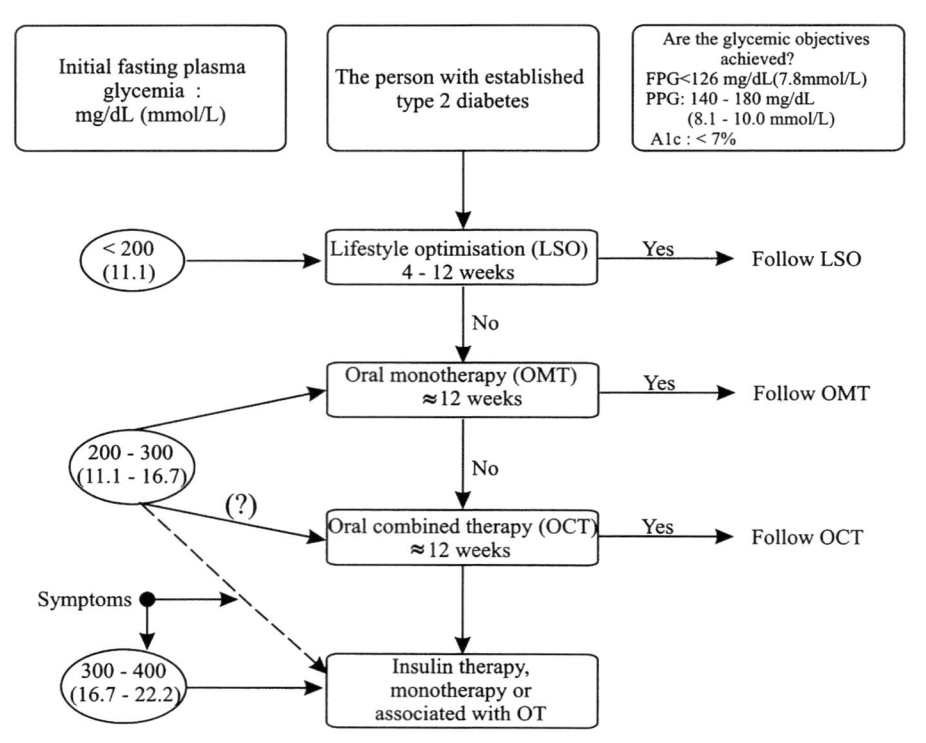

```
┌─────────────────────┐   ┌─────────────────────┐   ┌──────────────────────────┐
│ Initial fasting     │   │ The person with     │   │ Are the glycemic         │
│ plasma glycemia :   │   │ established type 2  │   │ objectives achieved?     │
│ mg/dL (mmol/L)      │   │ diabetes            │   │ FPG<126 mg/dL(7.8mmol/L) │
└─────────────────────┘   └─────────────────────┘   │ PPG: 140 - 180 mg/dL     │
                                                    │ (8.1 - 10.0 mmol/L)      │
                                                    │ A1c : < 7%               │
                                                    └──────────────────────────┘
```

Fig. 21.4. Step strategy suggested for glycemic control in type 2 diabetes. The initiation and duration of each step is determined by fasting glycemic values, glycemic related symptoms, global risk, achievement of glycemic objectives based on existing evidences and clinical judgement

There are some evidence (A, B and C level) regarding the possibilities to achieve the treatment targets and also to reduce the cardiovascular risk by controlling glycemia [5].

Management of Hypertension and Microalbuminuria

The goal of treatment is systolic blood pressure <130 mmHg (B–level of evidence) and diastolic blood pressure <80 mmHg (A–level of evidence) [9].

Patients with a blood pressure of 130–139/80–89 mmHg should be given lifestyle optimization therapy alone for a maximum of 3 months. If targets are not achieved, the pharmacotherapy should be initiated (A–level of evidence) [9]. It has been demonstrated that a reduction of blood pressure can be achieved by reduction of sodium intake and modest weight loss (A–level of evidence).

If the initial levels of blood pressure are ≥140/90 mmHg, drug therapy should be prescribed in addition to lifestyle optimization (A–level of evidence) [9].

The drugs of choice are [14]: ACE-inhibitors (particularly if microalbuminuria is present and/or in the presence of heart failure), calcium channel blockers, beta 1 – blockers (particularly in the presence of chronic coronary artery disease), alpha 1 –

blockers (particularly if dyslipidemia is present) and thiazide diuretics. As diuretic, indapamide can also be recommended.

The rational combinations suggested would be [14]: ACE-inhibitors + low-dose thiazides or calcium channel blockers, calcium channel blockers or alpha 1-blockers + beta 1-blockers and/or diuretics.

ACE-inhibitors seem to have additional benefits on cardiovascular events, metabolic abnormalities and microalbuminuria mainly in patients over the age of 55 with or without hypertension but with another cardiovascular risk factor (A-level of evidence) [9, 29, 60, 74].

The prescription of any drug or combination of drugs should be based on evidence and taking also into consideration their potential adverse events [87]. All of the major classes of antihypertensive drugs have limitations that complicate their use in persons with type 2 diabetes [87].

In individuals with microalbuminuria, reduction of protein intake to 0.8–1.0 g· kg^{-1}·wt^{-1} per day may slow the progression of nephropathy (C-level evidence) [9].

Weight Management

This must be a priority of any strategy. Practitioners should not forget the benefits that could be achieved by moderate weight loss and its maintenance (A and B evidence level) [5, 6]. Suggested guidelines are presented in Chapter 10.

Lipid Control

The *lipid objectives* for adults with diabetes are as follows [5]:

- LDL cholesterol <100 mg/dl (2.6 mmol/l) (B-level of evidence)
- HDL cholesterol in men: >45 mg/dl (1.15 mmol/l); in women: >55 mg/dl (1.40 mmol/l) (C-level of evidence)
- Triglycerides <150 mg/dl (1,7 mmol/l) (C-level of evidence)

Because diabetes mellitus is considered a coronary risk equivalent, the lipid objective is LDL cholesterol <100 mg/dl (<2.6 mmol/l) as lowering LDL cholesterol is associated with reduction in cardiovascular events (A-level of evidence), it represents the first priority of therapy [5, 7].

The *following recommendations* should be considered to achieve these objectives [5, 6]:

- Correcting the underlying metabolic abnormalities of diabetes with a good glucose control may play an important role in reversing dyslipidemia. In particular, triglycerides may be significantly reduced with optimal glucose lowering.
- Lifestyle optimization is an important step in any therapeutic program. The reduction of saturated fat (7–10% of energy intake), cholesterol (<300 mg/day), weight loss, and increased physical activity has been shown to improve the lipid profile in patients with diabetes (A-level evidence).
- If the lipid targets are not achieved with lifestyle modifications, the pharmacotherapy is indicated (A-level evidence).
- Statins should be used as first-line therapy for LDL lowering (A-level evidence).
- Fibrates should be considered in patients with low HDL cholesterol (A-level of evi-

dence). The therapy with fibrates has been shown to reduce cardiovascular events and progression of carotid intimal medial progression (A-level of evidence).
- Niacin is the best drug for raising HDL but may significantly deteriorate glycemic control [5].
- Bile-acid binding resins or fenofibrate are considered the second choice for LDL lowering.

The following *order of priorities for treatment* of dyslipidemia in adult with type 2 diabetes, should be considered [7, 55]:

- For LDL cholesterol lowering:
  - If the level is 100–129 mg/dl (2.6–3.3 mmol/l) lifestyle optimization should aggressively be given, or treatment with statins must be prescribed, mainly in the presence of atherosclerotic cardiovascular disease. If HDL cholesterol is < 40 mg/dl, fenofibrate might be used [7].
  - If the initial level is ≥ 130 mg/dl (3.3 mmol/l) statins and lifestyle modification treatment should concomitantly be used.
  - According to an expert opinion [110] statins should be initiated if the absolute coronary risk is ≥ 15 %.
- For HDL cholesterol rising, the lifestyle optimization and glycemic control may be useful. Statins modestly raise HDL. A greater increase is achieved with fibrates.
- For triglyceride lowering, the first priority is to achieve glycemic control. Fibrates (gemfibrozil, fenofibrate) are used in patients with high levels (≥ 400 mg/dl) of triglycerides. Statins at high doses are moderately effective in this respect.
- For combined hyperlipidemia the first choice is to improve glycemic control plus high dose statins. As second choice fibrates should be added to statins. The drugs for the third choice are resins plus fibrates or statins plus nicotinic acid. The association of hypolipidemic drugs can develop secondary effects such as myositis or deterioration of glycemic control. They must be monitored carefully [7].

Anti-aggregation Treatment

Acetylsalicilic acid should be used for both primary and secondary prevention according to ADA's [8] and AHA's recommendations [39] (see also Tables 21.19 and 21.22). In terms of "evidence" the following recommendations should be considered [5]:

- Therapy with aspirin (75–325 mg/day) in all adult patients with diabetes and macrovascular disease (A-level evidence)
- As primary prevention aspirin (75–325 mg/day) is indicated in patients ≥ 40 years of age, with diabetes and one or more other cardiovascular risk factors.

Special Groups and Conditions

While people with type 2 diabetes and multi risk factors are typical candidates for global cardiovascular risk control, there are also a few groups and certain conditions which deserve special care:

21 Global Approach to Cardiovascular Risk in Type 2 Diabetic Persons

- Women are no more protected against cardiovascular risk when they are diabetic. Consequently they must be treated with similar methods and intensity as men [39]. Hormonal replacement therapy (HRT) has to be considered in postmenopausal women if they show elevated LDL cholesterol levels [39, 93].
- The elderly ought to be treated according to their absolute risk, cardiovascular and renal status and life expectancy [39].
- Existing diabetic nephropathy should be treated accordingly [39]. In the case of dyslipidemia, the fibrates should be carefully prescribed, but statins have already proven their usefulness. Dialysis patients are under serious cardiovascuar risk and must be treated in centers with recognized expertise.
- As *depression* is considered by some authorities [1, 98] to be an independent cardiovascular risk factor in people with diabetes, it should be assessed and controlled through psychotherapy and antidepressant drugs [1]. Nevertheless the benefits have still to be proved.
- *Erectile dysfunction* is a frequent condition in type 2 diabetic men [102]. It does not only diminish the quality of life but it is also a marker for the development of cardiovascular disease. In addition, to make things worse, depression aggravates both cardiovascular risk and erectile dysfunction. Hence the erectile dysfunction should be carefully assessed and treated multidisciplinary. Sildenafil has offered very good results so far [94].
- Growing evidence suggests that the *postprandial state* represents a cardiovascular risk factor [4, 71, 82, 15, 57, 111, 17, 65, 46]. In fact, even in 1979 Zilversmith [111] considered atherogenesis a *postprandial phenomenon*. It has also been called by us *postprandial atherogenic state*. As it covers a great part of the nycthemeral period, its importance has to be recognized accordingly. Its main components are: postprandial glycemia with excessive glucose excursions, postprandial hyperlipidemia, prothrombotic factors and increased oxidative stress [4, 71, 82, 15, 57, 111, 17, 65, 46]. From these, only postprandial glycemia has been mentioned as a target objective for control. The investigation of the other parameters is not yet standardized. Consequently, repaglinide, alpha glucosidase inhibitors, metformin and rapid insulin analogues along with moderate physical exercise should be considered for postprandial glycemic control. Perhaps, other components should also be optimized.
- The *neglected* could represent a special group, which consists of people with so called *borderline* risk factors: LDL cholesterol 130–160 mg/dl, total cholesterol 200–250 mg/dl, triglycerides 150–250 mg/dl, HDL cholesterol 35–40 mg/dl, systolic blood pressure 130–139 mm Hg and diastolic 80–89 mm Hg, BMI 25–29 kg/m^2 with large waist (>80 cm for women and >94 cm for men), smoking less than 10 cigarettes/day, impaired fasting glucose (110–125 mg/dl). These factors are very often ignored in daily practice, which is a serious mistake. According to the concept of primary prevention, Table 21.20, these people would be candidates for long-term high-risk primary prevention [40].
- In the same group of the neglected, people with so called *hidden factors* such as: hyperhomocysteinemia, prothrombotic state, infections with chlamidia or other agents, Lp(a), LDL type B could be included. Because these factors are not currently explored, they remain hidden and they are not treated.

- Some people with type 2 diabetes could benefit from nutritional supplementation [1]: pyridoxine, vitamins B6, B12, folate-rich food in the diet to correct hyperhomocysteinemia; magnesium, in order to prevent the cardiovascular consequences of possible magnesium deficiency; vitamin E and ascorbic acid as antioxidants. The flavonoids from fruits, vegetables and red wine should not be forgotten because the *French paradox* is a reality.

But much work still has to be done to demonstrate the evidence in this field: until then, vigilance is a good rule to be followed [1].

Benefits and Costs

There is no multifactorial intervention trial on cardiovascular risk in persons with type 2 diabetes so far [21]. Few studies are ongoing. But the general benefits of such strategy could be predicted [73, 21] or at least extrapolated from the Steno type 2 randomized study [38]. This was an intensive multifactorial intervention in patients with type 2 diabetes and microalbuminuria which slows progression to nephropathy and progression of retinopathy and autonomic neuropathy [38]. However, a part of the endpoints considered in the ADDITION treatment study [73], could be suggested for practitioners involved in such interventions. Through those endpoints the benefits can be evaluated. They include the measuring of mortality and morbidity, macro and microvascular complications of diabetes, metabolic and hypertensive control and endpoints related to visits to outpatient clinics and hospital admission [73].

All large interventions which have focused on one or two factors in people with type 2 diabetes were cost – effective. This cannot yet be said regarding an intensive multifactorial strategy. However, the cost – effective data from UKPDS [99, 96] regarding the intensive glycemic or blood pressure control and also from lipid – lowering trials [42] could allow to think that global interventions are also justified from the economic point of view in people with type 2 diabetes. In addition, the results from DIGAMI study [108, 75, 3] clearly showed that intensive insulin treatment after acute myocardial infarction in persons with diabetes along with its favorable endpoints is also cost – effective.

Implementation of the Global Control

Knowledge is not enough for a good medical practice. Bridging the gap between theory and patients is essential in this respect. In order to implement the global control of cardiovascular risk in daily practice, some compulsory conditions should be followed, namely:

- Motivation of the patient through continued specific education.
- Increasing motivation of the practitioners for control by raising the awareness of cardiovascular risk.
- To plan stepwise actions and to evaluate the results of each step. The outcomes ought to help us to improve the next action.
- To organize an adequate setting for both short- and long-term interventions.
- To adopt the International Guidelines and to adapt them to the national or even local conditions. The slogan is *to think globally and act locally*.

- Tailoring the objectives and priorities of actions according to the person's possibilities, willingness and desire is also very important for success.
- To consider the global cardiovascular risk control as a typical *team approach action*. Consequently not only the specialists in diabetes but also general practitioners, cardiologists, angiologists and others should be involved in it. Importantly, they ought to collaborate in both top-down and bottom-up senses.

Although the strategy of global control of cardiovascular risk seems to be reasonably established and unanimously agreed, the achievements in this field are still far from what has been expected. Few barriers have been identified in this respect [37]. The first is due to the physician's failure to identify the major risk factors in the general population or in people with type 2 diabetes. The second barrier is poor data collection and interpretation. A global assessment of cardiovascular risk is only seldom used in practice despite the fact that there are few tools proposed, hence a practical plan of action is frequently overlooked.

The third fact is that even when the practitioners try to control the risk factors they fail to achieve target levels for optimal risk reduction. The survey data from Europe or US clearly show this sad aspect in both the general population and people with type 2 diabetes [83, 85, 72, 81].

We must also consider the person's responsibility in these unsuccessful aspects of the surveys. Due to low-motivation their adherence and compliance is also low. A very low adherence has been found typical to life style optimization and oral therapy either with antihyperglycemic, hypolipidemic or hypotensive drugs [22]. Hence it would be necessary to replace the concept of adherence or compliance with that of *concordance* namely a *therapeutic alliance* between the physician and patient [22]. Education has to empower the patient in the cardiovascular risk field to a greater intensity and it would be necessary to transform the self-neglected in self-controlled people. This would be an important moment in cardiovascular preventive strategies in type 2 diabetes.

Another important factor for successful implementation of global cardiovascular risk control is economic support from the government, insurance companies and even from pharmaceutical corporations. There are many countries where this education is not paid for and the drugs necessary for hypertension, dyslipidemia or obesity control are not reimbursed. Consequently, education is not performed and the drugs are insufficiently prescribed and used.

In conclusion, the lack of cardiovascular risk control both in the general population and type 2 diabetes, suggests that more intensive and extensive actions should be completed.

Certainly we know more than we do, but for sure we do less than we could [50].

Concluding Remarks

Type 2 diabetes has a high prevalence of cardiovascular events which are determined by multiple risk factors. This global cardiovascular risk can be stepwise approached as is suggested in Fig. 21.5.

A suggested flow chart to be used in clinical setting is shown in Fig. 21.6. It is worth

IDENTIFICATION OF:	INTERPRETATION OF:	INTERVENTION FOR:
☐ CARDIOVASCULAR RISK FACTORS	☐ GLOBAL CARDIOVAS-CULAR RISK: • scores • stratification	☐ ALL IDENTIFIED RISK FACTORS AND DISEASE WITH
☐ CARDIOVASCULAR DISEASES	☐ TYPE OF PREVENTION: • primary • secondary ☐ OBJECTIVES TO BE ACHIEVED	☐ APPROPRIATE CLINICAL MANAGEMENT: • lifestyle optimization • pharmacotherapy • therapeutical education • current monitoring • global evaluation

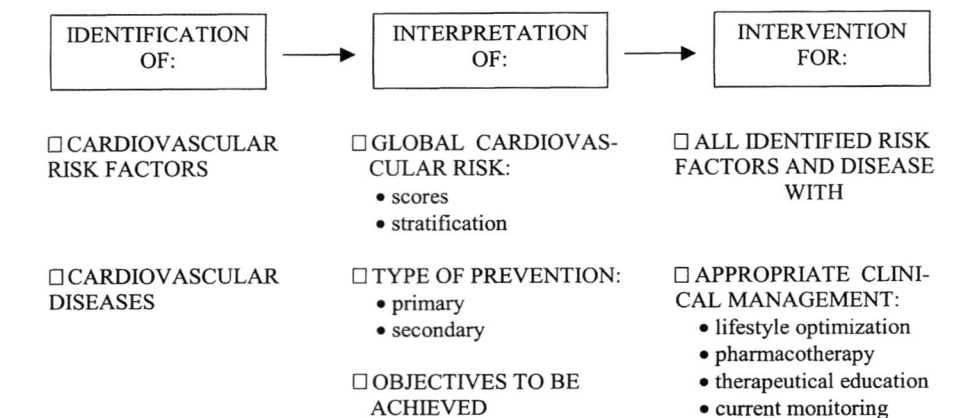

Fig. 21.5. The suggested stepwise approach of the global cardiovascular risk in persons with type 2 diabetes

to underline that all steps are important and all of them must be carefully accomplished. The practical approach to the global cardiovascular risk is a dynamic and flexible process. For instance the conclusions of global evaluation should be used for tailoring each method of clinical management.

The model of multiple cardiovascular risk factor intervention ought to be implemented in daily practice as much as possible. This offers a unique opportunity [21] to reduce the devastating cardiovascular morbidity and mortality in people with type 2 diabetes.

References

1. Arch Judith, Korytkowski Mary (1999) Strategies for preventing coronary heart disease in diabetes mellitus. Diabetes Spectrum 12:88–94
2. Assman G, Cullen P, Schulte H (1998) The Münster Heart Study (PROCAM). Results of follow-up at 8 years. European Heart Journal 19 (Suppl. A):A2-A11
3. Almbrad B et al (2000) Cost effectiveness of intense insulin treatment after acute myocardial infarction in patient with diabetes mellitus: results from DIGAMI study. European Heart Journal 21:733–739
4. American Diabetes Association (1999) Patient information: smoking and diabetes: kicking the habit is hard – but worth it. Diabetes Spectrum 12:101
5. American Diabetes Association (2002) Position statement: Standards of medical care for patients with diabetes mellitus. Diabetes Care 25 (Suppl. 1): S33-S49
6. American Diabetes Association (2002) Position statement: Evidence-based nutrition principles and recommendations for the treatment and prevention of diabetes and related complications. Diabetes Care 25 (Suppl. 1): S50-S61
7. American Diabetes Association (2002) Position statement: Management of dyslipidemia in adults with diabetes. Diabetes Care 25 (Suppl. 1): S70-S74
8. American Diabetes Association (2002) Position statement: Aspirin therapy in diabetes. Diabetes Care 25 (Suppl. 1): S78-S79
9. American Diabetes Association (2002) Position statement: Treatment of hypertension in adults with diabetes. Diabetes Care 25 (Suppl. 1): S71-S73

21 Global Approach to Cardiovascular Risk in Type 2 Diabetic Persons

First step: IDENTIFICATION OF:

♦ CARDIOVASCULAR RISK FACTORS

- Family history......
- Personal history.....
- Smoking..............
- Sedentarism.........
- Weight (kg)..........
- Waist(cm)...........
- BMI(kg/m²).........
- Blood pressure......
- Albuminuria.........
- Glycemia:
  fasting..................
  postprandial..........
- HbA₁c..................
- Triglycerides.........
- HDL Chol.............
- LDL Chol.............
- Chol/HDL.............
- Other...................

♦ CARDIOVASCULAR DISEASE

- Coronary heart disease (CHD)
- CHD equivalents:
  - Abdominal aortic aneurysm
  - Ischemia of the extremities
  - Carotid atherosclerosis
- Stroke

DIAGNOSIS: ....
....

Second step: INTERPRETATION OF:

♦ GLOBAL RISK SCORE .... STRATIFICATION:
- HIGH (≥20%)....................
- MEDIUM (10-20%)............
- LOW (<10%)....................

♦ TYPE OF PREVENTION:
- PRIMARY: SHORT THERM................. LONG THERM..................
- SECONDARY: ....

♦ OBJECTIVES (see the third step)

Third step: INTERVENTION OF:

METHODS \ OBJECTIVES	NON SMOKING	GLYCEMIA .... HbA₁c	BLOOD PRESURE	Chol........ TG.......... HDL........ LDL.........	Weight....... BMI.......... Waist.........	Prothrombotic syndrom	Other factor or disease
♦ Lifestyle: Diet Exercise Alcohol							
♦ DRUGS							
♦ EDUCATION							
♦ MONITORING: CURRENT							
♦ EVALUATION: GLOBAL							

REMARKS:
1. Planning the priorities
2. Feedback from global evaluation: new events, risk score, risk levels, tailored intervention
3. Drugs side effects or interactions
4. Adherence

Fig. 21.6. Suggested flow chart for stepwise approach of global cardiovascular risk in clinical setting

10. Betteridge J (2000) Diabetic dyslipidemia. Diabetes, Obesity and Metabolism 2 (Suppl. 1):S31-S36
11. Brown WV (2000) Risk factors for vascular disease in patients with diabetes. Diabetes, Obesity and Metabolism 2 (Suppl. 2):S11-S18
12. Buse JB (1999) Overview of current therapeutic options in type 2 diabetes. Diabetes Care 22 (Suppl. 3):C65-C70
13. Boyne MS, Saudek CD (1999) Effect of insulin therapy on macrovascular risk factors in type 2 diabetes. Diabetes Care 22 (Suppl. 3):C45-C53
14. Boulton AJ et al (2000) Recommendations for the management of patients with type 2 diabetes mellitus in the Central, Eastern and Southern European Region – Consensus statement. Int J Postgrad Training Med 8:3-26
15. Ceriello A (1998) The emerging role of post-prandial hyperglycaemic spikes in the pathogenesis of diabetic complications. Diabetic Medicine 15:188-193
16. Colwell JA (1997) Aspirin in diabetes. Diabetes Care 20:1767-1771
17. Coppack SW (1997) Postprandial lipoproteins in non-insulin-dependent diabetes mellitus. Diabetic Medicine 14 (Suppl. 3):S67-S74
18. Cooper Stephanie, Caldwell JH (1999) Coronary artery disease in people with diabetes: diagnostic and risk factor evaluation. Clinical Diabetes 17:58-70
19. Cockram C et al (2001) Diabetes and cardiovascular disease. International Diabetes Federation
20. Cullen P et al (1999) Dyslipidemia and cardiovascular risk in diabetes. Diabetes, Obesity and Metabolism 1:189-198
21. Cockroft JR, Wilkkionson IB, Yki-Järvinen H (2001) Multiple risk factor intervention in type 2 diabetes: an opportunity not to be missed. Diabetes, Obesity and Metabolism 3:1-8
22. Donnan PT, Brennan GM, Mac Donald TM, Morris AD (2000) Population-based adherence to prescribed medication in type 2 diabetes: a cause for concern (Abstr.) Diabetic Medicine 17(Suppl. 1):1
23. European Arterial Risk Policy Group on behalf of the International Diabetes Federation (European Region) (1997) A strategy for arterial risk assessment and management in type 2 (non-insulin-dependent) diabetes mellitus. Diabetic Medicine 14:611-621
24. European Diabetes Policy Group (1998-1999) A desktop guide to type 2 diabetes mellitus. International Diabetes Federation – European Region
25. Expert Panel on Third Report of the National Cholesterol Education Program (NCEP) (2001) Detection, evaluation and treatment of high blood cholesterol in adults (Adult Treatment Panel III). NIH Publication No 01-3670
26. Garber AJ (2000) Implications of cardiovascular risk in patients with type 2 diabetes who have abnormal lipid profiles: is lower enough? Diabetes, Obesity and Metabolism 2:263-270
27. Garber AJ (2000) Diabetes and vascular disease. Diabetes, Obesity and Metabolism 2 (Suppl. 2):S1-S5
28. Garber AJ (2002) Attenuating CV risk factors in patients with diabetes: clinical evidence to clinical practice. Diabetes, Obesity and Metabolism 4(Suppl. 1): S5-S12
29. Gerstein HC (2000) Cardiovascular and metabolic benefits of ACE inhibition. Diabetes Care 2:882-883
30. Glasgow RE (2000) Giving smoking cessation the attention that it deserves. Diabetes Care 23:1453-1454
31. Grundy SM (1997) Small LDL atherogenic dyslipidemia and the metabolic syndrome. Circulation 95:1-4
32. Grundy SM (1999) Primary prevention of coronary heart disease – integrating risk assessment with intervention. Circulation 100:988-998
33. Game FL, Jones AF (2001) Coronary heart disease risk assessment in diabetes mellitus – a comparison of PROCAM and Framingham risk assessment functions. Diabetic Medicine 18: 355-359
34. Gavin J, Kagan S (2000) Vascular disease prevention in patients with diabetes. Diabetes, Obesity and Metabolism 2 (Suppl. 2):S25-S36
35. Golay A, Assal JP (1999) Cardiovascular risk in diabetes and therapeutic patient education. Int J Metab 2:47

36. Grundy SM et al from AHA Task Force on risk reduction (1998) Primary prevention of coronary heart disease: guidance from Framingham. Circulation 97:1876–1887
37. Greenland P, Grundy S, Pasternak RC, Lenfant C (1998) Problems on the pathway from risk assessment to risk reduction. Circulation 97:1761–1762
38. Gaede P, Vedel P, Parving HH, Pedersen O (1999) Intensified multifactorial intervention in patients with type 2 diabetes mellitus and microalbuminuria: the Steno type 2 randomized study. Lancet 353:617–622
39. Grundy SM, Benjamin IJ, Burke GL, Chait A, Eckel RH, Howard BV, Mitch W, Smith SC, Sowers JR (1999) Diabetes and cardiovascular disease. A statement for health care professionals from the American Heart Association. Circulation 100:1134–1146
40. Grundy SM, Pasternak R, Greenland P, Smith S, Fuster U (1999) Assessment of cardiovascular risk by use of multiple-risk-factor assessment equations. A statement for health care professionals from the American Heart Association and the American College of Cardiology. Journal of American College of Cardiology 34:1348–1359
41. Gotto AM et al from ILIB (International Lipid Information Bureau) (2000) The ILIB Lipid Handbook for Clinical Practice. ILIB, New York
42. Grover SA, Coupal L, Zowall H, Alexander CM, Weiss TW, Gomes DRJ (2001) How cost-effective is the treatment of dyslipidaemia in patients with diabetes but without cardiovascular disease? Diabetes Care 24:45–50
43. Haffner SM (1997) The Scandinavian Simvastatin Survival Study (4 S) subgroup analysis of diabetic subjects: implications for the prevention of coronary heart disease. Diabetes Care 20:469–471
44. Haffner SM (1999) Evaluating the status of diabetes as risk factor for coronary artery disease. Acta Diabetologica 36 (Suppl. 3):S33-S34
45. Haffner SM (2000) Patients with type 2 diabetes: the case for primary prevention. Amer J Med 107 (2A):435–455
46. Haller H (1997) Postprandial glucose and vascular disease. Diabetic Medicine 14 (Suppl. 3):S50-S56
47. Hansson L (2000) The impact of antihypertensive therapy in type 2 diabetes. Diabetes, Obesity and Metabolism 2 (Suppl.1):S37-S41
48. Hauner H (1999) The impact of pharmacotherapy on weight management in type 2 diabetes. International Journal of Obesity 23 (Suppl.7):S12-S17
49. Heinig RE (2002) What should the role of ACE inhibitors be in the treatment of diabetes? Lessons from HOPE and MICRO-HOPE. Diabetes, Obesity and Metabolism 4 (Suppl. 1): S19-S26
50. Hâncu N (1999) Abordarea în practică a dislipidemiilor: necesităṭi, posibilităṭi, bariere. In: Dabelea Dana (Ed) Actualităṭi în lipidologie. Editura Mirton, Timi°oara, pp 184-189
51. Hâncu N for EPIDIAB Study Group (2000) First results of EPIDIAB Study in Romania. Poster presented at 37th EASD Congress, Glasgow, 2001
52. Hâncu N, De Leiva A (2001) La hiperglicemia como factor de riesgo cardiovascular. Cardiovascular Risk Factors 10:262–270
53. Hâncu N, De Leiva A (2001) Enfermedad cardiovascular en la diabetes mellitus: impacto sanitario y patogenia. Cardiovascular Risk Factors 10:251–262
54. Horvit PK, Garber AJ (1997) Diabetes and cerebrovascular disease. Clinical Diabetes 15:253–256
55. Henry RR, Saudek CD from International Consensus Group (2000) Managing dyslipidemia in patients with diabetes in the primary care settings – recommendations of an International Consensus Group. The John Hopkins University School of Medicine, Office of CME
56. Herbst KL, Hirsch IB (2002) Insulin strategies for primary care providers. Clin Diab 20: 11–17
57. Hanefeld M, Temelkova-Kurktschiev T (1997) The postprandial state and the risk of atherosclerosis. Diabetic Medicine 14 (Suppl. 3):S6-S11
58. Haffner SM, Lehto S, Rönnemaa T, Pyörälä K, Laakso M (1998) Mortality from coronary heart disease in subjects with type 2 diabetes and in non-diabetic subjects with and without prior myocardial infarction. New England Journal of Medicine 339:229-234
59. Hansson L, Zanchetti A, Capruthers SG et al. for the HOT Study Group (1998) Effects of intensive blood pressure lowering and low-dose aspirin in the patients with hypertension: principal results of the Hypertension Optimal Treatment (HOT) randomised trial. Lancet 351: 1755–1762

60. Heart Outcomes Prevention Evaluation (HOPE) Study Investigators (2000) Effects of an angiotensin-converting-enzyme inhibitor, ramipril, on cardiovascular events in high risk patients. New England Journal of Medicine 342:145–153
61. Heart Outcomes Prevention Evaluation (HOPE) Study Investigators (2000) Effects of ramipril on CV and microvascular outcomes in people with diabetes mellitus: results of HOPE study and MICRO-HOPE substudy. Lancet 355:252–259
62. International Diabetes Federation – European Region (1997) Hypertension in people with type 2 diabetes – knowledge-based diabetes specific guidelines. International Diabetes Federation (European Region)
63. International Task Force for Prevention of Coronary Heart Disease (1998) Coronary Heart Disease: reducing the risk. The scientific background for primary and secondary prevention of coronary heart disease. A worldwide view. Nutr Metab Cardiovasc Dis 8:205–271
64. Jenkins A, Lyons T (2000) Preventing vascular disease in Diabetes. Practical Diabetology 19:19–34
65. Karpe F (1997) Mechanisms of postprandial hyperlipidemia – remnants and coronary artery disease. Diabetic Medicine 14 (Suppl. 3):S60-S66
66. Kannel WB (1988) Contributions of the Framingham Study to the conquest of coronary artery disease. American Journal of Cardiology 62:1109–1112
67. Kelley DE (2002) Approaches to preventing mealtime hyperglycaemic excursions. Diabetes, Obesity and Metabolism 4: 11–18
68. Lebovitz HE (1999) Effects of oral antihyperglycemic agents in modifying macrovascular risk factors in type 2 diabetes. Diabetes Care 22:C41-C44
69. Lorber D (2000) Complicating matters. Practical Diabetology 19:35
70. Laakso M, Lehto S (1997) Epidemiology of macrovascular disease in diabetes. Diabetes Reviews 5:294–315
71. Lefèbvre PJ, Scheen AJ (1998) The postprandial state and risk of cardiovascular disease. Diabetic Medicine 15 (Suppl. 4):S63-S68
72. Leese GP et al (2000) Management of lipids: comparison between patients with diabetes and ischaemic heart disease. Practical Diabetes International 17:81–83
73. Lawritzen T, Griffin S, Borch-Johnsen K et al for the ADDITION Study Group (2000) The ADDITION Study: proposed trial of the cost-effectiveness of an intensive multifactorial intervention on morbidity and mortality among people with type 2 diabetes detected by screening. International Journal of Obesity 2000(Suppl.3):S6-S11
74. Mathiensen ER (2000) Effects of ACE inhibition on cardiovascular outcomes in people with diabetes mellitus. The findings of the HOPE study. International Diabetes Monitor 12:1–4
75. Malmberg K for the DIGAMI (Diabetes mellitus Insulin Glucose infusion in Acute Myocardial Infarction) study group. Prospective randomized study of intensive insulin treatment of long term survival after acute myocardial infarction in patients with diabetes mellitus. British Medical Journal 314:1512–1515
76. Mogensen CE (1997) The concept of intensified multifactorial treatment in diabetes. Medicographia 19:83–85
77. Mogensen CE (1998) Combined high blood pressure and glucose in type 2 diabetes: double jeopardy. British Medical Journal 317:693–694
78. Mommier L (1999) The role of blood glucose – lowering drugs in the light of the UKPDS. Diabetes, Obesity and Metabolism 1 (Suppl. 2):S14-S23
79. Maggio CA, Pi-Sunyer FX (1997) The prevention and treatment of obesity – application to type 2 diabetes. Diabetes Care 20:1744–1766
80. Miettinen H, Lehto S, Salomaa VV et al (1998) Impact of diabetes on mortality after the first myocardial infarction. Diabetes Care 21:69–75
81. Masting MG, Martch FM, Cove DH (2000) Cardiovascular disease risk reduction in patients with diabetes – is clinical practice effective? Practical Diabetes International 17:155–158
82. Passa P (1998) Reducing the cardiovascular consequences of diabetes mellitus. Diabetic Medicine 15 (Suppl. 4):S69-S72
83. Pearson TA (2000) The undertreatment of LDL-cholesterol: addressing the challenge. International Journal of Cardiology 74(Suppl. 1):S23-S28
84. Pozzili P, Leslie RDG (1999) Aspirin and diabetes. Practical Diabetes International 16:261–265

85. Pearson TA et al (2000) The lipid treatment assessment project (L-TAP). Archives of Internal Medicine 160:459–467
86. Reaven GM (2002) Multiple CHD risk factors in type 2 diabetes: beyond hyperglycemia. Diabetes, Obesity and Metabolism 4 (Suppl. 1): S13-S18
87. Standl E (1999) Cardiovascular risk in type 2 diabetes. Diabetes, Obesity and Metabolism 1 (Suppl. 2):S24-S36
88. Steiner G (2000) Lipid intervention trials in diabetes. Diabetes Care 23 (Suppl. 2):B49-B53
89. Scheen AJ, Lefebvre PJ (1999) Management of the obese diabetic patient. Diabetes Reviews 7:77–93
90. Savage PJ, Narayan Venkat KM (1999) Reducing cardiovascular complications of type 2 diabetes. Diabetes Care 22:1769–1770
91. Stamler J, Vaccaro O, Neaton JR, Wentworth D for the Multiple Risk Factor Intervention Trial Research Group (1993). Diabetes Care 16:434–444
92. Sacks FM, Pfeffer MA, Moye LA et al for the Cholesterol and Recurrent Events Trial Investigators (1996) The effects of pravastatin on coronary events after myocardial infarction in patients with average cholesterol levels: Cholesterol and Recurrent Events Trial Investigators. New England Journal of Medicine 335:1001–1009
93. Sattar N et al (1998) Hormone replacement therapy in type 2 diabetes mellitus: a cardiovascular perspective. Diabetic Medicine 15:631–633
94. Shabsigh R et al (1999) Erectile dysfunction and depression: a dynamic association. Sexual Dysfunction 1:42–45
95. Taskinen MR (1999) Strategies to treat CHD risk factor in type 2 diabetes patients. Acta Diabetologica 36 (Suppl. 3):S35-S38
96. Turner RC (1998) The U.K. Prospective Diabetes Study. Diabetes Care 21 (Suppl. 3):C35-C38
97. Turner RC, Millns H, Neil HAW, Stratton IM, Manley SE, Matthews DR, Holman PR for the UKPDS Group (1998) Risk factors for coronary artery disease in non-insulin dependent diabetes mellitus: United Kingdom Prospective Diabetes Study (UKPDS: 23). British Medical Journal 316:823–828
98. Talbot F, Nouwen A (2000) A review of the relationship between depression and diabetes in adults. Diabetes Care 23:1556–1562
99. UK Prospective Diabetes Study (UKPDS) (1998) Intensive blood-glucose control with sulphonylureas or insulin compared with conventional treatment and risk of complications in patients with type 2 diabetes (UKPDS 33) Lancet 352:837–853
100. UK Prospective Diabetes Study Group (1998) Tight blood pressure control and risk of macrovascular and microvascular complications in type 2 diabetes (UKPDS 38). British Medical Journal 317:703–713
101. UK Prospective Diabetes Study (UKPDS) Group(1998) Effect of intensive blood control with metformin on complications in overweight patients with type 2 diabetes (UKPDS 34). Lancet 352:854–865
102. Vinik A, Richardson D (1998) Erectile dysfunction in diabetes. Diabetes Reviews 6:16–33
103. Williams G (1999) Obesity and type 2 diabetes: a conflict of interests? International Journal of Obesity 23 (Suppl. 7):32–35
104. Wilson PWF, D'Agostino RB, Levy D, Belanger AM, Silbershatz H, Kannel WB (1998) Prediction of coronary heart disease using risk factor categories. Circulation 97:1837–1847
105. Wood D, De Backer G, Faergeman O, Graham I, Mancia G, Pyörälä K (1998) Prevention of coronary heart disease in clinical practice. Recommendations of the Second Joint Task Force of European and other Societies on Coronary Prevention. European Heart Journal 19:1434–1503
106. World Health Organization (1999) Definition, diagnosis and classification of diabetes mellitus and its complications. Part 1: diagnosis and classification of diabetes mellitus. WHO, Dept of Noncommunicable DiCare Surveillance. Geneva
107. World Health Organization – International Society of Hypertension (1999) Guidelines for the management of hypertension. Journal of Hypertension 17:151–183
108. Yudkin JS (1998) Managing the diabetic patient with acute myocardial infarction. Diabetic Medicine 15:276–281
109. Yudkin JS, Chaturvedi N (1999) Developing risk stratification charts for diabetic and nondiabetic subjects. Diabetic Medicine 16:219–227

110. Yeo WW, Rowland K Yeo (2001) Predicting CHD risk in patients with diabetes mellitus. Diabetic Medicine 18: 341-344
111. Zilversmith DB (1979) Atherogenesis: a postprandial phenomenon. Circulation 60:473-485

Addendum

Few months after the manuscript was submitted, the very important results of Heart Protection Study were published. [Heart Protection Study Collaborative Group (2002) MRC/BHV Heart Protection in 20536 high-risk individuals: randomized placebo-controlled trial. Lancet 360:7-22]. This impressive study clearly showed that lowering cholesterol with 40 mg Simvastatin daily, decreases the rates of major vascular events (coronary heart disease or stroke) in people of high-risk, totally independent of initial lipid values, even when LDL cholesterol is bellow 100 mg/dl (2.6 mmol/l).

In this study there are a large data about 5963 persons with diabetes, the largest cohort ever studied in this field. The benefits are equally impressive. Safety of Simvastatin 40 mg is „better than aspirin which is currently sold over the counter". The implication of these results could make life easier for physicians and individuals under treatment.

Probably we need neither to check the cholesterol level before the initiation of treatment nor to monitor the enzymes too often.

There is no doubt that the guidelines will be changed in this respect. As diabetes is defined as coronary risk equivalent, should all persons with diabetes be treated with simvastatin (statins?), irespective of their cholesterol levels?

In the same journal [Lancet 2002; 360:1-4] there is a nice commentary regarding Heart Protection Study: „Two decades of progress in preventing vascular disease", where Salim Yusuf wrote: „....in smoker with vascular disease, quitting smoking and use of four simple preventive strategy (aspirin, β-blockers, lipid lowering and ACE inhibitors) could theoretically have large potential benefit, say around 80 % relative-risk reduction". Regarding this optimistic though I would only say that probably it were true if at least 80 % of patients would adhere to smoking cessation and pharmacotherapy.

Subject Index

ACE-inhibitors 93–94, 264
acetylsalicilic acid 266
Action to Control Cardiovascular Risk in Diabetes (ACCORD) 209
actos (pioglitazone) 194
adhesion molecules 33
adipocytes 99
adiponectin 99
adipophilin 99
adipose tissue
- subcutaneous 119, 122–123, 128
- visceral 119–130
adipsin 99
adult treatment panel III (ATP III) 102, 257
AGE's (advanced glycosylation end-products) 16, 24, 29
aggregation 81
ALADIN study 189
albumin 86
- excretion rate (AER) 173, 176
- urinary (see there) 85–86, 88
albuminuria (see also microalbuminuria) 89
alcohol 63, 71, 73
aldose reductase 17
aldosterone 68
alleles 67
α_1-blocker 265
α-glucosidase inhibitor 266
amlodipine 77–19
amputation 64–65, 205
- peripheral 102
angiography/angiographic 236
- status 212
angiotensin
- converting enzyme (ACE) 206
- system 68, 74–75
- – angiotensin I 74
- – angiotensin II 76, 78
angiotensinogen 99
ankle systolic pressure 234–235
- ankle/arm systolic pressure index (AAI) 235
anti-aggregation treatment 265–266
antidiabetic agents 193

antioxidants 99, 141, 143–145
antiplatelet 81
antithrombin 164–167
- inactivation by nonenzymatic glycosylation 164
- thrombin-antithrombin complex formation 167
antithrombotic remedies 168
- anticoagulation 168
- antiplatelet therapy 168
aortic aneurysm 240
apolipoprotein (Apo)
- Apo B 56, 100, 250
- – atherogenetic metabolic triad 126, 129–131
- – secretion 56
- Apo E 56, 99
- – polymorphisms 56
apoprotein 90
arm, ankle/arm systolic pressure index (AAI) 235
aspirin 266
atenolol 74
atheriopathy, peripheral 240
atherogenesis/atherogenic 100
- lipoprotein phenotype (ALP) 55
- metabolic triad 129–130
- – Apo B 126, 129–131
- – hyperinsulinemia 123, 126, 129–130, 132
- – small LDL particles 125–126, 129–130
- process 94
atherosclerosis/atherosclerotic 11–13, 53, 58, 60, 63, 85, 88–89, 173, 175, 204, 209
- advanced lesion 13
- chronic inflammation 13
- fatty streak 12–13
- plaque 160, 166
- – atheromatous gruel 160
- – plaque disruption 160
- – sealing and healing of fissured plaque 160, 166
- – tissue factor realease 160
- response to injury hypothesis 13
- scavenger receptor 12

Subject Index

atorvastin 59
ATP (adult treatment panel)
- ATP III 102, 257
ATRAMI study 185
auscultation 233
autonomic
- nervous system 181–182
- neuropathy 181–189
- – clinical presentation 183–184
- – diagnosis 186–188
- – and glycaemic control 188
- – pathogenesis 182
- – prevalence and risk factors 182–183
- – risk stratification after myocardial infarction 184–186
- – therapy 188–189
avandia (rosiglitazone) 194

behavior/behavioural
- modification 154
- therapy 110
benfotiamine 189
β_2-blocker 264
β-cell
- function in type 2 diabetes 38
- modulation by repaglinide 38
- pancreatic 53
- stimulation by sulphonylureas 37, 40
biguanide 48
biopsy, endomyocardial 212, 224
blood
- flow, disturbed 160
- – increased blood viscosity 160
- – irregularities of exposed surface 160
- pressure 5–6, 50, 54, 91, 181–182, 205, 244
- – levels 90–91
- – nocturnal 91
- – response to sustained handgrip 186
- viscosity 100
BMI (body mass index) 98, 102–105
body fat distribution 118–121, 123
- android obesity 118
- gender differences 119
- gynoid obesity 118
- menopause 119, 121–122
- subcutaneous adipose tissue 119, 122–123, 128
- visceral adipose tissue 119–130
- waist circumference 121, 123, 127–128, 130–132

calcium channel blocker 93, 264
capillaries 68
captopril 74
carbohydrate 110
cardiac
- autonomic neuropathy (*see* autonomic) 181–189

- catheterization 213, 222
- exploration of diabetic patients 212–225
- function 195
- index 196
- output 68
- testing in diabetic patients, indications 213
cardiomyopathy, diabetic 212
cardiorespiratory arrests 183
cardiovascular
- complications 195–196
- death 204
- disease (CVD) 1, 22, 47, 57, 99, 104, 106, 120–121, 126, 151, 204
- – incidence 57
- factors/risk factors 4–5, 99, 101–105, 108, 240–241
- – blood pressure 5
- – cholesterol 5
- – HDL cholesterol 5
- – hyperglycemia 5
- – insulin resistance 5
- – obesity 5
- – thiazolidinediones effect on 196–197
- – triglycerides 5
- fitness 112
- mortality 57
- reflex test 186
- treatment of cardiovascular risk factors 6
- – blood pressure 6
- – dyslipidemia 6
- – hyperglycemia 6
carotidian echo-duplex 219–220
catecholamines 68
catheterization, cardiac 212, 222
CDH (coronary artery disease) 22, 87, 91, 212
cerebrovascular disease 103, 175, 240
CHD (coronary heart disease) 91, 101, 118, 120, 123, 125, 127–129, 132–133, 240
chlorpropamide 31
chlortalidone 73
cholesterol 5, 90, 247
- decreased removal of cholesterol from arterial wall 16
- dietary 111
- hypercholesterolemia 58
- HDL cholesterol (*see there*) 5, 49, 54, 56, 90–91, 100– 102, 108, 125–126, 129, 182, 196, 205, 241
- LDL cholesterol (*see there*) 49, 54, 56, 90, 108, 126, 129, 196, 205, 241
- National Chilesterol Education Program (NCEP) 102
- total 108
chronic inflammation 13, 93
cigarette smoking 205, 241
clamp 67

Subject Index

claudication, intermittent 232
clotting
- factors 166–167
- markers, activation of 166–167
- - activated protein Cα_1 antitrypsin complexes 167
- - D-dimers 167
- F 1–2 166–167
- fibrinopeptides (FpA, FpB) 167
- thrombin-antithrombin complexes 167
clustering 63–64
coagulation factors 100, 242
Collaborative Atorvastin Diabetes Study (CARDS) 206
compliance 38, 74
- mealtime regimens 38
- sulphonylureas 38
coronarography, selective 222
coronary
- acute coronary events 198
- artery disease (CDH) 22, 87, 91, 212
- heart disease (CHD) 91, 101, 118, 120, 123, 125, 127–129, 132–133, 240
C-peptide 41
C-protein C inhibitor 90
C-reactive protein 93
cystathionine-β-synthase 173, 174
cystathionine-γ-lyase 174
cytochrome 40
cytokines 93
- proinflammatory (*see there*) 160–163, 165

DEKAN study 189
depression 247
diabesity 98
diabetes/diabetic
- cardiomyopathy 212
- cardiovascular risk factors 151–152
- diabetic angiopathy and gliclazide 28–35
- dyslipidemia (*see there*) 14–15, 53–60, 90–92, 99, 102, 104
- medication 107
- metabolic abnormalities 53
- nephropathy 85
- prevalence 150–151
- and thrombosis (*see there*) 19
- type 2 diabetes 98, 101, 118–133, 150–157
Diabetes
- American Society (DAS) 213
- Atheroclerosis Intervention Study (DAIS) 206
- Control and Complication Trial (DCCT) 207
- International Research and Educational Cooperative Team (DIRECT) 209
- Mellitus Insulin – Glucose Infusion in Acute Myocardial Infarction (DIGAMI) 208

diacylglycerol and protein kinase C pathways 18
- diminished action of nitric oxide 18
- increased activity of vasopresor peptides 18
- vascular insulin resistance 18
dialysis 77–78
- haemodialysis 65
diastolic dysfunction 102
diet 99, 110–111, 153
- composition 110
- hypercaloric 99
- hypocaloric 110
- standard weight-reduction 110
- VLCD (very low caloric diet) 110–111
dippers, non-dippers 70
DLP (*see* dyslipidemia)
Doppler device 234, 236
doxazosin 73
drug therapy (*see* medication) 107–108, 113–114, 156
dysglycemia 208
dyslipidemia (DLP) 6, 14–15, 53–60, 90–92, 99, 102, 104, 240
- and cardiovascular risk in diabetes 53–60
- decreased removal of cholesterol from arterial wall 16
- large VLDL-1 15
- small dense LDL 15, 242

ECG (electrocardiogram/electrocardiography) 213–214
- exercise ECG 214
- *Holter* ECG monitoring 215
- resting ECG 214
echo-duplex, carotidian 219–220
education 109
electrocardiogram (*see* ECG) 213–214
enalapril 79–80
endocavitary electrophysiological investigation 224
endocrine organ 99
endomyocardial biopsy 212, 224
endothel/endothelium/endothelial 68
- activation 176
- cells 89
- damage/dysfunction 19, 28, 33, 88–90, 99–101, 160, 167, 231
- - exposing tissue factor 160
- - thromboembolic disorders 173
- - markers of endothelial dysfunction 167
- - release and/or secretion of *v*WF 164
- - releasing PAI-1 162
- function 48, 197–198
- loss of endothelial integrity 19
- oxidative stress and endothelium in diabetes 142–143
energy intake 107

environmental
- factor analysis   63, 67
- genetic-environmental interactions   154
epidemiological studies of PVD   229
- incidence   229
- prevalence   229
EPIDIAB program   103
erectile dysfunction   247
erythrocyte aggregability   100
estrogen   175
ethnic   65
Euro'98   252
EURODIAB IDDM complication studies   182, 186–187
evaluation   109
evidence based   69
exons   68

factor analysis   63
- environmental   63, 67
- factor VII   100, 162–163, 165, 247
- - in diabetic patients   162
- - increased postprandial activity   162–163
- factor VIIIC   164
- - increase in diabetic patients   164
- - normalization after intensive insulin therapy   168
fat   71
- abdominal   98
- body fat distribution (see there)   118–121, 123
- monounsaturated   110
- nonalcoholic fatty liver   101
- polyunsaturated   11
- saturated   110
- visceral   98
Fenofibrate Intervention and Event Lowering in Diabetes (FIELD)   206
FFA (free fatty acids)   55–57, 99
- efflux   56
fibrates   194, 266
fibres   99, 111
fibrin structure, gliclazide   30
fibrinogen   89, 93, 100, 163, 165–166, 242
- acute phase reactant   163
- role in platelet aggregation   166
fibrinolysis   30, 100–101
- gliclazide   30
- thrombotic/fibrinolytic systems   199
fibrinolytic activity   161
- α_2-antiplasmin   162, 165
- dilute blood clot lysin time   161
- factor XIII   161–162, 165–166
- PAI-1   162, 165, 168
fibrous cap   198
foam cells   100
folate treatment   173, 177
Fontaine stadialization   232

foot lesions   234
- neuroischemic   234
- neuropathic   234
- ulcerations   234
fosinopril   79
Framingham risk scores   252
free fatty acids (see FFA)   55–57, 99
free radicals   140–141, 145
- scavenging   31
furosemide   73

ganglia, sympathetic   182
gangrene   230
gene   67
- IRS-2   67
- GLUT 4   67
genetic
- defects   173
- predisposition   67
genetic-environmental interactions   154
glibenclamide   30, 40
- in comparison to repaglinide   41, 43–44
- pharmacology   40
gliclazide and diabetic angiopathy   28–35
- amino azabicyclo [3.3.0] octane ring   29
- fibrin structure   30
- fibrinolysis   30
- selectivity   29
glipizide   41
glitazone medication   114
glomerular function   60, 88
gluconeogenesis   39, 48
glucose
- clamp technique   54
- endogenous production   39
- exogenous load   39
- fasting   102, 108
- glucose-insulin homeostasis   121, 123, 125
- gluconeogenesis   39
- glycogenolysis   39
- hepatic glucose output   38
- impaired glucose tolerance (see IGT)   24, 65, 67, 71, 80, 245
- intolerance   101
- splanchnic sequestration   39
- transporters (see GLUT)   67, 99, 195
glucosidase inhibitor, α 267
GLUT-1   99, 195
GLUT-4   67, 99, 195
glutathione (see GSH, GSSG/GSH)   144
glycation   231
- non-enzymatic (see there)   16
glycemia/glycemic   250
- control   30
glycogen synthetasis   99
glycosaminoglycans   93
glycosylation end-products, advanced (AGE's)   16

Subject Index

GSH 145
GSSG/GSH 145
guidelines 69–71, 250

haemodialysis 65
haemorrheological distrubances 99
haemostasis disturbances 88–90
HbA1c 102, 108
- improvement 40–43
- - by metformin 41
- - by repaglinide 41
- - by troglitazone 43
Hcy
- metabolism 175
- plasma concentration 176–177
HDL cholesterol 5, 49, 53–54, 56, 90–91, 182, 196, 205, 241
- HDL-2 100
- HDL small and dense 100
- lipoprotein-lipid profile 125–126, 129
- low HDL 205
- total cholesterol/HDL cholesterol ratio 100
heart
- failure 102–103
- rate variability (HRV) 181, 185
- - in response to deep breathing 185
hemoglobin
- A1c 245
- glycosilated 77
hepatic
- failure 194
- glucose output 38, 193
- hypothesis about enhanced hepatic protein synthesis 165
- - excess flow of free fatty acids 165
- - hyperinsulinism 165
- - proinflammatory cytokines 165
hepatotoxicity with troglitazone 38
hexokinaza II 99
HMG-CoA 205
Holter 70
- ECG monitoring 215
HOMA$_{IR}$ index 101
homeostasis 68
homocysteine 173, 242
homocysteine/homocysteinemia 92–93
- homozygous 175
- metabolism 174
homocystinuria 173
HOPE studies 246
hormonal replacement therapy (HRT) 267
HOT studies 246
hydropiridines 72
- di-hydropiridines 72
- non-hydropiridines 72
hypercholesterolemia 58, 87, 102, 205
hypercoagulability 28, 100

hyperfiltration 67
hyperglycemia 5, 23, 56, 63, 85–86, 151, 181, 204–209, 241
- conventional risk factors 205206
- postprandial (*see there*) 23
hyperhomocysteinemia 92–93
- as cardiovascular risk factor 173–178
- - genetics of hyperhomocysteinemia 174
hyperinsulinaemia 47, 54, 63–64, 67, 85, 91–92, 101, 151, 165, 245
- atherogenic metabolic triad 123, 126, 129–130, 132
- euglycaemic clamp technique 54
hyperleptinaemia 101
hyperlipidaemia 109, 102
hypertension 47, 99, 101–102, 104, 152, 199, 245, 263
- oxidative stress 144–145
- postural 183
- systolic 93
- treatmet 93
hypertriglyceridaemia 53–54, 56, 87, 100–102, 205
- waist, hypertriglyceridemic 118, 130
hypertrophy, left ventricular 69, 72, 79, 102
hyperuricemia 85, 101
hypofibrinolysis 63
hypoglycaemia
- awareness of 44
- medication, hypoglycaemic 108
- renal dysfunction 38
- sulphonylureas as a cause of hypoglycaemia 37–38, 43
hypoinsulinemia, post-meal 206–207
hypokalaemia 73
hypotension, orthostatic 70, 79–80
hypothesis about enhanced hepatic protein synthesis (*see* hepatic) 165

IGF-1 (insulin-like growth factor -1) 99
IGT (impaired glucose tolerance) 24, 65, 67, 71, 80, 245
- hepatic production 80
- toxicity 64
IHD (*see* ischemic heart diseases)
indapamide 265
infarction, myocardial 23, 64, 73–75, 78, 85, 103, 175, 184–186, 204–207, 245
inflammation 231
- chronic 13, 93
- role of PPARγ 200
inspection 233
insulin 63–64, 67, 73–74, 81, 263
- association between insulin and lipid metabolism 55
- biphasic secretion 39
- exogenous treatment 38–39
- glucose-insulin homeostasis 121, 123, 125

- hyperinsulinaemia (*see there*)   47, 54, 63–64, 67, 85, 91–92, 101, 123, 126–132, 151, 165, 245
- hypoinsulinemia, post-meal   206–207
- IGF-1 (insulin-like growth factor -1)   99
- impaired insulin secretion   193
- medication   114
- modulation of secretion by sulphonylureas   40
- post-prandial insulin   55
- prandial response   39
- receptor   99
- resistance   5, 18, 47, 53–57, 85, 91–92, 99–101, 150, 193, 231, 242
- – acquired   54
- – genetic   54 IGF-1 (insulin-like growth factor -1)   99
- – and hyperinsulinemia   91–92
- – marker   54
- – syndrome   54, 63–64, 67–68, 72, 81, 126–127, 129, 132
- – vascular   18
- sensitising agents/sensitivity   38, 120, 122, 123, 125
- suppression test   54
insulinoma   67
interactions   40
interleukin (IL)
- IL-6   99, 200
intermittent claudication   232
invasive techniques   212
irbesartan   76–78
ischemic
- heart diseases (IHD)   85, 102–103, 205
- rest pain   232

Kumamoto study   29

labetalol   73
LDL
- cholesterol   49, 54, 56, 90, 108, 196, 241
- – high LDL   205
- dense   15, 100–102
- glycated   17
- lipoprotein-lipid profile   126, 129
- oxidated/LDL to oxidation   17, 141
- particles (sLDL-C)   196
- serum LDL   49
- small   15, 100–102, 242
- – atherogenic metabolic triad, small LDL particles   125–126, 129–130
- susceptibiltiy of LDL to oxidation   146
left ventricular hypertrophy   69, 72, 79, 102
leptin   99, 195
life expectancy   107
lifestyle
- and cardiovascular risk   150–157
- changes   107

- factors   63, 69, 81, 152–154
- – interventions that lower risk for CVD   154–156
- modification   154
- optimization   107, 109–110, 263
- sedentary   101
lipid   100, 245
- abnormalities   53, 90
- – dyslipidemia (*see there*)   6, 14–15, 53–60, 90–92
- control   264
- metablism   54–57
- oxidations   17
- – oxidants   17
lipid-lowering trials in diabetes   59
α-lipoic acid   189
lipoprotein   55, 58, 90, 241
- lipase (LPL)   55, 99
- triglycerides-rich (TG-rich)   58, 100
lipoprotein-lipid profile   120–123, 125–126
- cholesterol/HDL cholesterol   129–132
- HDL   125–126, 129
- LDL   126, 129
- triglycerides   125–126, 129–133
liver, nonalcoholic fatty liver   101
losartan   76, 78
LPL (*see* lipoprotein lipase)

macroalbuminuria   86
macrovascular
- complications   195
- disease   243, 246
markers
- clotting markers (*see there*)   166–167
- of endothelial dysfunction   167
- plasma   54, 88–89
matrix metalloproteinase-9   198
meal replacements   111
mealtime
- flexibility   39
- meal requirements with sulphonylureas   43
- missed meals   38, 43
- regimens, compliance   38
medial
- aterial calcification   245
- slerosis (*Monckeberg* disease)   228
medication/drug therapy   156
- diabetic   107
- glitazone   114
- hypoglycaemic   108
- insulin   114
- metformin   114
- sulphonylurea   114
- weight loss   113
meglitinides   193
menopause   119, 121–122
metabolism/metabolic
- abnormalities   53

Subject Index

- cellular 66
- Hcy metabolism 175
- MONW (metabolically obese, normal weight) 103
- syndrome 24, 243

metformin 31, 38–41, 193, 246
- in comparison to repaglinide 41
- in combination with repaglinide 41
- HbA1c 41
- medication 114
- renal dysfunction as a contraindication to metformin 38
- use in type 2 diabetes 38

methionine 173–174
methyldopa 73–74
methylene tetrahydrofolate reductase 173
metoprolol 74
microalbuminuria 64–65, 67, 70, 72–73, 76–77, 85–94, 101, 250, 263
- definition 85–86
- endothelial dysfunction and haemostasis disturbances 88–90
- epidemiology 86
- pathogenetic mechanisms 87–93
- treatment 93–94

microcirculation 228, 231
microHOPE studies 246
microvascular
- complications 47, 53, 195
- disease 246

Monckeberg disease (medial sclerosis) 228
monitoring 109
- *Holter* ECG monitoring 215
monocyte adesion 32, 92
monotherapy, oral 262
MONW (metabolically obese, normal weight) 103
morbidity 39, 64, 69, 73, 81, 85, 204–205, 213
mortality 64–65, 69, 73, 75, 79, 81, 85–87, 91, 108, 151, 175, 204–205, 213
MRA (magnetic resonance angiography) 236
multiple risk factor intervention trials (MRFIT) 175
muscle 63
- skeletal 63, 68
- smooth 68
mutation 68
myocardial
- contractility 181
- infarction 23, 64, 73–75, 78, 85, 103, 175, 184–186, 204–207, 245
- perfusion scintigraphy 221–222

nadolol 73
National Cholesterol Education Program (NCEP) 102, 261
nephropathy, diabetic 85, 91, 177, 267
nervous system, autonomic 181–182

neuropathy 178, 231
- autonomic 181–189, 212
NF-KB 33
nicotinic acid 266
nifedipine 72, 74, 79
nitric oxide 182, 223
- diminished action 18
nonalcoholic fatty liver 101
non-dipper phenomenon 183
non-enzymatic glycation 16
- advanced glycosylation end-products (AGE's) 16, 24, 29
- glycated LDL 17
- oxidated LDL 17
non-invasive methods/tests 214
noradrenaline reuptake inhibitor 113

obesity 5, 56, 63, 65, 68–69, 80–81, 92, 98, 118–119, 123, 153, 241
- android 118
- abdominal 101–102
- clinical management 107
- central 69
- gynoid 118
- MONW (metabolically obese, normal weight) 103
oral monotherapy 263
orlistat 113
overhydration 91
oxidative stress 28, 100, 140–147, 182, 231
- and aging 145
- and endothelium 142–143
- as pathogenetic factor of hypertension in diabetes 144–145
- pathogenetic implication 145–147
oxygen measurement, transcutaneous 236

PAI-1 (plasminogen activator inhibitor 1) 50, 85, 99–100, 199, 241
- decreasing 50
- increased 19
pain, ischemic rest pain 232
palpation 233
pancreatic
- beta cells 53
- lipase inhibitor 113
peripheral
- atheriopathy 240
- resistance 196
- vascular disease (*see* PVD) 199, 204, 227–237, 240
peroxisome proliferator-activated receptor (PPAR) 68, 194
- PPARγ 194
phosphatidylinositol 3-kinase (p85-a Pl3K) 195
physical
- activity 99, 112

- inactivity 153
pioglitazone 196
pioglitazone (actos) 194
piridoxine 173, 177
plaque
- atherosclerotic (see there) 160, 166
- rupture 198
plasminogen activator
- inhibitor I (PAI-I) 50, 85, 99–100, 199, 241
- tissue antigen (tPA) 100
platelets 165–168
- aggregation 166
- enhanced binding of fibrinogen 166
- glycation of platelet membrane proteins 166
- hyperreactive in diabetic patients 165–166
- platelet β-thrombomodulin 167
pleiotropic factor 92
pletismography 235
polyol-myoinositol pathway 17
- aldose reductase 17
- sorbitol 17–18
postprandial hyperglycemia 23, 39, 206
- as a cause of mortality and morbidity 39
potassium 71, 73
- channels 40
PPAR (see peroxisome proliferator-activated receptor)
pravastatin 59
prazosin 74
prediabetic state 3
prevalence 63–64, 67
prevention 241
procoagulation factors 100
proinflammatory cytokines 160–163, 165
- and endothelial dysfunction 160
- intraabdominal tissue dereived 163
- stimulation of PAI-1 synthesis 162, 165
- stimulation of vWF secretion 164
propranolol 73
prostaglandins 99
protein 111
- kinase C pathways (see also diacylglycerol) 18
- protein C system 164–165
- restriction 71
proteinuria 85–86
prothrombotic
- status 89, 99
- syndrome 159–168
pulse volume recordings 227
PVD (peripheral vascular disease) 204, 227–237, 240
- characteristics 228
- clinical assessments 232–237
- epidemiological studies (see there) 229
pyridoxine 175

QT interval prolongation 183
Quebec cardiovascular study (QCS) 129

radioisotopic techniques 212
ramipril 75
30:15 ratio 186
Ratschow procedure 233
receptor, agonists 73
- blocker of ATP-II 76
- subtype AT1, AT2 76
reflex test, cardiovascular 186
renal
- artery stenosis 74, 79
- chronic renal failure 173
- dysfunction 38–40
- - as a cause of hypoglycaemia 38
- - as a contraindication to metformin 38
- - use of repaglinidine in 40
renin-angiotensin 102
repaglinide 38–41, 267
- β-cell 38
- HbA1c 41
- metformin 38–41
- - in comparison to repaglinide 41
- - in combination with repaglinide 41
- renal dysfunction 40
- sulphonylureas in comparison to 41
- troglitazone
- - in combination with 41–43
- - in comparison to 41
resins 266
resistin 68, 99
respiratory
- cardiorespiratory arrests 183
- spontaneously respiratory arrest 181
retinopathy 34, 65, 74–75
revascularization 75
risk/risk factors 4–6, 22
- cardiovascular (see there) 4–5, 99, 101–105, 108, 240–241
- clinical class 104
- equivalents 243
- Framingham risk scores 252
rosiglitazone (avandia) 194–196

scintigraphy, myocardial perfusion scintigraphy 221–222
self-control 114
self-observation 114
serotonin (5-HT) reuptake inhibitor 113
sibutramine 113
sildenafil 267
simvastatin 94, 205
skeletal muscle 63, 68
smoking 102, 230
- and health 205
socioeconomic status 153
splanchnic sequestration 39

Subject Index

sR (soluble receptors)   99
statins   246
steno hypothesis   88
stenosis, renal artery   74, 79
steroids   99
stimulus control   114
strokes   102
- stroke volume index   196
sulphonylurea/sulfonylurea   29, 37–38, 43, 193, 208, 245
- accumulation   38
- as a cause of hypoglycaemia   37–38, 43
- compliance   38
- in comparison to repaglinide   41
- ethical considerations in clinical trials   43
- food requirements   43
- insulin modulation of secretion by   40
- mealtime, meal requirements with sulphonylureas   43
- medication   114
- pharmacokinetics   37
- pharmacology   40
- stimulation of beta-cells   37
superoxide
- anion (O_2)   141
- generations   141
surgery   109
- bariatric   113
- gastric-reduction   110
- vertical banded gastroplacy   114
sympathetic nervous system   100
syndrome
- dysmetabolic   101
- metabolic X   99, 101
- X-syndrome   85, 92

tachycardia   181
- resting   183
THEME programes   109
therapeutic education   110–111
therapy   109
- behavioural   110
- medication/drug therapy (see there)
- treatment of high risk abdominally obese men weight loss   122–123
thiazides   72–73, 81, 265
thiazolidinediones   38, 193–201
- effect on the vascular wall   198
thromboembolic disorders   173
- endothelial dysfunction   173
thrombogenic factors   241
thrombomodulin
- plasma concentration   176
- platelet   167
thrombosis and diabetes   19
- endothelial dysfunction (see there)
- increased PAI-I   19
- loss of endothelial integrity   19

- venous thrombosis   175
thrombotic/fibrinolytic systems   199
timolol   75
tissue factor   99
TNF-α (tumor necrosis factor-α)   99
toe, systolic pressure   235
tolbutamide   31
- plasminogen activator inhibitor (PAI-1)   31
- tissue-type plasminogen activator (t-PA)   31
tPA (plasminogen activator tissue antigen)   100
treatment (see therapy)
triamterene   73
triglycerides   5, 108, 206, 242
triglycerides-rich (TG-rich) lipoproteins   58, 100
troglitazone   38–43, 194
- in comparison to repaglinidine   41
- in combination with repaglinidine   41–43
- HbA1c   43
- hepatotoxicity   38
- use in type 2 diabetes   38
type B phenotype   55

UAC (urinary albumin concentration)   86
UAER (urinary albumin excretion rate)   85, 88
UK'99   255
UKPDS   29, 188

Valsalva manoeuvre   181, 186
vascular
- insulin resistance   18
- peripheral vascular disease (see PVD)
vasoconstriction   68
vasodilatation   68, 76
vasopresor peptides, increased activity   18
VCAM-1   89
VDLD-apoB phenotype   55
VDLD-TG, plasma   55, 57
venous filling   233
ventricular hypertrophy   69, 72, 79, 91
ventriculography   222
Veterans Affairs Diabetes Trial (VADT)   209
visceral
- adipose tissue   119–130
- obesity   47
vitamin
- vitamin B_6 174–175
- vitamin B_{12} 173, 176–177
- vitamin E   141, 143, 145–146
VLCD (very low caloric diet)   110–111
VLDL   15, 50, 90
- large VLDL-1, diabetic dislipidemia   15
VWF   88

waist 99, 102
- body fat distribution 120–133
- - waist circumference 121, 123. 127–128, 130–132
- - waist-to-hip ratio (WHR) 120–121, 123, 125, 127–128, 132–133
weight 67, 70–71, 264
- gain of 39, 41, 49, 107
- loss/weight reduction 106, 108, 110–111, 155
- - benefits 107
- - long-term 108
- - treatment of high risk abdominally obese men weight loss 122–123
- maintenance 107–109, 111–112
- medication for weight loss 113
- reasonable 107, 109
- standard weight-reduction 110
von Willebrand factor 88–89, 100
Winsor index 235
WOSCOPS data 59

X-syndrome 85, 92

Printed in Great Britain
by Amazon